FROM MEDICINE TO MANUSCRIPT

FROM MEDICINE TO MANUSCRIPT

Doctors with a Literary Legacy

Seymour I. Schwartz

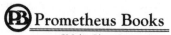

Prometheus Books

59 John Glenn Drive
Amherst, New York 14228

Published 2018 by Prometheus Books

Cover design by Jacqueline Nasso Cooke
Cover design © Prometheus Books

Inquiries should be addressed to
Prometheus Books
59 John Glenn Drive
Amherst, New York 14228
VOICE: 716–691–0133 • FAX: 716–691–0137
WWW.PROMETHEUSBOOKS.COM

22 21 20 19 18   5 4 3 2 1

Library of Congress Cataloging-in-Publication Data

Names: Schwartz, Seymour I., 1928- , author.
Title: From medicine to manuscript : doctors with a literary legacy / by Seymour I.
    Schwartz.
Description: Amherst, New York : Prometheus Books, 2018. | Includes bibliographical
    references.
Identifiers: LCCN 2018012149 (print) | LCCN 2018013529 (ebook) |
    ISBN 9781633884342 (ebook) | ISBN 9781633884335 (hardback)
Subjects: | MESH: Physicians | Authorship | History, Medieval | History, Early Modern
    1451-1600 | History, Modern 1601- | Biography
Classification: LCC R690 (ebook) | LCC R690 (print) | NLM WZ 112 |
    DDC 610.69/5—dc23
LC record available at https://lccn.loc.gov/2018012149

Printed in the United States of America

CONTENTS

CONTENTS

CONTENTS

PART II: THE PRESENT

FOREWORD

Gertrude Stein, one of America's most intriguing and noteworthy authors, launched her literary career as a medical student. As a senior at Radcliffe, Stein asked her mentor, William James, for career advice. Quoting Oliver Wendell Holmes, James told her, "A medical education opens all doors." Stein went on to medical school at Johns Hopkins University, leaving in her fourth year bound for Europe and an extraordinary life journey marked by literary contributions ranging from *The Making of Americans* to *The Autobiography of Alice B. Toklas*.

With *From Medicine to Manuscript: Doctors with a Literary Legacy*, Dr. Seymour I. Schwartz shows us how many doors a medical education can open as he reviews the contributions of physician authors dating from the ancient times to the present. Dr. Schwartz—Sy to his friends—is a most appropriate curator of this veritable museum of physician authors. He reached the pinnacle of the surgical profession as professor and chairman of surgery at the University of Rochester, and as president of the American College of Surgeons, but he is also the coauthor of *Principles of Surgery*, the most-referenced textbook of its time, and the author of ten other books on topics spanning map drawings to the saints of medicine.

In this book, Schwartz takes us on a grand tour of the canon created by polymathic physicians as authors, poets, playwrights, satirists, philosophers, and political and social commentators. He examines his physician subjects with thoughtful perspectives on their work, their lives, and their most famous quotes. And he does so with an easy and inviting style, almost as if he is providing us with a briefing on a guest soon to arrive at our dinner party.

And what a dinner party it is! Awaiting you in Schwartz's serious but engaging book is an introduction to physicians who have lived, or are today living, most interesting lives. You will undoubtedly learn something about them you didn't know before—perhaps even discovering they were physicians—and you will certainly enjoy their company.

Last but not least, I must confess a bias about Schwartz's work. I was his student forty-five years ago. For me and many others, he not only opened doors, but he encouraged us to bravely walk through them and discover what lies beyond. For Dr. Schwartz's guidance and support, I will always be grateful.

—Bernard T. Ferrari, MD, JD, MBA, professor and dean, Johns Hopkins University Carey Business School

APOLOGIA

The genesis of a series of essays concerning the lives of individuals who have combined medical experience with literary notability was a personal quest for an explanation. I had recently delivered a quasi-autobiographical talk entitled "Scribo Ergo Sum," implying an absolute necessity to write. I asked myself, "Does such a compulsion exist?"

During my youth, I had little interest in literature or composition, and throughout my early education, as well as my undergraduate and medical schooling, that lack of interest persisted. As an aspiring academic surgeon, I had published basic scientific research articles and clinical considerations in peer-reviewed journals. At the same time, I had developed a concentrated interest in liver surgery, a recently evolving field. I avidly read the literature of past accomplishments related to liver surgery, and became aware that there was no inclusive work on the subject.

Reinforced by the dictum proposed by Francis Bacon in the seventeenth century that "reading maketh a full man, conference a ready man, and writing an exact man," I presumptuously compiled the first textbook in English on the subject, *Surgical Diseases of the Liver* (1964). The publisher of that book, shortly thereafter, embarked on the production of a new textbook of surgery and selected me to head the editorial board. *Principles of Surgery* appeared in 1969, and I subsequently shepherded the textbook through seven editions. During that period, I also edited *The Yearbook of Surgery* and a monthly journal, *Contemporary Surgery*, each issue of which called for me to compose a historical, philosophical, or otherwise titillating essay. Representative essays were compiled and published as *Surgical Reflections* (1993).

On the occasion of my achieving tenure as an academic surgeon at my university, my wife pointed out that I was "monolithic" and suggested that I needed a hobby. I asked that she find one for me, and, the next day, she handed me a secondhand book on the history of cartography, indicating that the subject might capture my interest. I became a collector of early maps pertaining to America and embarked on scholarship regarding the subject. Once again, I concluded that a vacuum existed in that there was no definitive book on the subject. This led to *The Mapping of America* (1979), coauthored with Ralph Ehrenberg. My continued interest in cartography led to the publications of *The French and Indian War* (1995), *An Englishman's Journey along America's Eastern Waterways* (2000), *This Land Is Your Land* (2000), *The Mis-Mapping of America* (2003), and *Putting "America" on the Map* (2007).

In 2005, my career as an operating surgeon came to an end. This, coupled with the completion of an eleven-year period of serving as chair of surgery and surgeon in chief of my university's hospital, allowed for more leisure time. The void was filled with an increased dedication to scholarship, writing, and more diversification. Several books of more panoramic scope resulted. *Gifted Hands: America's Most Significant Contributions to Surgery* (2009), *Holystic Medicine: The Patron Saints of Medicine* (2011), *Cadwallader Colden: A Biography* (2013), and *The Anatomist, the Barber-Surgeon, and the King* (2015) were published.

Having come to the conclusion that I have harbored a compulsion to write, one that has intensified with time, I sought an answer to the question "why?" I reached out to more significant and notable kindred souls who have combined medicine with literary productivity. Perhaps a study of their lives would help to determine if there is a pattern or an explanation.

The journey has been long and arduous, but, also, informative and entertaining. I have made many new acquaintances and accumulated many new heroes. I soon realized that each of the individuals whose life and writings I investigated was unique. The investigation, which extended from the distant past to more modern times and into the present, has uncovered a broad spectrum of individuals. Some bear names that are well known; some names are eponymous, and some have faded into obscurity. Diversity dominates, while the question that served as the stimulus for this project remains unanswered.

INTRODUCTION

Medicine is currently characterized by constant scientific and technological expansion. The imprecise conjectures and therapeutic nostrums of the past now reside in the realm of obscurity. Today's biopsychosocial model of the practice of medicine has become heavily weighted by established facts that have evolved as a consequence of scientific investigation. The computer has been interposed between the patient and the physician. The medical heroes of today have unraveled the double helix, defined the genome, prevented and successfully cured several cancers, replaced joints and limbs, transplanted vital organs, and minimized surgical trauma. But, while science and technology have become pervasive and dominant, the humanistic aspect of medicine has become less apparent.

The heritage of medicine, from its very beginnings through modernity, has included humanism, defined as a concern with the interests and ideals of people. Literature, which offers a mirror of society, contributes to the development of humanism. Among those who have penned the prose and poetry are individuals who had either actively practiced medicine or prepared themselves for a medical career. They have either changed direction from medicine to authorship or incorporated their writings as part of their daily activities.

The combination of medicine and literature predated the written word. During the time of oral dissemination of mythology, Apollo, the son of Zeus and Leto, was identified as the god of medicine, music, poetry, and intellectual inquiry. As thoughts gained permanence by pen or stylus, in early Christianity, the fourth book of the Gospels was written by Saint Luke the Evangelist, whose name derives from Latin, meaning "bringer of light." Luke studied medicine in Antioch and Tarsus, and was referred to by Saint Paul as his "most dear physician."

The Gospel according to Luke, a doctor, is unique in that it includes accounts of Christ's birth, infancy, and childhood. It is also notable for the parable of the Good Samaritan and that of the Prodigal Son, and three of the sayings of Christ on the cross: "Father forgive them," "Thou shalt be with me in Paradise," and "Father, into Thy hands I commend my spirit." Luke's

Gospel, which takes up more pages in the New Testament than the writings of any other author, emphasizes Christ's compassion for sinners, unhappy individuals, outcasts, lepers, and the poor.

As time passed, the contributions of doctors to the literature of the age increased. Proceeding along chronological lines, the conjunction of medicine, literature, and causative factors will be considered by detailing the lives and writings of authors who have journeyed from medicine to manuscripts.

PART I

THE PAST

1

MAIMONIDES

A Beacon in a Dark Age

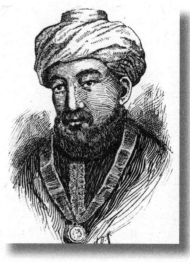

T he period in European history that extended from 500 to 1500 CE has been referred to as the Middle Ages or medieval period. Positioned between the rich Greco-Roman classical period and the Renaissance, which refers to the "rebirth" of the past artistic and intellectual advancements, the Middle Ages were characterized by stagnation and retrogression. Consequently, the bracketed thousand years is often referred to as the Dark Ages.

The early Middle Ages (500–1000 CE) were preceded by the disruption of the Roman Empire, followed by the mass migration of ethnic groups into the lands that had been occupied by the Roman Empire, and the rise and rapid growth of Islam. In the late Middle Ages (1300–1500 CE), although education continued to be focused on the training of the clergy, the development of universities spread throughout Europe. During the late Middle Ages, Dante Alighieri (d. 1321), Giovanni Boccaccio (d. 1375), Geoffrey Chaucer (d. 1400), and François Villon (d. 1463) contributed to the rise of vernacular literature.

In the so-called high Middle Ages (1000–1300 CE), science was stagnant, and those interested in intellectual inquiry were entrapped in atmospheric doldrums. During the high Middle Ages, one individual who produced notable literary works and gained an unrivaled reputation as a physician flourished. That man, whose literary contributions to the interpretation of Jewish law earned him the acronymic name of "the Rambam" (Rabbi Moses ben Maimon), is considered the most notable postbiblical Jewish personality. At the same time, he served as personal physician to the sultan of Egypt and provided medical care for countless followers of Islam. He was deemed to be equivalent to the most highly regarded of the medieval Arab physicians.

Moses ben Maimon, best known by his Hellenized name, Maimonides, was born in Cordoba, Spain, on March 30, 1138. At the time, Cordoba was part of an Islamic empire that permitted non-Muslims to live in harmony. Maimonides's father, Maimon, a judge of the rabbinical court of Cordoba, was a member of a distinguished family, which, for seven generations, produced leaders of the Jewish community in Spain. Young Maimonides was educated, mainly, by his father. His education included the Jewish laws and history, astronomy, mathematics, philosophy, and rhetoric.

It is likely that Maimonides was exposed to the classical medical writings of Galen, because of the firm Jewish conviction that health must be maintained to allow for unimpeded pursuit of the knowledge of God and the acquisition of virtues. Although there was early evidence of Maimonides's precocity as a student, his scholarly development was gradual.

The family's life was dramatically disrupted in 1148 when the Almohads, a violent and intolerant fundamentalist Muslim sect, gained control of the Iberian Peninsula. Rather than accept a mandatory conversion to the Muslim religion, the family escaped to Almeria in southeastern Spain, which had not submitted to the Almohads at the time. Three years later, the Almohads occupied southeastern Spain and the Maimon family was forced to seek asylum in several small towns until 1160, when they gained permission to sail to Fez in Morocco.

During the prolonged period of constant wandering in Spain, Maimonides continued to enhance his education, and, at the same time, he began to give his ideas permanence when he wrote a series of treatises on logic and metaphysics, comments on the Bible, and a consideration of the astronomical and mathematical aspects of the Jewish calendar. One year before leaving Spain for North Africa, Maimonides embarked on his first major literary project, in which he devoted the ensuing ten years to an interpretation of the *Mishnah*, which Rabbi Judah ha Nasi had written around 200 CE as a compilation of the laws by which Jews lived.

Fez offered Maimonides the opportunity to extend his studies and to associate with respected physicians. The Muslim leadership of the area insisted that the Jews articulate a formula for conversion and outwardly conform to

Islam. In 1162, Maimonides wrote *Letter on Conversion*, in which he cited the Talmud (Jewish book of laws) stating that it was permissible to save one's life by reciting the Muslim formula for conversion. While in Fez, the Maimon family displayed no evidence of being Jewish, and Maimonides adopted the Arabic name abu Imran Musa ibn Maimon, a name that he would maintain for his authorship of medical and philosophical works written in Arabic.

After spending five years in Fez, Maimonides had become a marked man. He was arrested but saved by the intervention of a Muslim poet. The family left Fez on April 18, 1165, and arrived at Acre, the largest Jewish community in Palestine, then known as the Kingdom of Jerusalem. The region was under the control of Christians, who permitted civil freedom for all. But dissatisfaction with the opportunities and social relationships in Palestine led the Maimon family to shorten their stay and move to Egypt, where Jews enjoyed the greatest freedom. Rabbi Maimon died shortly after the family arrived at Alexandria in 1165. In 1168, Maimonides published *Commentary on the Mishnah* and moved to Fustat, a small city near Cairo, the Egyptian capital.

Commentary on the Mishnah, Maimonides's first great literary work, is a fusion of several facets of his scholarship and an entwining of his philosophy of Judaism with Aristotelian precepts. The Mishnah is made up of six orders (*sederim* in Hebrew), divided into chapters, paragraphs, and verses. They deal with prayers, blessings, tithes, the Sabbath, holy days, celebrations, marriage, divorce, oaths, civil and criminal law, sacrificial rites, the Temple, and dietary laws, including those related to both a physical and a spiritual purity and impurity.

Maimonides began each section with a discussion of the oral law on which the written law (the Mishnah) had been based. Written in Arabic and using the Hebrew alphabet, the work was directed at a broad population of Arabic-speaking Jews. The author invoked the Greeks' golden mean between immorality and self-righteousness. He indicated his opposition to the concepts of predestination and an all-satisfying afterlife. Maimonides presented Thirteen Principles of Faith, the lack of adherence to any one of which constituted a breach of contract with Judaism.

Maimonides, in this work and in his subsequent writings, emphasized that the words of the Torah (the Pentateuch) and Talmud (written laws, a combination of the Mishnah and Gemar, the second part of the Talmud) were not always to be taken literally. *Commentary on the Mishnah* was written not only to clarify Jewish law, but also as a solution to ensure the survival of the Jews that, at the time, was in jeopardy. In 1171, Maimonides wrote *Sefar ha-Mitzvot* (*The Book of Commandments*) in anticipation of producing his major work, *Mishnah Torah*. *Sefar ha-Mitzvot* is a consideration of the 613 commandments decreed in the Pentateuch and also those that had been added subsequently. In his writing, Maimonides offered a personal assertion of the validity of each commandment.

By 1171, Maimonides was being referred to as the head of the Jews by the Muslim leaders. That year, a political transformation occurred that had a significant impact on his life. Saladin became the leader of Egypt and assumed the title of sultan and reigned from 1174 till 1193. At roughly the same time, Sunnism, a more tolerant sect of Islam, became dominant.

Shortly thereafter, Maimonides's reputation was enhanced by a situation related to Yemen, on the Arabian Peninsula. Earlier, in 1172, the leader of the Jewish community in Yemen wrote to Maimonides, informing him of a dire situation in that country. The Shiites had gained power, and, in keeping with their overt intolerance of any other faith, they demanded of the Jews either conversion or death. Conversion became widespread, and the Yemenite Jewish leader feared that his people would be annihilated. Maimonides's letter in response, known as *Petah Tikvah* (*Gate of Hope*), which was later circulated throughout the Jewish populace of the Arab world, reassured the Jewish Yemenites that they would survive and that the efforts to destroy them were doomed to failure. About a year after Maimonides's response, the brother of Saladin, the sultan of Egypt, gained control of Yemen and, in keeping with the Egyptian policy, reinstated religious freedom for the Jews.

In contrast to the usual scenario, in which literary productivity followed medical involvement, Maimonides's emergence as a notable physician occurred after his reputation as an author had been established. While Maimonides pursued his scholarship and gained appreciation for his leadership throughout the known world's Jewish communities, his younger brother, David, ran the gem-trading business that sustained the entire Maimon family. In 1174, David drowned when his ship sank during a business voyage to India, and the thirty-six-year-old Maimonides became responsible for financially providing for the entire family.

There had been a tradition among Jewish religious leaders that monetary reward should not be a consequence of religious service. The Babylonian sage Hillel (c. 110 BCE −7 CE) stressed that whoever derived a profit for himself from the words of the Torah was contributing to his own destruction.

Given the importance of health in the path to spiritual satisfaction, rabbis were often also skilled and respected physicians sought after by Muslim and Christian leaders. Maimonides began his practice of medicine in 1175 with a background of years of studying medicine at a time when the sole domain of medical literature resided in Arabic texts.

The medicine that Maimonides practiced had been established about one thousand years previously, in the second century CE, by the Greek physician Galen of Pergamon. All disease was systemic and was based on an imbalance of four bodily humors: blood, yellow bile, black bile, and phlegm. The relative dominance of the four humors resulted in the four temperaments of sanguine, choleric, melancholic, and phlegmatic, respectively. An appreciation of human anatomy was a consequence of dissection of nonhuman animals. As the Roman Empire declined and intellectual torpor spread throughout the Christian world, a vacuum developed in the practice of medicine. When the Muslim influence expanded into Europe in the eighth century, the classical Greek writings, including those of Hippocrates and Galen, were translated into Arabic texts, which became the repository for medical knowledge during medieval Christendom.

Maimonides drew from the works of Rhazes (of the ninth to the tenth century), Haly Abbas (tenth century), Avicenna (the tenth to the eleventh century), Albucasis (the tenth to the eleventh century), and Avenzoar (the tenth to the eleventh century), all of whom essentially interpreted and adhered to the postulates of Galen. By the end of his career, Maimonides's name would be positioned alongside his distinguished predecessors.

Maimonides practiced as a Galenist. Among his ten medical writings, the largest and most famous is *The Medical Aphorisms of Moses Maimonides*. It is based on Galen's work, but it uniquely brings into focus forty errors made by Galen and the contradictions of several Galenic assertions that Maimonides discovered. The book, written in Arabic, was soon translated into Hebrew, and five Latin editions were ultimately published in Europe.

Another of Maimonides's medical works, titled *The Extracts*, consists of selected works of Galen, presented specifically for the use of Maimonides's students. A third Maimonides work, titled *Aphorisms*, critically addresses the writings of Hippocrates. Maimonides also wrote treatises on hemorrhoids, poisons and bites, and asthma as well as works titled *On Sexual Intercourse, Glossary of Drug Names, Discourse on the Explanation of Fits*, and *The Preservation of Youth*.

In the realm of medicine, Maimonides made no scientific discoveries or original clinical contributions. Rather, he was recognized as a wise and skilled physician, who uniquely incorporated an appreciation of psychosocial and spiritual issues in his treatment of patients.

Maimonides's medical reputation was achieved at a time when European medicine was almost nonexistent, as evidenced by the fact that, in 1215, Cannon 22 of the Fourth Council of Lateran decreed, "Before prescribing for the sick, physicians shall be bound, under pain of exclusion from the Church, to exhort their patients to call in a priest and thus provide for their spiritual welfare." Moses Maimonides was a leading physician during his time with a large and diverse group of patients, which included the Egyptian vizier el Fadil. In 1198, five years after the sultan Saladin died, and his son, al Afdal, succeeded him, Maimonides was appointed chief physician.

Returning to Maimonides as a literary figure, the most highly regarded of his written works is *Mishnah Torah*, meaning "repetition of the Torah." It was directed at Jews throughout the world, and, therefore, unlike *Commentary on the Mishnah* that was written in Judeo-Arabic, *Mishnah Torah* was written in Hebrew. This work, which consisted of fourteen volumes containing one thousand chapters, was completed in 1180 after ten years of work.

Mishnah Torah provides a complete, concise, well-organized, readily understandable resolution of the points of Jewish law. The applicable Hebraic word for the set of Jewish laws is *halakah*, which derives from several sources, mainly from the Torah, but also from laws subsequently instituted by rabbis, and from laws consequent to established customs. *Mishnah Torah*, which has been hailed as a literary, theological, and legalistic masterpiece, offers a universal statement of how Jews should conduct their lives and worship their god. It discusses rituals and ethical behavior, considers contemporary concerns, and offers a pathway for the future of all Jews.

The publication of the work raised the pedestal on which Maimonides already stood. He became the most prestigious Jewish scholar in the world and its most notable Jew. And still, he would rise to greater heights. In 1187, the year that he was named chief rabbi of all the lands controlled by the sultan Saladin, Maimonides began work on a treatise that was destined to become his most famous work.

The Guide for the Perplexed, which was completed in 1190, was written in Arabic and directed toward an audience that differed distinctly from the anticipated readership of *Mishnah Torah*. While the latter work was written for ordinary people, it was anticipated that *The Guide for the Perplexed* would be read and digested by enlightened scholars. The essence of the work is an expression of the view that faith and reason do not require reconciliation because they actually share a common ground. The author indicates that not all the words of faith are to be taken literally, but rather may represent allegorical or meta-phoric presentations. Also, Maimonides deemed it appropriate to incorporate classical Greek philosophical concepts into an interpretation of scripture.

Almost one thousand years after the completion of *The Guide for the Perplexed*, Dr. Francis Sellers Collins, an esteemed researcher in the field of genetics, director of the Human Genome Project, and subsequently director of the National Institutes of Health, provided a pertinent analogy. His 2006 publication, *The Language of God: A Scientist Presents Evidence for Belief*, which appeared on the *New York Times* best-seller list, offered the perspective that Christianity can be reconciled with evolution and science.

After completion of *The Guide for the Perplexed*, Maimonides continued to maintain a busy and demanding life, divided between widespread rabbinical involvements and a continuously expanding medical practice. Maimonides died on December 13, 1204. An assessment of his life gives testament to the fact that there was a time in history in which one man, the Rambam, Moses Maimonides, simultaneously was the most renowned writer *and* the most renowned physician in the world.

We are left with his statements: "Truth does not become more true by virtue of the fact that the entire world agrees with it, nor less so even if the whole world disagrees with it," and "The physician should not treat the disease but the patient who is suffering from it."

SOURCES

Collins, Francis S. *The Language of God: A Scientist Presents Evidence for Belief.* New York: Free Press, 2006.
Nuland, Sherwin. *Maimonides.* New York: Nextbook Schocken, 2005.

2

THOMAS LINACRE

Health and Humanism

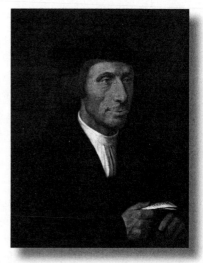

In 1962, a new constituent college was established at the University of Oxford. It was named Linacre College to honor a physician, classicist, and humanist, who founded the Royal College of Physicians. The honoree, a presence during the Renaissance of England, made sufficiently diverse and meaningful contributions to merit the current appellation of "a true Renaissance man."

Thomas Linacre was born circa 1460 at Brampton, Chesterfield, in Derbyshire and was initially educated at the Canterbury Cathedral school under the tutelage of William Tilly of Selling, a Benedictine prior of Christ Church, Canterbury, and a notable humanist who became a member of All Souls College, Oxford. Linacre studied at Oxford from 1480 to 1484 and was elected a fellow of All Souls College. While at Oxford, Linacre established friendships with scholars William Grocyn and William Latimer of All Souls College. The three names remain recognized as an Oxford triumvirate that developed English scholarship and humanism. Thomas More entered Canterbury in 1497 and indicated that he owed his knowledge of Greek to Linacre.

In 1484, Tilly was sent by Henry VII as an envoy to Pope Innocent VIII, and Linacre joined the train in order to capture the opportunity of visiting Italy, where the Renaissance had reached its height. In Florence, Linacre became a pupil of Angelo Poliziano (Politian) and shared instruction with the sons of Lorenzo de' Medici. Linacre moved to Padua, where he received the degree of doctor of medicine in 1496. He was among the earliest Englishmen to receive a medical degree from the University of Padua, where Andreas Vesalius would produce *De humani corporis fabrica* in 1543, and where William Harvey would receive his medical degree in 1602.

After Linacre received his medical degree, he returned to Oxford, where he translated an astronomical treatise, *De sphaera* (*Of Spheres*), by Proclus. The book was printed in Venice in 1499 by the great scholar and printer Aldus Manutius, whose editions of the classics are monumental. In the dedication of the work to Arthur, the Prince of Wales, the son of Henry VII of England, Aldus pays tribute to the scholarship of Linacre. The book was the first translation of a Greek author produced in England and earned for Linacre recognition as the restorer of Greek literature in that country.

In 1499, Desiderius Erasmus of Rotterdam, Holland, first met Linacre, with whom he studied Greek. Linacre also cared for Erasmus medically, and the two men would remain identified as allied humanists. In the early part of the sixteenth century, Linacre moved to London and became a member of the court of Henry VII as well as the tutor of the Prince of Wales. In 1509, on the accession of Henry VIII, Linacre was designated physician to the king. This post brought him such notable patients as Princess Mary, Sir Thomas More, Cardinal Thomas Wolsey, Archbishop William Warham, and Bishop Richard Fox.

Linacre's most significant and lasting contribution to medicine and science was the founding of the College of Physicians, now called the Royal College of Physicians of London. In 1518, with the aid of the then lord chancellor Wolsey, a royal charter was granted, and Linacre was elected the first president, a position he held until he died in 1524. The college was preceded only by the Royal College of Surgeons as the oldest English-speaking medical society, and was formed to grant licenses to those who fulfilled specific qualifications and to punish those who conducted malpractice. For close to one hundred years, the meetings were conducted in the house on Knight Rider Street where Linacre had resided. The house and its library were bequeathed by Linacre to the college; regrettably, both were destroyed by the Great Fire of London of 1666.

In October 1524, only eight days before his death, Linacre made provision for two lectureships at Oxford and one at Cambridge to encourage the study and teaching of medicine. In the original deed, nothing was said as to the subject of the lecture. The Statutes of Queen Elizabeth in 1580 directed that the lecturer was to be a master of arts versed in the works of Aristotle and Galen. The Statutes of Queen Victoria in 1849 indicated that the lecturer was to deliver courses about foods and drugs, on the care of health, on methods of healing, on forensic medicine, and other subjects approved by the master.

In 1592, Henry Briggs, a distinguished mathematician and later Savilian Professor of Astronomy at Oxford, gave the lecture. In 1625, Briggs published a map of North America that defined California as a large island, a representation that appears on almost all maps for almost one hundred years. William Heberden, known as the English Celsus, was Linacre lecturer from 1734 to 1748, and Sir Thomas Watson, who compiled a popular textbook of medicine, lectured from 1822 to 1826.

Linacre is included in the list of humanists of the Renaissance. His emphasis on human interests rather than the natural world or religion was pervasive, and was enthusiastically shared with those of equal mind. The English humanists were concerned with activating the revival of classic learning in England. In Linacre's field of medicine, the classic writings in Greek and Latin had disappeared from Western civilization and become sequestered in the Arabic world after the fall of the Roman Empire during the fourth and fifth centuries. In the Middle Ages, the teachings of Islamic physicians, such as Rhazes and Avicenna, were influential throughout the Muslim world and also dominant in Europe.

The medical humanists of the Renaissance were dedicated to resurrecting the scholastic period of Greek medicine. During his stay in Italy, Linacre had been exposed to the manuscripts of Galen and others, and was committed to disseminating them so that the principles enunciated within them formed the basis of practice. Linacre's literary contributions were mainly Latin translations of Greek works. The first to appear was a Paris 1517 publication of Galen's *De Sanitate Tuenda* (*On Maintaining Health*). The work was dedicated to Henry VIII and was sufficiently popular to appear in over five editions. A copy on vellum with a manuscript dedicated to Cardinal Wolsey is housed in the British Library. Linacre's second book, *Methodus Medendi* (*The Method of Healing*), was a folio published in Paris in 1519, and was also dedicated to Henry VIII.

The third of Linacre's translations, a small quarto, titled *De Temperamentis et de Inaequali Intemperie* (*On the Temperaments and on Excess*), was an early Cambridge press publication in 1521. That work was inscribed to Pope Leo X, who was Giovanni, the younger son of Lorenzo de' Medici, with whom Linacre lived while he was in Florence. Linacre had studied with the young Giovanni under Politian and also acted as Giovanni's tutor.

Three other translations of Galen by Linacre were published in London: *De Naturalibus Facultatibus* (*On the Natural Faculties*), *De Pulsuum Usu* (*On the Use of the Pulse*), and *De Symptomatum Differentis et Causis* (*On the Differences and Causes of Symptoms*). The last was published after Linacre's death.

Two months after Linacre died, his most significant literary contribution was published. That work, *De Emendata Structura Latini Sermonis* (*On the Correct Form of the Latin Language*), established his reputation as a grammarian. Previously, at the time that he was tutoring Princess Mary, Linacre published two elementary grammars in English. The first, a copy of which is housed in the British Library, is thought to be a grammar prepared for St. Paul's School, but rejected by Jean Collet, the humanist dean of St. Paul's Cathedral. The publication includes verses by Linacre, Sir Thomas More, and the celebrated grammarian and first master of the St. Paul's School, William Lily.

The second Latin grammar, *Rudimenta Grammatices* (*The Rudiments of Grammar*), was dedicated to Princess Mary, for whose health and education Linacre was responsible. Linacre's major grammatical opus, *De Emendata Structura Latini Sermonis*, and its author are—according to William Osler's biography on Linacre—generally believed to be the subjects referred to in Erasmus's *Praise of Folly*: "I knew an old Sophister that a Grecian, a Latinist, a mathematician, a philosopher, a physician, and all to the greatest perfection, who after three score years of experience in the world had spent the last twenty of them only in drudging to conquer the criticisms of grammar, and made it the chief parts of his prayers that his life might be so spared till he had learned how rightly to distinguish betwixt the eight parts of speech, which no grammarian whether Greek or Latin had yet accurately done."

In 1520, Linacre retired from his medical practice but maintained his activities related to the Royal College of Physicians. At some time between 1510 and 1520, he took the orders of a priest and, in 1519, was designated rector at the parish of Wigan in Lancashire. He died on October 20, 1524, of complications related to bladder stones.

In 1557, Dr. John Caius, then president of the Royal College of Physicians, whose name was attached to Gonville College, Cambridge, that year, had, at his own expense, a monument erected in St. Paul's Cathedral near Linacre's grave. Beneath the statue of a phoenix, a tablet bore this inscription:

Thomas Linacre, physician of King Henry VIII, a man most learned in Greek and Latin as well in medicine, restored to life many who during their lifetime were languishing and who had lost heart. He translated many of the works of Galen [from Greek] into Latin with astonishing and singular eloquence. At the request of his friends, a little before his death, he composed an outstanding work on the correct form of Latin speech. He gave two public lectures at Oxford and one at Cambridge *in perpetuum* for those zealous of medical study. In this city [London] by his diligence was established the College of Physicians, of which he was elected president. Detesting deceit and artifice, faithful to his friends, he was distinguished among every rank. Some years before he died he was ordained to the priesthood. Full of years, he departed this life much missed, in the year of Our Lord 1524, on the 20th day of October. His reputation survives his death.

The memorial remained until the Great Fire of London in 1666. As time has passed, it has been questioned whether Linacre was a better Latinist or Grecian, a better grammarian or physician, a better scholar or man for his moral qualifications.

SOURCES

Dictionary of National Biography (1993), s.v. "Linacre, Thomas."
Johnson, John Noble. *The Life of Thomas Linacre*. London: Edward Lumley, 1835.
Osler, William. *Thomas Linacre*. Cambridge: Cambridge University Press, 1908.

3

FRANÇOIS RABELAIS

Mirth as Medicine

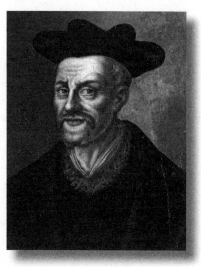

F rançois Rabelais was a Renaissance French physician who has been credited with a literary impact that placed him in a category alongside Homer, Dante, Shakespeare, and Cervantes. Rabelais, who was a prime developer of the French literary tongue and had a profound influence on the world's subsequent literature, was born sometime between 1483 and 1494 in Chinon in the Loire Valley, where his father practiced law. As a youth, Rabelais dedicated himself to scholastics, including Greek, Latin, the classics, and law. Between 1510 and 1511, he became a monk in the Franciscan order and entered the monastery of Le Puy Saint-Martin in Fontenay-le-Comte, located in the Pays de La Loire region in France. While at that locale, the earliest of his extant literary productions, a letter dated March 1521, and written to the French humanist Guillaume Budé, was composed. Rabelais's classical studies and early writings were criticized by his Franciscan colleagues because his conclusions were deemed to be contrary to the accepted biblical interpretation by the Franciscan order. Rabelais was made to feel uncomfortable at the monastery, whereupon he received permission from Pope Clement VII to transfer to the less restrictive Benedictine order at Saint-Pierre-de-Maillezais in the Ven dé Ee, France. That order was led by Bishop Geoffrey d'Estissac, who became Rabelais's patron.

In 1526, Rabelais decided to study medicine, which meant he had to abandon his life as a monk because the clergy were not allowed to practice medicine. Initially, he may have studied in Paris between 1526 and 1529. In 1529, he is known to have matriculated as a medical student at the University of Montpellier, the oldest continuously functioning medical school in western Europe. At the time, medicine was considered to be the center of all natural sciences and humanities, and was incorporated in philosophy. In 1531, Rabelais taught a course at Montpellier on the Greek text of Hippocrates.

In 1532, Rabelais settled in Lyons, where he received a prestigious appointment at the Hôtel-Dieu hospital. That year, he published French editions of several classical medical works by Hippocrates and Galen. In 1534, he went to Rome for three months with Bishop Jean du Bellay, who later became a cardinal. Rabelais made several trips as a traveling companion with the cardinal to Rome, and lived for a while with the cardinal's brother in Turin.

Rabelais taught medicine at Montpellier in 1537 and 1538, during which time he lectured on Hippocrates's *Prognostics*. He translated the works of Hippocrates and Galen from the Greek and, in 1537, published a translation of *The Aphorisms of Hippocrates*. Also, in 1538, it is recorded that he performed an autopsy, accompanied by a scientific explanation, on a man who had been hanged. The University of Montpellier continues to honor Rabelais with a monument in its Jardin des Plantes, with the tradition in which the graduating doctors take an oath under Rabelais's robe, and by the continued use of the students' cap, a *faluche*, styled in the fashion of the one that Rabelais wore.

Between 1545 and 1547, Rabelais lived in Metz in northeast France, which at the time was a free city and republic. This allowed him to escape the wrath of the Sorbonne, which his writings had brought about because of their scatological and bawdy descriptions. In 1547, Rabelais became curate of St. Christophe de Jambe and of Meudon. He resigned those positions before he died in Paris in 1553. Just prior to his death, he is reputed to have said, "I go to see a great perhaps."

Rabelais's seminal contribution to fiction consists of four books: *Pantagruel* (1532), *Gargantua* (1534), *Tiers Livre* (1546), and *Quart Livre* (1548). Several other works of comic fiction attributed to Rabelais were published posthumously, but the authenticity of his authorship of those works has been disputed. The four books he is known to have written constitute a continuum. As such, *Gargantua*, the name of the royal giant who fathered Pantagruel, the central character of the other three books, is usually presented first in modern publications of the series, although it was published second. *Gargantua*'s name persists in the English language to connote something that is immense.

Perhaps in anticipation of controversy, Rabelais initially maintained anonymity as the author of his fictional works. The author of his first publication, *Pantagruel*, was listed as Alcofribas Nasier, an anagram of François Rabelais. Similarly, Rabelais's anagram appears as the author of the second book, *Gargantua*.

Gargantua consists of a series of tales about Pantagruel's father's life. It is a political and religious satire and an endorsement of a tolerant Christianity that incorporates classical Greek philosophical concepts. The work is significantly more sophisticated than *Pantagruel*, in that, although it is also comic, it evidences the knowledge and experience of an ex-monk and a physician and offers a meaningful message from a humanist. In the final chapters of *Gargantua*, devoted to the Abbey of Thelema, Rabelais champions religious freedom and denigrates poverty and monastic chastity. At the Utopian abbey, men and women live together in equality, harmony, and beauty.

Pantagruel, the first of Rabelais's works of fiction to be published and the most popular of his books, is a topical satire of the extremes of lifestyle in France and the time of carnival that also incorporates evidence of scholarly learning and enthusiasm for humanism. It attracted critical attention because of the previously unparalleled pervasive presence of obscenities as well as fecal and genital references. Both *Pantagruel* and *Gargantua* were condemned by the Sorbonne, acting as the church's office of censorship.

Despite the church's condemnation, Rabelais's *Tiers Livre de Pantagruel* was published with the "Royal Privilege of Francis" included on the title page and was dedicated to the king's sister, Queen Margaret of Navarre. The book is the least comic and most learned of Rabelais's four works. It includes a dialogue in which the rational humanism of Pantagruel is contrasted with the hedonistic attitude of his companion, Panurge, who champions debt and questions the value of marriage. In the narrative, the assertions of scholars, a theologian, a doctor, and a philosopher are invoked for support in the arguments. The *Quart Livre* uses masterful comic writing to advocate the incorporation of ancient Jewish and classical wisdom into Renaissance Christianity.

Rabelais's literary works were highly regarded by his contemporaries, but by the eighteenth century they fell into disrepute because scatological and sexual descriptions were no longer considered to be appropriate writings. Voltaire wrote, "Only a few eccentric persons pride themselves on understanding and esteeming his work, as a whole; the rest of the nations . . . hold his book in contempt. . . . He is regarded as chief among buffoons . . . he is a drunken philosopher who wrote only when he was drunk." A century later, leading

FROM MEDICINE TO MANUSCRIPT

French romanticists François-René Chateaubriand and Victor Hugo praised Rabelais as an initiator and genius. At present, he is referred to as the least popular and least appreciated of the great writers.

Rabelais was a physician who considered laughter to be beneficial for health. During his time, health and disease were the consequence of the balance between the four humors: blood, yellow bile, black bile, and phlegm. Organ pathology was not considered to be causative. Laughter was ascribed as the potential to heal and regenerate by affecting the humoral balance. Rabelais's many references to feces are in keeping with the Hippocratic and Galenic assignment of importance to the assessment of bodily excretions in order to define and treat diseases.

Rabelais targeted, as his opposition, the dogma, rigidity, authoritarianism, and serious tone of the ecclesiastical and feudal culture of the time. The conflict between carnival and Lent was allegorical. Carnival represented freedom and humanism that occurred during a period of revelry and celebration, while Lent stood for ecclesiastical and feudal restrictions. He espoused the humor of the carnival and the common marketplace, using grotesque images, indecent language, profanities, and oaths to denigrate the staid, immutable, and confining society to which the populace was exposed.

Although Rabelais's readers were, in general, learned, they were well acquainted with carnival as well as marketplace and comic folk language. Carnival involved all people, and all were considered equal during carnival. The other relevance concerning the author's use of the grotesque realism of carnival is the positive message of metamorphosis and regeneration.

This author of extraordinary comic literature has left us with such memorable statements as "Nature abhors a vacuum," "He always looked a given horse in its mouth," "Robbing Peter to pay Paul," "Hit the nail on the head," and "Everything comes to those that can wait." This physician and writer, who was also a prime inventor of the French literary vernacular, is now more frequently remembered merely as an adjective, Rabelaisian, "connoting ribald, bawdy, or indecent writings or statements."

SOURCES

Bakhtin, Mikhail. *Rabelais and His World*. Cambridge, MA: MIT Press, 1968.
Screech, M. A. *Rabelais*. Ithaca, NY: Cornell University Press, 1979.

4

MICHEL DE NOSTREDAME

Potions and Prognostications

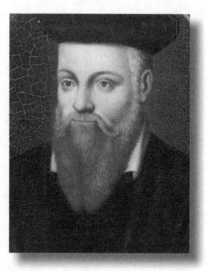

In the classical era, Greek and Roman writers were traditionally mononymous, in other words, recognized by a single name of distinction. In the medical literature, Hippocrates and Galen are representative examples. In the field of epic history, Homer and Thucydides stand out, while in philosophy, Socrates, Plato, and Aristotle are most notable. The three most popular Greek tragedians were Aeschylus, Socrates, and Euripides. In the Renaissance, sporadic evidence of single-name authors returned. The philosopher Erasmus comes to mind, while the most blatant was the Swiss German physician, astrologer, and alchemist Philippus Aureolus Bombastus Von Hohenheim, who used the pseudonym Paracelsus to imply that he was the equal of the famous Roman chronicler of medicine, Celsus. Yet another poignant example from the Renaissance is the physician, and most memorable of all prognosticators, Nostradamus, who used a Latinized variant of his French surname to add gravitas to his publications.

Michel de Nostredame was born about December 23, 1503, according to the Gregorian calendar, at Saint-Remy in Provence, France. Both his maternal and paternal grandfathers were physicians who attended the nobility. In 1501, Louis XII of France issued an edict that all Jews were to be baptized or were required to leave Provence. Consequently, Nostradamus's parents—his father a successful notary—and both his grandfathers were baptized, as was Nostradamus.

Nostradamus received his early education at the home of his maternal grandfather and, subsequently, that of his paternal grandfather. The youngster proceeded to the city of Avignon to study the liberal arts, and, while conducting his studies, he evidenced an early interest in astrology. In 1522, Nostradamus enrolled at the University of Montpellier, where he studied medicine for three years and received a baccalauréat, or bachelor's degree. This was followed by a rigorous examination and the awarding of a license to practice medicine by the bishop of Montpellier.

In 1525, the year in which Nostradamus received his license, an outbreak of the plague occurred throughout southern France. He abandoned the university's program, in which he was registered to obtain a doctorate in medicine, in order to care for victims. He established a reputation as a capable physician with the citizens of Montpellier and throughout the countryside of southern France. The records of the university indicate that he returned in October 1529 as a candidate for a doctorate, which he was awarded that year. He joined the faculty and remained there until 1532. There is no evidence that Nostradamus and Rabelais ever met at the university they attended, or communicated about medical matters.

Another biographer, John Houge, who represents the minority, presents a disparate chronicle of Nostradamus's medical education. Houge indicates that, from 1521 to 1529, Nostradamus traveled widely, researching herbal remedies and acting as an apothecary. In 1529, he entered the university at Montpellier to study for a doctorate in medicine. Shortly thereafter, it was discovered that he had been an apothecary, a trade that was specifically banned by the university's rules. Nostradamus was consequently expelled, and documentation of the action, allegedly, exists in the university's archives.

In 1532, Nostradamus responded to an invitation from Jules-César Scalinger, a physician/mathematician, botanist, and philosopher/poet, who was considered to be one of the most learned men in Europe, to join him. Nostradamus settled in Agen near Scalinger, developed a lucrative medical practice, and married a woman "of high estate" with whom he had two children. His idyllic life came to an end when his wife and two children died, and his relationship with Scalinger became antagonistic. In 1538, Nostradamus set out on a six-year period of travel in France, but which extended as far east as Venice. He sought to add to his knowledge of astrology, pharmacology, and medicine, but there is no evidence that he visited the University of Padua.

When Nostradamus completed his travels in 1544, he participated in the treatment of victims of a new outburst of the plague in Marseilles, France. Two years later, he treated plague victims in Aix-en-Provence. In both locations he ascribed cures to the use of his own concoction of pills, which he produced by crushing red roses. To his credit, he refrained from bleeding or purging patients, and, in appreciation of his efforts, he was awarded a lifetime pension by the French Parlement.

In 1546, Nostradamus settled in Salon de Provence, which would remain his home for the rest of his life. He married a wealthy widow with whom he would parent several children, six of whom would survive him. In Salon, he devoted most of his time to developing cosmetics for a wealthy clientele, and enhancing his interest in astrology. From the time of his arrival in Salon and throughout the remainder of his life, there is little evidence of his practicing medicine.

Nostradamus's first publication, featuring astrological predictions, appeared in 1550. Doubtless, it was quatrain 35, which appeared in *Les Prophéties de Mr Michel Nostradamus (The Prophecies of Mr. Michel Nostradamus*, also known as *Centuries I*, published in Lyons in 1555), that raised his visibility among the French royalty. The reaction to Nostradamus's predictions was mixed. The most learned individuals discounted them. The uneducated masses thought they were foolish or a tool of the devil to be feared. But the nobility of France constituted a receptive audience. None was a greater devotee than Catherine de' Medici, the wife of French king Henry II.

Astrology enjoyed widespread acceptance in Florence, Italy, beginning with Cosimo de' Medici, the first of the Medici political dynasty. In 1536, after Henry of Valois was elevated to the position of heir apparent to the throne of France, his young wife, Catherine de' Medici, sought the prediction of the most famous Italian astrologer, Luca Gaurico, regarding her husband's future. Gaurico's forecast indicated that Henry would become king of France, and that his regency would be marked by a duel that would end his reign and result in his death.

In July 1556, Catherine de' Medici summoned Nostradamus to Paris. Although the champions of Nostradamus's prognostications would point out that his writings can be interpreted as predicting the adverse circumstances that would subsequently affect her children, Nostradamus could only relate to Catherine that all her sons would be kings, which could be interpreted as constituting a truth. Nostradamus's reputation was enhanced by the consultation.

On July 1, 1559, while celebrating the marriage of his daughter to Philip II of Spain and his sister's marriage to Emmanuel Philibert, Duke of Savoy,

Henry II engaged in a joust with the captain of his Scots Guards. The king sustained a mortal blow when his opponent's lance broke, raised the king's visor, and pierced his right eye. Nostradamus's famous quatrain 35 was retrospectively interpreted as precisely predicting the unusual event, further enhancing the prognosticator's reputation.

In October 1559, the Duke of Savoy stopped at Salon on his way home and was later joined by his bride. Nostradamus was commissioned to compose an inscription for the arches honoring the visiting royalty. In 1564, Catherine de' Medici led a royal progress to expose the populace to the young, recently enthroned Charles VIII of France. When the progress passed through Provence, Catherine visited Nostradamus. Charles VIII honored Nostradamus by giving him a financial gift and appointing him counselor and physician in ordinary. In June 1566, Nostradamus died in Salon. His tomb is located in the Church of St. Lawrence in Salon.

Nostradamus's first publication was an almanac that appeared in 1550. The almanac, which appeared almost every year until his death, contained prophecies for only the year to come. Cumulatively, the almanacs contained over six thousand predictions. In 1552, his publication of *Traité des fardemens et confitures (Treatise of Cosmetics and Preservatives)* appeared, which was a combination of descriptions of recipes for cosmetics, preserves, and concoctions to prevent and treat the plague. His only other publication related to medicine, *Paraphrase de C. Galen sur L'exortation de Menodote, aux Estudes des Bonnes Artz, Mesmement Medecine. Traduict de Latin en Francoys par M. Nostradamus*, was printed in 1557. Both medical books were of little consequence.

Nostradamus is best known for the publications of *Les Propheties de M. Michel Nostradamus*, which was translated into several languages and has rarely been out of print. Over two hundred editions have appeared. Nostradamus planned an ongoing project that was to include prophecies for more than two thousand years, until 3797. Each publication was to contain a collection of one hundred quatrains (four line verses), thus accounting for the assigned name, "the Centuries."

The first edition contained 353 quatrains, three groups of one hundred, and the fourth containing fifty-three quatrains. A second edition, containing 640 quatrains, appeared in 1557. After Nostradamus died in 1566, a compendium of two parts was published. It contains 942 quatrains, assembled in nine sets of one hundred or "Centuries" and one of forty-two.

The most notable quatrain appears in the first edition as number 35.

The young lion will overcome the old one
On the field of battle in single combat:
He will put out his eyes in a cage of gold:
Two fleets (wounds) one, then to die a cruel death.

Published in 1555, the quatrain was touted as having predicted, with extraordinary specificity, the fatal joust of Henry II of France in 1559. Post hoc analysis concluded that 1) the "young lion" referred to the fact that the opponent, who accidentally administered the blow to the king, was almost twenty years younger than Henry II, 2) "the field of battle in single combat" described a joust, 3) "put out his eyes" described the site of the wound, 4) "cage of gold" denoted the king's gilded helmet with a visor, and 5) "two fleets" (wounds) referred to injuries to the eye and the brain. Henry II was thought to have been identified by his gold helmet and his lion crest.

Nostradamus never ascribed to himself the powers of a prophet. The appeal of his writings resides in their focus on a panoply of disasters. Interpretations of the implications of his verses continue to appear. The implications of his predictions are recurrent subjects of attention of a variety of recent books, television documentaries, and websites.

SOURCES

Hogue, John. *Nostradamus: Life and Myth*. London: HarperCollins, 2003.
Leoni, Edgar. *Nostradamus and His Prophecies*. New York: Bell Publishing, 1982.

5

SIR THOMAS BROWNE

Favorite of the Future

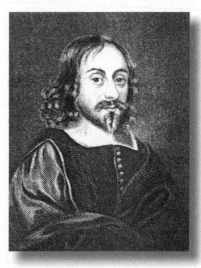

O ne seventeenth-century physician and literary figure was
knighted for his contributions, and has
been cited over the ensuing centuries for his
erudition and literary productions. During
the nineteenth and twentieth centuries, he
became a focus of study and adulation
by two of the most highly regarded physician bibliophiles of modern times—Sir
William Osler and Sir Geoffrey Keynes,
two men whose own productivity merit
inclusion within this work.

This object of high regard was
Thomas Browne, the dominant English
literary personality of the seventeenth century. The son of a London silk merchant, whose name he bore as the eldest child, Thomas was born on October
19, 1605, in Cheapside (a location in London). His father died when he was
eight years old, and three years later, young Thomas began an eight-year study
period at Winchester College, which is the oldest of the English public schools.
It was established as a feeder or source of future students for New College,
Oxford, in 1382. Anthony Ashley Cooper, the Earl of Shaftesbury, who
was influential in the life of the social and political philosopher John Locke,
attended Winchester College shortly after Browne. The curriculum consisted
of prayers, coupled with Latin and Greek exercises, and was devoid of the
natural sciences. It was oriented to the preparation of future clerics.

Browne failed to receive a scholarship at New College, Oxford, and in
1623, he enrolled at Broadgates Hall, later to become Pembroke College,

Oxford, as a commoner paying his own way. This circumstance contributed to Browne's eventual selection of a medical career because Pembroke College was the center of medical and anatomical studies at Oxford. In 1623, on the occasion of the death of William Camden, who had played a significant role in the modernization of Oxford, Browne authored a poem, "Camdeni Insignia," which became Browne's first printed work. He so impressed the leaders at Broadgates in his first year there that he was selected to give the opening oration, in 1624, at the founding of Pembroke College.

At Pembroke College, Master Thomas Clayton was the most influential of Browne's teachers in that, as a professor of medicine, he emphasized reconciliation between physical and spiritual medicine. Browne received a master's degree from Pembroke in 1629, having received his bachelor's degree two years previously. While at Oxford, Browne had been exposed to the works of Vesalius, Fallopius, and Aquapendente in anatomy, and in 1628, he was introduced to the revolutionary publication on the circulation of blood by William Harvey.

At the time Browne completed his studies at Oxford, it was widely believed that the best medical education was offered on the European continent. In a desire to expand his medical knowledge, he spent the next three years sequentially at Montpellier in France, at Padua in Italy, and at Leiden in Holland. At Montpellier, where Rabelais and Nostradamus had received their medical education, and John Locke would later visit, Browne used Rabelais's Latin translation of Hippocrates's *Aphorisms*.

During Browne's stay on the Continent, the medical school at Montpellier had begun to decline in reputation, while Padua was at its peak, and Leiden was in ascent. Although Browne never formally matriculated, he entered the fall term at Montpellier in 1631. The curriculum stressed plant remedies and used a magnificent botanical garden as an educational facility. Browne's interest in the anatomy and diseases of the brain were stimulated at Montpellier.

He spent a period from the second half of 1632 through the first half of 1633 at Padua, twenty-two years after Galileo ended his eighteen years of teaching at that university. For students at Padua, the three premier attractions were anatomy lectures, botanical demonstrations, and clinical experiences, particularly at the Hospital of St. Francis.

Browne began his studies at the University of Leiden on December 3, 1633, and received his MD on December 21, 1633. The brevity of the period between the two events was not unusual. The doctoral candidate was only required to pass an examination covering the fundamentals of medicine, offer a defense of two selected Hippocratic aphorisms, and present a thesis. Browne defended his thesis on smallpox.

Browne returned to England in 1634 and spent the first three years in the provincial town of Halifax, West Yorkshire, a center of England's woolen manufacture. The town had gained some notoriety for the Halifax Gibbet, an early guillotine that had been installed during the sixteenth century and was used until 1650. Browne's selection of a provincial site was necessitated by the limitation of the locations for his practice between his obligatory conversion fourteen years between his enrollment at Oxford and the conversion of his Leiden MD into an Oxford doctorate.

Little is known of his medical presence in Halifax. *A Dictionary of English County Physicians, 1603–1643* lists none active in Halifax. A 1708 publication, titled *Halifax and Its Gibbet-Law Placed in a True Light*, by Samuel Midgley, stated that "the learned Dr. Browne . . . in his Juvenal Years, he fixed himself in the Populous, and rich Trading Place, wherein he shew his Skill, and gain Respect in the World; And that during his Residence amongst us, and his vacant Hours he writ his admired Piece, called by him *Religio Medici*." Browne himself indicates that he composed his *Religio Medici* (*The Religion of a Physician*) around 1634–35. There are eight extant manuscripts of the work, the earliest of which is dated 1639.

In 1637, Browne moved to the town of Norwich in the county of Norfolk. Norwich, with a population of about thirty thousand, was second only in number to London at the time. The main encouragement for the move came from one of Browne's Oxford tutors, the Reverend Thomas Lushington, who had assumed the post of chaplain to the bishop of Norwich the previous year. Five years after Browne's arrival, he married Dorothy Mileham, who was seventeen years his junior. The couple had twelve children, eight of whom predeceased them. Edward, the one son who survived, became physician to St. Bartholomew's Hospital and was president of the Royal College of Physicians of London from 1704 until his death in 1708.

The information available regarding Thomas Browne's medical practice has been compiled and published in the four-volume *The Works of Sir Thomas Browne* (1964). Browne was regarded as the leading physician throughout East Anglia in the mid-eastern region of England. He served both as a consultant to his medical colleagues and physician for the leading families in Norfolk County. He often traveled long distances on horseback and remained absent from his home for long periods when he was providing medical care. He is known to have provided care to the poor at no charge and with disregard for the patients' religious or political status.

During his time in Norwich, patients suffering from smallpox and the plague were prevalent. There were four outbreaks of the plague in that period. In 1665–66, over two thousand people died. Although Browne sent his family to a distant village during the outbreaks, unlike many other physicians, he remained to offer service. He also cared for patients with malaria, which was common in the region at the time.

Bladder stones were also a common affliction. Norfolk had a higher incidence than any other English county. Browne treated several dignitaries of the church and Parliament, employing marshmallow and other bland remedies. He treated patients suffering from phthisis (tuberculosis) gout, asthma, venereal disease, and rickets; his records indicate that he practiced obstetrics and gynecology, but performed no surgery. His case records include several patients who were more than one hundred years old. One 102-year-old lady manifested the classic symptoms of hyperthyroidism and compulsive eating. Another of his case records describes a patient with hydropneumothorax, for whom he recommended drainage. Browne employed the common medical practices of purging (use of laxatives) and bloodletting, and recommended "taking the waters" at Bath and Epson for generalized aching.

One of the unique aspects of Browne's medical care was his awareness of psychological disturbances and the influence of emotions on disease. He stressed the importance of treating patients as whole human beings rather than as bodies with "excessive or impeded humours." He pointed out that the physician's service may span not only medical but also religious and moral roles, and may have a social context. He indicated that the management of a patient should involve the patient's family. An evaluation by a modern American psychiatrist, J. M. Schneck, offers evidence that Browne recognized the unconscious aspect of the superego, the correlation between dream content and illness, and the psychopathology associated with senility.

Although he made no scientific or clinical discoveries, Browne has been credited with the first account of adipocere, i.e., the liquefaction of human and animal muscle after death, the first suggestion that rabies may be transmitted from one animal to another.

Although Browne maintained a belief in witchcraft and the efficacy of the king's touch to cure scrofula, he recognized the importance of William Harvey's contribution regarding the circulation of blood. Browne continually attempted to keep abreast of medical advances. In 1664, he was elected as an honorary fellow of the Royal College of Physicians of London.

By the mid-seventeenth century, Thomas Browne had become one of the most highly regarded intellectuals not only in England but throughout Western civilization. His correspondence was widespread, and he was frequently visited by other learned men.

The springboard that initially propelled Browne to a rarified realm of intellectual eminence was the publication of *Religio Medici*. Browne wrote that the work was not intended for publication, but "was composed at leisurable hours for his private exercise and satisfaction." Several manuscript copies were distributed among his friends. One of these fell into the hands of a publisher who published the work in 1642 without the author's permission or identification. Browne felt compelled to correct the inaccuracies that were presented in print, leading to the publication of "a true and full coppy," which was published under the author's name in 1643. The book was an immediate success, translated into several languages, including Latin, and has never been out of print.

The book is one of the earliest attempts to reconcile religion and "natural philosophy," the precursor of modern science. For Browne, religion was based on the virtues of faith, hope, and charity. Browne rejected the authority of the church or the papacy and religious realism in favor of reason and the Scripture. He regarded an individual's faith to be the dominant element, and he presented science as being in agreement with religious belief. He not only was concerned with erasing the conflicts between religion and science, but also promoted tolerance in religious belief. *Religio Medici* was referred to by Sir William Osler, the "father of modern medicine" as "the most precious book" in his library.

Browne's second, most encyclopedic, and his personal favorite publication, *Pseudodoxia Epidemica [An Epidemic of False Doctrines]: or, Enquiries into Very Many Received Tenents and Commonly Presumed Truths*, was published as a small folio in 1646. The work consists of seven books, arranged in the Renaissance concept of the scale of creation: Book 1—an essay on the nature of error, Book 2—fallacies in the fields of mineral and vegetable, Book 3—the animal kingdom, Book 4—errors about Man, Book 5—art, Book 6—geography and history, and Book 7—astronomy and cosmos.

Errors are assessed according to the three criteria of reason, sense, and authority. The descriptions include examples of empiricism, formulation of hypotheses, and experiments on electricity and magnetism. Browne sets forth the argument that nature never does anything in vain, and readers are urged to trust God.

In 1658, Browne's *Hydriotaphia, Urn-Buriall* (a discourse of sepulchral urn) and *The Garden of Cyrus* were published together within the binding of a single octavo. The study of cremation urns and plant life, respectively, presents a crystallization of Browne's antiquarianism and the concept of plants as a representation of natural philosophy. The recent discovery of a Roman urn burial in the county of Norfolk stimulated Browne to describe burial and funerary methods of the past and current times and consider the human struggle with death.

The Garden of Cyrus represents Browne's interconnection between the plants and herbs of nature and art and hermetism, which is based on the concept that there is a single theology, given by God, and present in all religions. Browne uses the quincunx pattern of five units (five dots arranged in a cross like the number five on a die) to demonstrate Platonic forms in nature and how God uses geometric forms. Nature is shown to have five-sided physical patterns and quintuple phenomena throughout the animal and plant kingdoms, e.g., honey combs, snake skin, fish scales, etc. In both *Hydriotaphia, Urn-Buriall* and *The Garden of Cyrus*, Browne stresses the value of detailed and precise description for both the antiquarian and natural historian.

Two of Browne's literary works were published posthumously. *A Letter to a Friend*, which was written in 1656 and published in 1690, was prompted by the death of a patient with consumption (tuberculosis) who had died at a young age. The work includes some of Browne's most often referred to philosophical quotations. It discusses Browne's assessment of the value of dreams and the importance of signs in establishing a medical diagnosis. Within the nineteen paragraphs of text is Browne's fullest description of a Christian physician in action and the complex problems encountered, related to religious, moral, and medical issues, and their social context faced with the care of patients.

Christian Morals was written during the last decade of Browne's life and was published in 1716. The work is an extension of *Religio Medici* and consists of Browne's more mature considerations about Christian conduct. With the emphasis on a positive attitude rather than contempt for the world, Browne indicates that the goal is to live meaningfully and completely, make the best of adversity, offer charity and maintain humility, while functioning based on reason rather than passion.

In September 1671, King Charles II, with the queen and a large entourage, visited Norwich. As reported in the *London Gazette*, "There the *King* knighted the so famous *Brown*, Whose worth & learning to the world are known." Browne lived out his life in Norwich, where he died at the age of seventy-seven on his birthday, October 19, in 1682. His body was buried in his parish church. During repairs to the church, his skull was removed, only to be deposited five years later by a local physician in Norfolk and Norwich Hospital. In 1900, Osler paid to have a case, inscribed with silver plates, made to contain and display the skull. Twenty-two years later, the skull in its casket was reinterred in the church.

Browne is considered to have been one of the most significant English writers of prose. The stateliness and eloquence of his prose has not appealed to modern readers. But, if one filters his ponderous style, there are many examples of Browne's profundity and literary craftsmanship. These continue to be quoted.

From *Religio Medici*:

> "We carry with us the wonders, we seek without us."
> "Obstinacy in a bad cause, is but constancy in a good."
> "Persecution is a bad and indirect way to plant Religion."
> "No man can justly or condemn another, because indeed no man truly knows another."
> "We all labour against our own cure, for the death is the cure of all diseases.

From *Pseudodoxia*:

> "If reason is a rebel unto faith, so is passion unto reason."

From *Hydriotaphia*:

> "The long habit of living indisposeth us from dying."

From *A Letter to a Friend*:

> "Be charitable before Wealth makes thee covetous."

Browne's ingenuity remains manifest in the latest edition of the *Oxford English Dictionary*, where he ranks at number seventy on the list of top cited sources.

He has over eight hundred entries, is quoted in over 3,600 entries, and is credited as the first source for more than seven hundred words, including "ambidextrous," "analogous," "anomalous," "approximate," "archetype," "ascetic," "carnivorous," "coexistence," "coma," "compensate," "computer," "cryptography," "cylindrical," "disruption," "electricity," "exhaustion," "ferocious," "follicle," "generator," "gymnastic," "herbaceous," "indigenous," "insecurity," "jocularity," "literary," "locomotion," "medical," "migrant," "mucous," "polarity," "prairie," "precocious," "prostate," "pubescent," "suicide," "therapeutic," "ulterior," "ultimate," and "veterinarian."

SOURCES

Buston, R.W. "Sir Thomas Browne and the Religio Medici." *Surgery, Gynaecology & Obstetrics* 131, no. 6 (1970): 1164–70.

Keynes, G, ed. *The Works of Sir Thomas Browne*. London: Faber and Faber, 1968.

Osler, William. *An Alabama Student and Other Biographical Essays*. Oxford, England: Oxford University Press, 1908.

Schneck, J. M. "Sir Thomas Browne, Religio Medici, and the History of Psychiatry." *American Journal of Psychiatry* 114, no. 7 (1958): 657–60.

6

JOHN LOCKE

Premier Physician/Philosopher During the Enlightenment in England

By the end of the sixteenth century, England's political stature had risen, in large part related to its defeat of the armada of Spain, which was Europe's leading power. Under Elizabeth I's rule, England had initiated its quest for a Northwest Passage in the Western Hemisphere to facilitate access and trade with Asia, and efforts to colonize North America were entertained. Sir Francis Bacon championed the scientific method of acquiring knowledge, thereby opening upon whole new areas of intellectual exploration. In the early part of the seventeenth century, after James I succeeded Elizabeth, successful

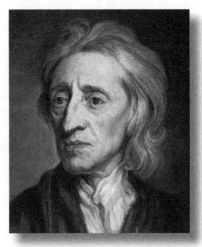

Portrait by Sir Godfrey Kneller.

English colonization of America began with Jamestown in 1607, followed in Massachusetts by the founding of Plymouth in 1620 and Salem in 1630. In the field of medicine the most significant contribution was William Harvey's 1628 publication of *De Mortu Cordis* (*On the Motion of the Heart and Blood*), which provided a complete description of the circulatory system for the first time.

Four years after the publication of that monumental work, one of the most influential Enlightenment philosophers, and a highly regarded physician, was born. His literary and philosophical contributions led Voltaire to recognize him as among the greatest philosophers, as well as the ablest writers, of their age. His influence would have a significant impact on defining the principles of liberalism and religious tolerance in colonial America.

John Locke was born in Somerset, England, on August 29, 1632. Sponsored by a member of Parliament and friend of the family, Locke began his education at the prestigious Westminster School in London. As a twenty-year-old, he entered Christ College, Oxford, with about forty other undergraduates. He graduated in 1656, and two years later was awarded an MA degree. He then intensified his studies of medicine that he had initiated several years previously.

In 1666, Locke composed a speculative essay, "Morbus" ("Disease"), on the cause of disease. He suggested that "small and subtle parcels of matter which are apt to transmute far greater portions of matter into a new nature" were the likely cause of disease, but he confessed that he could not define the process by which the small "ferments" worked.

At the time, Oxford's requirements for attaining a bachelor of medicine degree, which was sufficient for licensure, consisted of three years of formal courses. In 1666, Locke petitioned to receive a medical doctorate without previously becoming a bachelor. He failed, but associated himself with a practitioner in the community of Oxford and received a license to carry out that activity as a community medical practitioner. In 1674, he would eventually receive a bachelor of medicine degree from Oxford, but never receiving his doctorate.

During Locke's stay at Oxford, his interest in chemistry was stimulated by Robert Boyle, who continually offered advice to Locke regarding research. Boyle's book *Memoirs for the Natural History of Human Blood* (1684) includes Locke's experimental work on the action of acids, alkalis, and volatile spirits on blood.

In 1666, a chance meeting with Lord Anthony Ashley Cooper would alter Locke's life. Cooper had, at the time, an undefined medical ailment for which he sought the mineral waters from a village near Oxford. Cooper traveled to Oxford to visit his son, who was a student at Trinity College, and, while there, he planned to acquire a supply of the desired waters. In the absence of the senior physician with whom he was associated, Locke met with Cooper, and an immediate mutual attraction occurred. As a consequence, Locke was invited to become part of Lord Anthony Ashley Cooper's retinue at Exeter House in London. In 1667, Locke moved to London, where he became involved in Cooper's political activities, tutored the lord's young son, and served as a physician to the household.

In that latter capacity, Locke developed an association with Dr. Thomas Sydenham, who had attended Exeter House on medical matters. Sydenham, whose name remains attached to a type of chorea or nervous disorder marked by spasms, was England's most notable physician. He has been assigned the appellation "the English Hippocrates," based on his insistence that careful observation of the individual patient should determine therapy rather than a formulaic approach.

In 1668, Locke wrote an article entitled "Anatomie," in which the influence of Sydenham is apparent. Locke contended that anatomy does not provide an insight into the workings of the body. He, like Sydenham, argued for empirical rather than theoretical bases for treating diseases and patients. He echoed Sydenham's insistence that experience and diligent observation should form the protocols for effecting cures.

Locke practiced together with Sydenham, accompanying him on rounds. In 1668, the second edition of Sydenham's *Methodus Curandi Febres* (*Methods of Curing Fever*) was prefaced by a poem of Locke's praising Sydenham's approach to the management of febrile patients, endorsing cooling rather than heating of the patient's body, and emphasizing the importance of continually observing the individual patient.

The most notable case with which Locke was associated involved his patron, Anthony Ashley Cooper. The disorder first manifested itself with intense abdominal pain when Cooper was eighteen years old. It was the disorder that brought Locke together with his patron as the latter sought mineral waters. In May 1668, Cooper experienced serious abdominal pain and excessive vomiting. He was initially purged by the Cambridge professor of physick, Francis Glisson (whose name is affixed to the liver capsule). In June, a soft tumor became palpable in the right upper quadrant of Cooper's abdomen. Locke called several physicians and surgeons in for consultation, and drainage was performed. The description of the drainage is convincingly compatible with the diagnosis of a hydatid cyst of the liver caused by a parasite.

H. R. Fox Bourne, the nineteenth-century biographer of John Locke, wrote, "The operation was performed, and Ashley's life was saved, by Locke." Both Locke and Sydenham offered the opinion that the silver pipe, which had been inserted to effect drainage, should be left in place as long as there was drainage. Sir Anthony Ashley Cooper continued to wear the drain for the rest of his life, and he was often referred to as "Tapski."

Locke's second unusual case also involved a member of the nobility, Lady Northumberland, of whom Locke described a classic symptom complex of trigeminal neuralgia or tic douloureux (intense pain along the distribution of the fifth cranial nerve), and treated the patient palliatively. Locke planned to write a treatise on the philosophy of medicine and another work on anatomy, but neither ever came to fruition.

From January 1676 through March 1677, Locke was at Montpellier, which was thought to have a climate beneficial to a chronic respiratory condition that he presumed he had. He was well received by the famous university's medical dignitaries, and his medical judgment was valued by members of the profession throughout the remainder of his life. However, although Locke never became "in any orderly way a physician," he was generally referred to as Dr. Locke. Throughout much of his adult life, he awaited the opportunity of devoting himself to his favorite occupation, that of a physician.

Among physicians who have made literary contributions unrelated to medicine, John Locke maintains an unchallenged supremacy in regard to profundity: his works were both diverse and provocative. His publications, which transcend metaphysics, epistemology, theology, education, economics, and political philosophy continue to evoke admiration, and are included in the current curricula of a liberal education.

Locke's first publication was produced by a Dutch press while he was residing in Holland and the United Dutch Provinces because he felt endangered in England, as a consequence of his relationship with the political views of Lord Shaftesbury, Anthony Ashley Cooper. The seeds of the publication were sown in 1667 when Locke composed *An Essay Concerning Toleration*. Two years later, the *Fundamental Constitutions of Carolina* were adopted by the eight Lords Proprietor of the Province of Carolina. Locke is credited with authorship of the passage that underscored the need for religious freedom. It stated,

> Since the natives of that place, who will be concerned in our plantation, are utterly strangers to Christianity, whose idolatry, ignorance, or mistake gives us no right to expel or use them ill; and those who remove from other parts to plant there will unavoidable be of different opinions concerning matters of religion . . . it will not be reasonable for us on this account to keep them out . . . and also Jews, heathens and other dissenters from the purity of Christian religion may not be scared and kept at a distance from it . . . therefore, any seven or more persons agreeing in any religion, shall constitute a church or profession.

John Locke's *A Letter Concerning Toleration* was initially published in Latin as *Epistola de Tolerantia* in 1689, and was immediately translated into English. Locke contended that government and religion serve separate functions and must be considered separate. The government should not mandate religious belief. Only churches that espouse toleration should be allowed in society. In the publication, Locke wrote, "No-one is by nature bound to any particular church or sect; everyone voluntarily joins the society in which he thinks he has found the creed and mode of worship that is truly acceptable to God," and "No private person has any right to encroach in any way on another person's civil goods because he declares his allegiance to another church or religion."

In 1690, three books by Locke were published in London. *Two Treatises of Government* consists of two parts. The first is a rebuttal of a publication that asserted an absolute, divinely instituted, regal authority to rule, and that obedience of subjects to the government was mandatory. In the second part, Locke argues that men are born free of political authority, and are at liberty to choose those who govern them. The governors, in turn, have no absolute authority; rather they are answerable to those who have chosen them. Locke wrote, "Men being, as has been said, by nature, all free, equal, and independent, no one can be put off this estate, and subjected to the political power of another, without his own consent," and "The end of law is not to abolish or restrain, but to preserve and enlarge freedom."

Locke's *An Essay on Human Understanding* established his reputation as a philosopher and leading empiricist. He conceived of the human mind to be at birth devoid of knowledge, but which evolves throughout life by virtue of sensory experiences and reflections. He wrote, "Let us then suppose the mind to be, as we say, white paper [tabula rasa], void of all characters, without any idea; How comes it to be furnished? Whence comes it by that vast store which the busy and boundless fancy of man has painted on it with almost endless variety? To this I answer, in one word, from 'experience.'" He emphasized, "No man's knowledge can go beyond his experience."

For Locke, simple ideas, passively acquired through the senses, form the building blocks for complex ideas, comparisons, and relationships. Locke's aim was "to find out those measures whereby a rational creature, put in that state which man is in this world, may and ought to govern his opinions and actions depending thereon." *An Essay on Human Understanding* includes a consideration of words and verbal language as a unique attribute of the human being. Locke contends that words can be abused and contribute to the obfuscation of ideas.

A Second Letter Concerting Toleration was the third book by Locke to be published in 1690. It was an intense rebuttal of a brief pamphlet published anonymously by an Anglican clergyman named Jonas Proast, who doubted that religion could gain anything by exercising toleration. Two years later, Locke published his *Third Letter of Toleration*, which expressed concern with the historical evidence for miracles. He argued against the premise that Anglicanism was the only "true religion."

The diversity of Locke's intellectual inquiry is evidenced by *Some Considerations of the Consequences of the Lowering of Interest and Raising the Value of Money*, published in 1692, and *Further Considerations Concerning Raising the Value of Money*, published in 1695. Locke's thoughts on the subject of economic theory can be traced to 1668, when his patron, Lord Anthony Ashley Cooper was Chancellor of the Exchequer. In response to a publication that advocated for a reduction of the official interest rate from 6 percent to 4 percent, arguing that it would stimulate trade, investment, and the circulation of money, Locke composed a rebuttal.

Locke argued that reducing the interest rate would reduce trade both domestically and that exports would suffer, the circulation of money would decrease, and land values would fall. He emphasized that a country's wealth is based on its ownership of precious metals. Circulation of money and production of goods are increased by the import of precious metals for coining money. Locke incorporated these ideas in his later publications, in which he stated, "For it is to be remembered, That no man borrows Money, or pays Use, out of mere Pleasure," and, as evidence of his belief in the law of supply and demand, "Now I think the Natural Interest of Money is raised two ways; First, When the Money of a Country is but little in proportion to the Debts of the inhabitants one amongst another."

The most oft-quoted of Locke's writings is to be found in *Some Thoughts Concerning Education*, published in 1693. In it he wrote, "The only fence against the world is a thorough knowledge of it"; "Children (nay, and men too) do most by example"; "Virtue is harder to get than knowledge of the world"; "He that will have his son have a respect of him and his orders, must himself have a great reverence for his son"; and "Knowledge is grateful to the understanding, as light to the eyes."

Locke firmly believed that education, both formal and informal, forms the main basis for what a person becomes. He stressed the importance of a healthy body to house an expanding mind and a virtuous nature, and curiosity should be encouraged. Although John Locke never married or had any children, his principles of education were applied by the tutors of the sons of Lord Anthony Ashley Cooper and the son of Edward Clarke, a barrister and trustee of Cooper's estates.

Locke did not recommend the Bible for reading by children. "The promiscuous reading of it, through by chapters as they lie in order, is so far from any advantage to children, either for the pleasure of reading, or principling their religion, that perhaps a worse could not be found." Locke's thoughts about religion as expressed in *The Reasonableness of Christianity, as Delivered in the Scriptures* (1695), *A Vindication of the Reasonableness of Christianity* (1695), and *A Second Vindication of the Reasonableness of Christianity* (1697) were among his last publications.

Locke asserted that the fundamental tenet that defined an individual as a Christian was that Jesus was the Messiah. He did not believe that humanity inherited Adam's original sin, but we do suffer the consequences of eventual mortality. After the publication of *The Reasonableness of Christianity*, he was accused of being a Socinian, namely, believing in God and adherence to Christian Scriptures but denying the divinity of Christ and the Trinity. Locke was of the mind that "the law of faith, being a covenant of free grace, God alone can appoint what shall be necessarily believed by everyone whom He will justify. . . . And therefore He alone can set the measures of it: and what he has so appointed and declared is alone Necessary. No-body can add to these fundamental articles of faith. . . ." The publications of *A Vindication of the Reasonableness of Christianity* and *A Second Vindication of the Reasonableness of Christianity* were specifically produced by Locke to rebut the charges made against his religious beliefs.

Though John Locke died on October 28, 1704, he continued to exert a profound influence well beyond his lifetime. Within the century following his death, his arguments concerning liberty and social obligations influenced the Founding Fathers of the United States. Thomas Jefferson placed Locke amid Bacon and Newton as "the three greatest men that have ever lived, without exception, as having laid the foundation of those superstructures which have been raised in the Physical and Moral sciences."

A passage from Locke's *Second Treatise* is incorporated, verbatim, in the Declaration of Independence. Many scholars trace the origin of "life, liberty, and the pursuit of happiness" in the Declaration of Independence to Locke's expression of his theory of rights. He maintains his stature as one of the important figures of the Enlightenment for his empiricism, for his epistemology, and for his liberalism.

SOURCES

Osler, William. "John Locke as a Physician." In *William Osler, An Alabama Student and Other Biographical Essays*. New York: Oxford University Press, American Branch, 1908.

Woolhouse, Roger. *Locke: A Biography*. Cambridge: Cambridge University Press, 2007.

7

CADWALLADER COLDEN

Epistles and Exaggerated Expertise

Famed, flawed, and forgotten are three adjectives assigned to Cadwallader Colden, who was one of about a dozen American colonial physicians who had been formally educated and earned a doctor of medicine degree. Although he never developed a successful medical practice, he maintained an interest in medicine throughout his adult life, championing continued medical education, the examination for licensure, public health measures, and the establishment of the first hospital in New York. His literary contributions were varied, spanning the history of Native Americans, farming, botany, philosophy, and Newtonian science. Also,

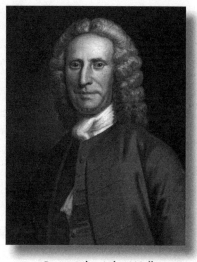

Portrait by John Wollaston.

he produced a large corpus of correspondence with the most notable scientists and thoughtful men, both in America and on the other side of the Atlantic Ocean, all while serving the Province of New York for fifty-eight years, longer than any other individual.

Cadwallader Colden was born in Ireland on February 7, 1688, to Scottish parents while his father, Reverend Alexander Colden, was stationed at a parish in Wexford, Ireland. A year after Cadwallader's birth, the family moved to the Presbytery of Duns, Scotland, about thirty miles from Edinburgh, where his parents would remain for the rest of their lives. Cadwallader enrolled at the University of Edinburgh in February 1703 as a second-year student because of his proficiency in Latin and Greek. The curriculum exposed him to botany, general physics, and Newtonian science. Colden graduated with a MA in 1705, at which time he forsook his father's plan for him to join the ministry, and elected to study medicine in London for five years. After completing his medical studies, he attempted to establish a practice in London, but was unsuccessful.

As a result, in 1710, he accepted the invitation of his mother's widowed sister to join her in Philadelphia, where he would conduct a medical practice and assist his aunt in her mercantile business with the Caribbean trade. While in Philadelphia, although he was unable to attract many patients, he is credited with the first attempt to establish a systematic course of medical lectures in the American colonies, but the Pennsylvania Assembly failed to endorse or fund the project. During Colden's time in Philadelphia, he briefly returned to Scotland to marry. While away, Colden presented a paper titled "Animal Secretions" to the prestigious Royal Society in London.

In 1718, at the invitation of a fellow Scot, Governor Robert Hunter, Colden moved to New York with an appointment as surveyor general and master of chancery in the judiciary system. Within three years, Colden was made a member of the governor's twelve-man council, a position he would hold for over half a century. Colden became a polarizing political figure early in his career, creating foes on the council and in the New York Assembly. Initially, Colden concentrated on creating order out of the chaos and corruption in the activities of the surveyor general's offices.

During the first decade of service as surveyor general, Colden spent much of his time in the Mohawk Valley, the Catskills, and the region around Orange and Ulster Counties. He developed an appreciation of the Five Nations of the Iroquois Confederacy, and he was held in high regard for protecting the rights of Native Americans. He was made an honorary member of the Mohawk tribe. One significant consequence of his association with Native Americans was his construction of "A Map of the Countrey of THE FIVE NATIONS," which was the first map to be published in the colony of New York.

But Colden's more significant contribution related to Native Americans was his book *The History of the Five Indian Nations*, which was published in New York in 1727. The printing of five hundred copies quickly sold out to a colonial, English, and European audience, and established Colden's literary reputation. Lawrence C. Wroth, the librarian of the John Carter Brown Library, deemed the work to be an important part of the corpus of colonial literature. The work consists of six segments of history that occurred in the seventeenth century, which had an impact on the Five Nations and their relationship with the English and French colonists. It drew from two previously published French books, which Colden credited, and incorporates none of Colden's personal knowledge or experience. A second edition of Colden's work was published in 1747, but that printing failed to sell and was remaindered. The second edition included Colden's "Papers Relating to the Indian Trade of New York," originally published in 1724.

In 1738, Governor Robert Burnet was replaced by Governor John Montgomerie, and Colden realized that his political influence would be minimized, and that of his opponents would increase. Therefore, Colden and his family moved their residence from New York City to Orange County, where he had been granted three thousand acres of land, which he named Coldengham at time of his employment by the colony of New York. When Colden started to work the farm, he began to compile a journal that chronicled his activities. That manuscript, which is currently housed in the Rosenbach Museum and Library in Philadelphia, is the earliest extant farm journal for the Hudson Valley.

One of the unique aspects of the farm was the construction of a canal, which had as its point of origin an enlarged pond and allowed horse-pulled barges to transport material through the property. Colden, prescient for the development of the Erie Canal, suggested that a direct link should be established between the Mohawk River and Lake Ontario and the other Great Lakes.

His activities during the decade from 1739 to1748, when he was in his fifties, reflect the multifaceted aspects of his life. He devoted an increased amount of time to correspondence. He exchanged letters with educated fellow physicians and with Benjamin Franklin regarding shared scientific interests, and with writer and lexicographer Dr. Samuel Johnson, an Anglican minister, who became the first president of King's (later to become Columbia) College. Colden corresponded with horticulturalist Peter Collinson in London, botanist Carolus Linnaeus in Sweden, and with Johannes Frederick Gronovius in Leiden about botany.

After Colden became acquainted with the Linnaean taxonomy of plants based on sexual characteristics, he wrote a catalogue, using that system, to classify the plants in the vicinity of Coldengham. Colden, always interested in applying his own imprimatur, suggested that there were imperfections in the Linnaean categorization. Linnaeus, subsequently, published Colden's catalogue as "Plantae Coldenhamiae in Provincia Novaboracensi Americanes . . ." ("Coldenghamiae Plants in North America"). When Linnaeus published *Species*

Plantarum in 1753, he referred to "C. Colden" as a source of his knowledge of New World flora. The name "Coldenia" was later assigned by Linnaeus to a specific plant.

Colden's focus on botany was replaced with his interest in Isaac Newton's theories regarding matter, motion, and gravity. Whereas Newton, who had formulated the laws by which the effects of gravity could be predicted, specifically indicated that he could not define the cause, Colden considered himself qualified to disagree with some of Newton's postulates and to offer an explanation of the cause of gravity. Colden's *An Explication of the First Causes of Action in Matter; and of the Cause of Gravitation* was published in New York in 1746, and represents the first scientific publication in colonial America. The leading mathematicians and scientists in Europe deemed Colden's dissertation to be "absurd."

A literary byproduct of Colden's interest in Newtonian science earned him the designation as "the only important American materialist philosopher prior to the American Revolution." According to Colden, all ideas, which human beings have of external entities, come from action on the human senses. Thinking is a distinct kind of action. Matter possesses a distinctive force. Action of matter is determined by external causes. Matter is a sublimated force; mind is a spiritual matter. Both possess the common denominator of a diffused, uniform, and elastic ether. Colden's digression from physics to metaphysics exists as an unpublished draft, entitled "First Principles of Morality, or of the Actions of Intelligent Human Beings." The work appears in manuscript form in the Rosenbach Museum and Library of Philadelphia.

During the decade of the 1740s, Colden maintained his interest in medical matters. In 1741, his "Essay on the Iliac Passion" was printed by Benjamin Franklin. Colden's attention was drawn to public health issues and sanitation in New York City. In 1743 and 1744, he published articles on seasonal fevers that affected those people who lived in the city, while sparing the inhabitants of rural areas. Colden is credited as being the first individual to deal with public health in New York by having the council adopt stringent regulations regarding it and having them enforced. He chronicled his observations on the effect of a rattlesnake bite on a steer, and the benefit achieved by pouring heated hog's lard into the steer's stomach. He wrote that yaws (a bacterial infection) and lues venerea (syphilis) were two distinct diseases, the former with an African origin, while the latter originated in America prior to the arrival of Europeans. Colden also published on the effects of tar water to treat a variety of diseases.

As a sexagenarian, Colden continued his interest in medicine. In 1751, he published in *Gentlemen's Magazine* an article on the value of pokeweed as a cure for cancer. He also published on the efficacy of bloodletting and medicine extracted from moss as a cure for hydrophobia (rabies) due to a dog bite. But much of Colden's time was spent defending his 1745 forty-eight-page publication on action in matter and gravitation. In 1751, he published a revised and enlarged (215-page) English edition with a new title, *The Principles of the Action in Matter, the Gravitation of Bodies and the Motion of the Planets, Explained from these Principles.* The result was a continuation of adverse criticism.

While in his seventies, Colden reached his political peak, but his reputation decreased to its low point. From the time that he was designated surveyor general of New York in 1718, continuing through his membership on the Governor's Council, Colden stood in opposition to the New York City mercantile faction. The New York Assembly referred to Colden as "a person obnoxious to the house." In 1760, Colden was the major force behind the passage of a bill to regulate the practice of "physic and medicine." The bill, which specified that passing an examination was required by those aspiring to practice, was the first to regulate the practice of medicine in the American colonies. But it was limited to New York City and excused all those who were currently in practice. Also in 1760, when his major opponent, Lieutenant Governor James Delancey died, Colden, being the senior member of the council, became president of the council and commander in chief of the Province of New York. A year later, he received his formal commission as lieutenant governor.

In 1765, Colden gained a reputation as the ultimate Loyalist and enemy of the people. In his role as lieutenant governor, he took an oath to endorse the Stamp Act. Shortly thereafter, he received a threatening letter, indicating that he would be hanged. His two sleighs, his sedan chair, and several carriages were burned by a mob that hanged him in effigy. Despite his political turmoil, that same year Colden published his *Treatise on Wounds and Fevers*, the most notable of his medical works. It was considered to be authoritative and was referred to for several decades.

When in his eighties, Colden continued to serve effectively for the last eight years of his life, running the colony of New York in the absence of the governor. His last activity related to medicine took place in 1771, when as lieutenant governor he signed the charter for the New York Hospital, which would become the second-oldest hospital in the United States. On September 20, 1776, the eighty-eight-year-old Cadwallader Colden died in Flushing, Long Island, where he had resided since 1757.

Colden's correspondence with members of his family, political figures in the American colonies, members of the British Parliament, three notable formally trained physicians in the American colonies, botanists both in the American colonies and across the Atlantic Ocean, and Benjamin Franklin comprises nine volumes, consisting of about 4,500 pages, which was published between 1917 and 1923 by the New York Historical Society. Colden's last published letter was a report of the affairs in the Province of New York, and was addressed to the Earl of Dartmouth, New York's secretary of state, on July 3, 1775. It was written to inform the British leaders in London that George Washington had been appointed commander in chief of the Continental Army.

In considering the legacy of Cadwallader Colden, it is surprising that his name does not appear in the *Autobiography of Benjamin Franklin*, in spite of the extensive correspondence between the two men. This was probably a deliberate disassociation by Franklin, the man credited with the formation of America's first learned society, the American Philosophical Society, and despite the fact that Colden was one of the first New Yorkers to be asked to join. To Franklin, the same Colden, who had been referred to as the "most learned man in the colonies," was overshadowed by his reputation as an unwitting provocateur of the American Revolution.

SOURCES

Schwartz, Seymour. *Cadwallader Colden: A Biography*. Amherst, NY: Prometheus Books, 2013.

8

ALBRECHT von HALLER

Prodigy, Physiologist, Physician, Poetry, and Prose

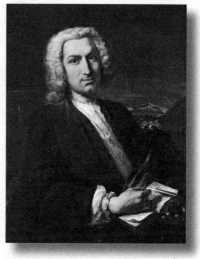

Portrait by
Johann Rudolph Huber.

The rarest of individuals are those who contribute equally to disparate fields of endeavor. Albrecht von Haller, by virtue of being acknowledged as "the father of modern physiology," and coupled with the historical impact of his epic poem *Ode sur les Alpes* (*Ode to the Alps*) and other writings, merits recognition as the medical and literary figure most worthy of the description "the epitome of dual distinction."

Haller was born on October 16, 1708, in Bern, which at the time was a canton in the Swiss Confederacy. He was the youngest of five children. His father was an inconsequential jurist, and his mother died when he was young. He was raised by his stepmother and educated at public school. As a child, he had a delicate constitution and suffered ill health, which was offset by a precocious mind. At age four, he read and explained the Bible to the family's servants. During his childhood, he collated a Hebrew and Greek vocabulary, and outlined the grammar of Chaldee, the Aramaic vernacular that was the original language of parts of the Bible.

While a youth, he replicated the seventeenth-century *Grande Dictionaire Historique* (*Great Historical Dictionary*) by compiling the biographies of over a thousand men and women. He translated several Latin classics, wrote a history of the origin of the Swiss Confederacy, and authored dramas and poems, all in his youth. He burned all the writings of his youth in 1729.

From 1722 to 1723, after his father died, Haller lived with his step-uncle, who was a physician, and it was during that time that Haller decided to prepare himself for a career in medicine. From January 1724 to April 1725, Haller studied medicine at Tübingen in Baden-Würtemberg. He later transferred to the medical program at Leiden, where Hermann Boorhave—a founder of clinical teaching—and Bernard Siegfried Albinus—the author of an anatomy textbook—were the main attractions. In May 1727, Haller graduated with a doctorate of medicine, after he defended his thesis, which proved that the alleged salivary duct recently discovered by Professor Coschwitz was actually a lingual vein supplying the tongue.

Shortly thereafter, Haller traveled to England and academic centers in Europe to expand his knowledge. In London, he met Sir Hans Sloane, the first English physician to be made a baronet, whose collection and library, after his death, became the initial core of the British Museum. Haller visited William Cheselden, the author of an anatomy text and a lithotomist at St. Thomas' Hospital. In Edinburgh, Haller initiated a lifelong friendship with Sir John Pringle, who later gained a reputation as the father of military medicine and is credited with the concept that evolved into the International Red Cross. In Paris, Haller became acquainted with Jakob B. Winslow, an anatomist, who had written on the origin, insertion, and nomenclature of muscles. Haller ended his tour in Basel, Switzerland, where he studied mathematics under famed mathematician Jacob Bernoulli.

In 1728, Haller journeyed through the Swiss cantons and the Alps, where he began a collection of flora and enhanced his knowledge of botany, which remained a continuous interest and intellectual pursuit throughout his life. Following the pattern, which he evidenced as a youth, he aimed to create an encyclopedia of Swiss flora and a comprehensive and all-inclusive taxonomy. Having corresponded with Carl Linnaeus, Haller rejected the Linnaean sexual system of classification and the consequent binary nomenclature.

In 1729, Haller returned to Bern, where he practiced as a physician while maintaining research in botany and anatomy. In 1736, he was appointed professor of anatomy, botany, medicine, and surgery at the newly founded University of Göttingen in Lower Saxony. In that capacity, he established the university's botanical garden (Alte Botanische Garten der Universität Göttingen). In 1742, he published his first work on botany, *Enumeratio Methodica*

Stirpium Helvetiae Indigenarum (*A Methodic Enumeration of Plants Indigenous to Switzerland*). An expansion of that work was published in 1768 as *Historia Stirpium Indigenarum Helvetiae Inchoate* (*An Initial Attempt at a History of the Indigenous Plants of Switzerland*), a major treatise on Swiss flora. The expansion provided a geographical description of the country, a description of the changing vegetation as influenced by climate, and magnificent illustrations. It was well received by botanists around the world, and Linnaeus honored Haller by attaching the name *Halleria* to a South African shrub. Haller's last botanical publication, the two-volume *Bibliotheca Botanica*, appeared in 1771–1772.

The literary product of Haller's initial trek through the Alps was his poem entitled "Die Alpen," which he had completed in 1729 and was first published anonymously with nine other poems in 1732, in *Versuch Schweizerischer Gedichten* (*Attempt at Swiss Poems*). "Die Alpen" consisted of forty-nine stanzas of ten lines with a rhyme sequence. Footnotes offer the Latin description of plants. The poem is one of the earliest expressions of an appreciation for the mountains as a physical entity as well as a sociological comparison between mountain life and life in more crowded areas. The relative merits of the natural and artificial elements were stressed. The simple and moral life of the mountain dwellers was contrasted with the turmoil, corruption, and decadence of more heavily populated regions.

Eleven additional editions, in which his authorship was recognized, were published during Haller's lifetime. The work was translated into Latin, French, Italian, and English. Haller's resulting fame as a poet preceded his recognition as a scholar and scientist.

Haller's other literary contributions were written during the last decade of his life. He published three romances: *Usong. Eine Morgenländische Geschichte (Usong, An Oriental Story)* in 1771; *Alfred, König der Angel-Sachsen (Alfred, King of the Anglosaxons)* in 1773; and *Fabrius und Cato, ein Stück der Romanischen Gechichte (Fabrius and Cato, a Piece of Roman History)* in 1774. The trilogy was a vehicle for Haller to express his political philosophy. The first book of the trilogy depicts an absolute monarchy. The third book deals with a republican form of government. The second book, *Alfred, King of the Anglosaxons*, represents the condition of a country with a limited monarchy. The book was Haller's plea for a monarchy that included representation not only from the nobility but also the people as a whole.

During Haller's seventeen years as an academician in Göttingen, from 1736 to 1753, he considered anatomy and physiology to be a unit, referring to physiology as "anatomia animate." This concept anticipated the approach in current medical education, in which structure and function are deliberately intertwined in the curriculum. In his embryologic studies, Haller demonstrated that blood flows from right to left through the foramen ovale in the interatrial septum between the right and left atrium. He showed that the branches of the fetal umbilical veins become the branches of the portal vein. By analyzing data quantitatively, he was the first to conclude that fetal growth is maximal in its early stages and reduces over time. However, he erroneously persisted in siding with the evolutionists in insisting that the organism developed from a preformed structure within the egg, in contrast to the epigenesists who ascribed to the theory that there was new formation of all parts during the development of the embryo.

Haller's studies of embryology led to his investigation of the human gonads. He is credited with the first correct description of the rete testis (a network of anastomosing tubules in the middle of the testis), which bears the term "rete testis Halleria." Haller used injection techniques to study the distribution of the smaller blood vessels. He demonstrated that there are more veins (Thebesian veins) that open into the atrial cavity from the atrial and auricular walls than had been described. He showed that the coronary arteries fill during contraction of the ventricles (the ejection of the blood).

As part of his investigation of respiration, Haller performed studies on the structure of the human diaphragm, and in 1744, he was the first to present an accurate description of it. He also demonstrated experimentally that the pleural cavity surrounding the lungs contained no air. Haller defined the effects of respiration on the motion of the circulating blood. His findings disproved previous interpretations regarding blood flow in the brain.

Haller's most significant physiologic experiments related to the nervous system, which led to him being called "the father of neurology" as well as "the father of modern physiology." He demonstrated that muscle contained the specific property of "irritability," or the ability to contract. A slight stimulus, regardless of the type, caused a sharp contraction. He applied the term "sensibility" to the property of nerves. He also showed that, when a stimulus was applied to a nerve connected to muscle, contraction of that muscle occurred while the nerve did not change perceptibly. This also implied that nerves carry impulses of sensation.

Haller's conclusions were based on extensive experimentation. Investigating all parts of the body that manifest contraction, he classified those parts on a scale of high to low "irritability." One of his most important contributions was demonstrating the self-regulatory contractility of the heart, associated with the marked irritability of the cardiac muscles stimulated by the filling of each chamber with blood. The combination of his studies of the propulsion of the blood in the heart and through blood vessels led to him being considered "der Begründer der modernen Hämodynamik" ("the founder of modern Hemodynamics").

Haller's propensity for writing, which was manifested early in his life, intensified with his scientific productivity. Among his more important publications was *Hermanni Boerhaave Praelectiones Academicae* (*The Academic Lectures of Herman Boerhaave*) in seven volumes (1739–1744), an extension of the lectures of Herman Boerhaave, the chair of practical medicine at the University of Leiden. Haller's anatomical studies were published in the elegantly illustrated *Icones Anatomicae* (*Anatomical Illustrations*) in 1743–1754. Haller's name was attached by subsequent anatomists to dozens of anatomic structures, including items in the nervous and vascular, glandular, and muscular skeletal systems.

Haller is credited with advancing the theory that inguinal hernia may have a congenital origin, related to the descent of the testis and the persistence of a patent *processus vaginalis*. In a discussion of intussusception (a telescoping of one portion of the intestine into the subsequent segment), he stated that reduction of the involved segment of intestine could sometimes be achieved by blowing air into the distal bowel, thereby anticipating a modern technique.

His physiological considerations were published in *Elementa Physiologiae Corporis Humani* (*Elements of the Physiology of the Human Body*) in eight volumes (1757–1766). Haller regarded this to be his major work. The first two volumes deal with the anatomy and the function of the heart and blood vessels, and include a defense of William Harvey's conclusions regarding the circulation of blood. Anatomy and physiology were combined in *Bibliotheca Anatomica qua Scripta ad Anatomen et Physiologiam* (*An Anatomical*) in two volumes (1774–1777).

Haller edited a monthly journal titled *Göttingische Zeitungen von gelehrten Anzeigen* (*Göttingische Zeitungen News of Scholarship*), from 1747 to 1753, and continued to contribute to it in his later years. It is estimated that he provided over twelve thousand articles on a wide variety of subjects.

After Haller left Göttingen, be began compiling *Bibliotheca Medica*, which included an extensive number of references, accompanied by biographical notes on the authors. The first *Bibliotheca* to be completed was *Botanica* (*Botany*) in 1771, followed by *Chirurgica* (*Surgery*) in 1774, *Anatomica* (*Anatomy*) also in 1774, and *Medica* (*Medicine*) in 1776. This compendium represented a forerunner to *Index Catalogue* and *Index Medicus*, which were initiated by John Shaw Billings and Robert Fletcher in the United States Surgeon General's Library in 1872. According to Sir William Osler, Haller's accomplishments as a "bio-bibliographer" were so significant that he "stood out above all his predecessors."

FROM MEDICINE TO MANUSCRIPT

At times Haller's behavior was aberrant. It has been suggested that he was addicted to opium prior to his move to Göttingen, as a consequence of being plagued by a variety of symptoms and disorders during his youth and early adulthood. He was irritable, impatient, and had few friends. He married three times and had eight children, all of whom survived to maturity. He remained religious throughout his life and followed the reformed theology promulgated by Huldrych Zwingli, who denied that the body of Jesus was in the Eucharist.

While still a member of the faculty at Göttingen, Haller was elected to the council of Bern in 1745. On April 23, 1749, he was ennobled by Kaiser Franz I of Austria, adding the "von" to Haller's name. It was hoped that this would entice Haller to remain in Göttingen. In 1753, he resigned from his academic position and moved to Bern, where he practiced as a physician and combined scientific and literary activities with public service. From 1758 to 1764, he lived in the rural community of Roche and directed the Bern saltworks. He continued to maintain his literary productivity until his death on December 12, 1777.

History has judged Haller to be one of the most important medical figures of the eighteenth century. Haller considered himself mainly a man of science. In a preface to a friend's collection of poems, Haller wrote, "A poet diverts for a quarter of an hour, a physician improves the condition of a whole lifetime." In his writings, there is frequent expression that religion is a motivating force behind Haller's dedication to science. He believed that scientific work was a form of worship: "God did not make the marvels of nature to be known by beasts . . . this beautiful spectacle was destined for man."

As a physician, Haller was concerned with improving people's physical health and regarded science as the vehicle with which this could be achieved. He also recognized the importance of science for its own sake and realized that his inquisitive and fertile mind constantly needed a topic or question to work on. He was a relatively unique scientist in admitting to selfish motivations and a desire for reward, but he ascribed the quest for recognition to the divine plan of making the wonders of creation known. "Nature never jests," he wrote.

SOURCES

Siegrist, Christoph. *Albrecht von Haller*. Stuttgart: J. B. Metzlersche
    Verlagsbuchhandlung, 1967.

9

TOBIAS GEORGE SMOLLETT

Picaresque Primacy

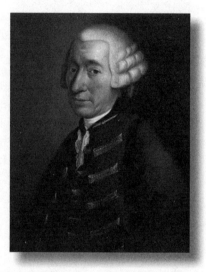

Scholars have ascribed the birth of the English novel in the seventeenth century to several authors. Daniel Dafoe (*Robinson Crusoe*, 1719, and *Moll Flanders*, 1722), followed by Samuel Richardson (*Pamela, or Virtue Rewarded*, 1740), Henry Fielding (*The History of Tom Jones, a Foundling*, 1749), and Tobias Smollett, who is identified by a series of picaresque novels with improbable titles, have all been credited. Sir Walter Scott articulated the significant influence that Smollett had on his own writing. *Select Works of Tobias Smollett . . . with a Memoir of the Life and Writings of the Author, by Sir Walter Scott* ends with this assertion: "that we readily grant to Smollett an equal rank with his great rival Fielding, while we place both far above any of their successors in the same line of fictitious composition."

Tobias George Smollett was born on or about March 16, 1721, near the village of Renton, Dunbartonshire, Scotland, into a prominent family. As a fourteen-year-old, he went to Glasgow University for medical training. He worked in a dispensary in Glasgow, and, in 1736, he was apprenticed for five years to surgeons John Gordon and William Stirling. Smollett ended his apprenticeship three years later. Rather, with a newly crafted tragedy titled *The Regicide* in hand, Smollett went to London to seek a career as a dramatist. When no one would produce his play, he was forced to embark upon a medical career in order to sustain himself.

In 1740, he was commissioned as a surgeon's second mate aboard the

Chichester, which participated in the attempt to capture the Spanish base at Cartagena in Colombia. The mission was a disastrous failure, but Smollett performed most favorably in providing medical care for wounded and infirm sailors during the battle. He specifically described the ship fever, which was encountered. His ship returned to England after a year at sea, and he remained on the naval payroll until February 1742. On a return trip to the Caribbean, he met in Jamaica the woman he would marry. Once back in London in 1744, Smollett established a medical practice in Downing Street. Unable to develop a sustaining practice there, he moved to Chapel Street, Mayfair, in 1746, but his medical practice failed to improve.

As a consequence of his medical interests, Smollett enjoyed engaging in discourse with several leading physicians of the time, including William Hunter, whose greatest work was an atlas of the pregnant uterus, and William Smellie, who developed new forceps for the delivery of babies. In 1750, Smollett was awarded the doctor of medicine degree by Marischal College in Aberdeen, Scotland. He attempted once more to set up a practice, this time in Chelsea, but, once again, he failed to attract patients.

In 1751, Smollett published a review, in which he extolled Smellie's *Treatise on the Theory and Practice of Midwifery*. A year later, he published in a medical journal "An Essay on the External Use of Water," in which he questioned the benefit of mineral water baths, while considering the application of cold water as a cure for some disorders. Later, Smollett drew from his medical experiences to satirize the seamy side of medicine, and medical issues appear in many of his literary works, as evidenced by the inclusion of about two dozen quotations from those works in a modern compendium of significant medical quotations.

Smollett's literary career was launched with resounding success in 1748, with the publication of *The Adventures of Roderick Random*. This action-packed narrative was written in eight months and, according to its author, was "intended as a satire on mankind." In the preface, Smollett acknowledges the influence of the Spanish author Miguel de Cervantes and French novelist Alain-Rene Lesages's *Gil Blas*. In his novel, Smollett portrays the envy, greed, and snobbery of the upper and middle classes. He also draws from his naval military experience to expose the incompetence and brutal injustices of the Royal Navy. He is considered to be the first to focus on a *sailor* as a major character in English fiction. The work, which abounds with amusing incidents and eccentric comic characters, is regarded by most critics as Smollett's masterpiece.

In 1749, with his reputation established and a readership eager for more of his writing, Smollett published his tragedy *The Regicide*. Two years later, *The Adventures of Peregrine Pickle* was published. This being the second of Smollett's satirical picaresque novels, it is more expansive and more finished but perhaps falls slightly shy of the level of his first work, yet it was very well received by readers. The plot and characters present a comic and scathing analysis of the manners and customs of eighteenth-century European society. Human greed, which generates cruelty to others, was a dominant element in the narrative. Personal satires of the thespian David Garrick and Smollett's main literary competitor, Henry Fielding, were incorporated in the narrative. These personal criticisms were excluded when the book was revised and reissued in 1758.

Smollett's third novel, *The Adventures of Ferdinand Count Fathom*, was published in 1753. The principal character is treacherous and amoral to such an extent that Sir Walter Scott commented, "The picture of moral depravity presented in the character of Count Fathom is a disgusting pollution of the imagination." In *Select Works of Tobias Smollett*, the author goes on to state, "Condemning, however, the plan and tendency of the work, it is impossible to deny our applause to the wonderful knowledge of life and manners, which is evinced in the tale of Count Fathom, as much as any of Smollett's works."

Interposed between Smollett's second and third novels was the second of his plays, *The Reprisals, or the Tars of Old England*, which was written and produced in 1751 to energize the British populace against the French with whom they were at war. As was the case with Smollett's first drama, *The Regicide*, *The Reprisals* was regarded as having little merit.

In 1755, Smollett published a translation of Miguel de Cervantes's *Don Quixote*. The following year, he assumed the editorship of the *Critical Review*, a periodical that was established by the Tory Party to counter the *Monthly Review*, which expressed the views of the opposition Whigs. He held the position until 1763. In 1758, Smollett published his *Complete History of England, Deduced from the Descent of Julius Caesar to the Treaty of Aix-La-Chapelle, in 1748*.

After a hiatus of seven years following the publication of *The Adventures of Ferdinand Count Fathom* in 1753, Smollett returned to writing a novel. *The Life and Adventures of Sir Launcelot Greaves* initially appeared in serial form in the *British Magazine*, which Smollett was editing. It was the first illustrated serial novel published in England, and the first novel to be published in serial form by an established novelist. Charles Dickens, who regarded Smollett as a major influence on his own style, and William Makepeace Thackeray would follow suit in the nineteenth century with serialized novels of their own. The first installment of Smollett's work appeared in 1760, continued as a serial through twenty-five issues, and was published as a book in 1762. Having been patterned after *Don Quixote*, Smollett's novel gained little popularity.

The fifth and final volume of Smollett's *Continuation of the Complete History* was published in 1765. Sir Walter Scott wrote, "Upon the whole, with all its faults and deficiencies, it may well be long ere we have a better History of Britain, during this latter period, than is to be found in the pages of Smollett." In 1766, using the epistolary form (a novel written as a series of letters), Smollett published *Travels through France and Italy*. He resided in those two countries for two years between November 1763 and April 1765.

In 1769, Smollett's sociopolitical satire, *The History and Adventures of an Atom*, was published. The novel was set in Japan and is an allegorical attack on the British political and military leaders during the Seven Years War, known in America as the French and Indian War. The work is replete with Rabelaisian humor (see chapter on Rabelais).

The last of Smollett's novels was published in 1771, the year the author died. *The Expedition of Humphry Clinker* was well received by the public. This epistolary novel is considered by many to be Smollett's most humorous, most pleasing, and most accomplished work. In keeping with the author's previous novels, it exposes disintegrating elements of contemporary society and satirizes politicians.

Although Smollett's first publication, "The Tears of Scotland," was a poem about the Battle of Culloden in the Scottish highlands, he is regarded as a major writer of prose but a minor poet. Three of his novels contain poems, the most memorable of which is "Ode to Leven-Water" in *The Expedition of Humphry Clinker*. He did publish two major poems, "Advice" and "Reproof: A Satire" in 1766. The first, a satirical dialogue between a poet and his friend, is a scathing attack on corruption and the decline of morality. The second poem continues as a dialogue between a poet and his friend, and satirizes both social customs and individuals who had offended Smollett. *The Complete Works of Tobias Smollett* also includes fourteen minor poems.

The eighteenth-century British literary critic George Gillflan wrote, "Smollett's poetry need not detain us long." But then he added, "In fiction he is undoubtedly a great original. He had no model, and has no imitator." Smollett, who wrote, "Facts are stubborn things," certainly merits recognition as the first physician to achieve stature as a significant contributor and innovator of English literature.

SOURCES

Simpson, Kenneth. "Smollett, Tobias George (1721–1771)." In *Oxford Dictionary of National Biography*. Oxford University Press, 2004; online ed., 2018. http://www.oxforddnb.com/view/10.1093/ref:odnb/9780198614128.001.0001/odnb-9780198614128-e-25947.

Smollett, T., and Sir Walter Scott. *Select Works of Tobias Smollett*. Philadelphia: Carey, Lea & Blanchard, 1848.

10

OLIVER GOLDSMITH

A Questionable Inclusion

There is little question that Oliver Goldsmith was one of the earliest Anglo-Irish writers to gain international acclaim among eighteenth-century literary figures. However, there is disagreement as to whether he had completed an academic degree in medicine and whether he is to be regarded as having truly practiced as a physician. The intrigue related to Goldsmith's association with medicine coupled with the importance of his literary contributions led me to include him in this panoply of physician/writers.

Oliver Goldsmith was born on November 10, 1728, either in Pallas, near Ballymahon, County Longford, Ireland,

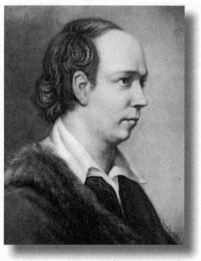

Portrait by P. Krämer.

where his father was curate to the rector of Kilkenny West, or at his maternal grandparents' home in County Roscommon. He was the fifth of eight children. In 1730, his father became rector of Kilkenny West. After attending a series of local schools, Oliver entered Trinity College in June 1744 as a sizar, which refers to a student of limited means with a scholarship. His academic performance was marginal, and he received an AB degree in February 1749.

Goldsmith's uncle had suggested that he study for a career in medicine, and the young man may, perhaps, have taken a course in anatomy at Dublin. Goldsmith moved to Edinburgh in autumn of 1752. A letter, which he wrote the following year, indicates that he "appreciated" the course in anatomy given by Alexander Munro, but had little regard for the other courses. Bishop Percy,

Goldsmith's contemporary biographer, wrote that Goldsmith's studies at Edinburgh were "irregular and mixed with dissipation."

In 1754, Goldsmith proceeded to Leiden, intending to continue his medical studies. At that time he wrote, thoughtfully, "Such sciences enlarge our understanding, and sharpen our sagacity; and what is a physician without both an empiric, for never yet was a disorder found entirely the same in two patients. . . . But the skillful physician distinguished the symptoms; manures the sterility of nature or prunes her luxuriance; nor does he depend so much on the efficacy of medicines, as on their proper application."

Goldsmith was disappointed with the education at Leiden and left after about one year without receiving a degree. Instead, he traveled to Louvain, Paris, and then Padua before returning to England. There is no evidence that he received a medical degree from Padua or any other university. The only suggestion that Goldsmith received a degree related to medicine stems from Bishop Percy's memoir. In that work it is written, "In February 1769, Dr. Goldsmith made an excursion to Oxford with Dr. [Samuel] Johnson, and was admitted in that celebrated University *ad eundem gradum* (granting academic standing or a degree based on work done elsewhere), which he said was that of M.B."

This was strengthened by the contemporary report of the Regius Professor of Medicine of Oxford in *Jackson's Oxford Journal*, dated February 18, 1769: "Yesterday Oliver Goldsmith, Esq. Bachelor of Physick in the University of Dublin, author of 'The Traveler, a Poem,' of the 'Present State of Polite Learning in Europe,' and of several other learned and ingenious Performances, was admitted in Congregation to the same Degree in this University." Goldsmith had never received a degree in "Physick" from Dublin!

As we come back to the chronicle of Goldsmith's life, he had returned to England penniless in February 1756. After securing temporary employment as a journeyman to an apothecary, he emerged as a "physician in a humble way" in Bankside, Southwark. This is the first appearance of Goldsmith as a physician. It is likely that he assumed a fictitious degree. Shortly thereafter, he accepted a position as a reader and corrector at a printing establishment. At the end of December 1757, he wrote his brother-in-law, "By a very little practice as a physician, and a very little reputation as a poet, I make shift to live."

In 1758, Goldsmith toyed with accepting an appointment as a physician and surgeon to one of the British factories in India, but this never came to fruition. In December of that year, he presented himself to Surgeons Hall for examination by the Royal College of Surgeons of London. The record states,

"Oliver Goldsmith was found not qualified for ditto [surgery]." From that point on, Goldsmith devoted himself to literary pursuits, but he did not repudiate his alleged medical degree, and was often alluded to as "Oliver Goldsmith, M.B." and "Dr. Goldsmith."

In 1764, *The Traveler* was published with the author listed as "Oliver Goldsmith M.B." Dr. Samuel Johnson referred to "Dr. Goldsmith" in his writing, and Sir Joshua Reynolds, who painted Goldsmith's portrait, suggested in 1765 that Goldsmith make a medical call on a man of social status. In 1774, Goldsmith's last medical involvement concerned his own terminal medical ailment, in which he prescribed for himself.

Actually, Goldsmith's literary career began in 1757, when he joined the employ of a bookseller named Griffiths, who was the owner of the *Monthly Review*, a popular periodical of the day. Goldsmith contributed a large number of articles and translations of French works to that review. In April 1759, his first book, *Enquiry into the Present State of Polite Learning in Europe*, appeared. It offered a pessimistic view, which was, in part, attributed to the poor remuneration of authors. While editing the proofs of the book, Goldsmith met the Reverend Thomas Percy, at the time rector of Whitby in Northamptonshire, who would became a close friend and, as previously noted, Goldsmith's biographer.

That year, Goldsmith started a new magazine, the *Bee*, which included book reviews, reviews of theatrical productions, translations of foreign articles, and tales of various types, but the periodical lasted for only eight issues. He later edited *Lady's Magazine*. Goldsmith's essay on the life of Voltaire appeared in the 1761 edition of that annual work. His reputation was significantly expanded with the anonymous publication of the two volumes of *Citizens of the World* in 1762. These were a series of essays that provided the perspectives of English customs and lifestyle, as noted by a fictional Chinese traveler.

Goldsmith gained the acquaintance of essayist and lexicographer Samuel Johnson, as well as artist Joshua Reynolds, and became one of the nine original members of "the Club" in 1764. The Club met one evening a week at the Turk's Hill Inn in London's Soho district. Irish statesman and political philosopher Edmund Burke, who had been contemporary of Goldsmith's at Trinity College, was also an original member, as was John Hawkins, who authored the first English-language history of music.

In December 1764, *The Traveller; a Prospect of Society* was published. This broadened Goldsmith's popularity, beyond the cognoscenti, to the entire public. The work was Goldsmith's first long poem, a philosophical piece that attempted to demonstrate, through the author's travels, that happiness can be achieved in different countries, cultures, and venues. Goldsmith followed, shortly, in a poetic mode with the ballad "The Hermit," which he initially had printed for a countess as "Edwin and Angelina." The romantic poem was first published as "A Ballad" sung by a character in *The Vicar of Wakefield*.

The Vicar of Wakefield was published in 1766. The public was not impressed, and the immediate sales were unrewarding. But, over the course of time, the book's popularity increased. It has been translated into many languages and has maintained its position as a representative eighteenth-century English novel. The plot and characters depict innate goodness unfettered by recurrent Job-like afflictions incurred by a sinful world. The same year, his ironic poem "An Elegy on the Death of a Mad Dog" was published.

Goldsmith next tried his hand at a theatrical comedy. In 1767, he completed *The Good-Natured Man*, which opened at the Covent Garden Theatre in January 1768. The interweaving of the main plot and the subplot offers a warning against overgenerosity. A year later, Goldsmith's *Roman History*, a readable compilation and evaluation of standard histories, was published.

Goldsmith's reputation was significantly enhanced by the publication of "The Deserted Village" in 1770. The poem is an expression of sociological concern for the depopulation of the countryside and rural areas coupled with the greed of the wealthy landowners. Reference is made to the immigration to America as a contributing factor. The last of Goldsmith's major works to be published during his life was *She Stoops to Conquer*, a comedy that was first performed on the stage in 1773 and is still performed today.

Goldsmith was known for the extravagance of his lifestyle, which included frequent gambling and living beyond his means. After he died at the age of forty-three, there was no public funeral, and he was simply buried in the Temple Church Burial Ground.

Among his quoted words are the following: "Success consists of getting up just one more time than you fall"; "Every absurdity has a champion to defend it"; "Where wealth accumulates, men decay"; and "A great source of calamity is regret and anticipation; therefore, a person is wise who thinks of the present alone, regardless of the past or future."

In Westminster Abbey in the Poets' Corner, Samuel Johnson's epitaph for Goldsmith, which is written in Latin, appears on a marble slab over a doorway, and translates as "Oliver Goldsmith: A Poet, Naturalist, and Historian, who left scarcely any style of writing untouched, and touched nothing that he did not adorn. Of all the passions, whether smiles were to move tears, a powerful yet gentle master. Ingenius, vivid, versatile, sublime. In style, clear, elevated, elegant."

SOURCES

Crawford, Raymond. "Oliver Goldsmith and Medicine." *Proceedings of the Royal Society of Medicine* 8 (1915): 7–26.

Dictionary of National Biography (1890), s.v. "Goldsmith, Oliver."

Sells, A. Lytton. *Oliver Goldsmith: His Life and Works*. New York: Barnes & Noble, 1974.

11

ERASMUS DARWIN

A Grand Grandfather—
Progenitor of the Man and His "Ism"

C harles Darwin was and remains one of the most recognizable names of the nineteenth century. His *On the Origin of Species by Means of Natural Selection, The Descent of Man,* and *Selection in Relation to Sex* transformed natural philosophy and engrained the concept of evolution, which has also become known as "Darwinism" throughout the years. It has been suggested that "the greatest of Darwin's predecessors as an evolutionary thinker, though, was his grandfather, Erasmus Darwin." Dr. Erasmus Darwin certainly qualifies as a physician, who gained fame in the literary world.

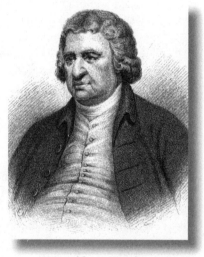

Painted by J. Rawlinson and engraved by R. Cooper.

Erasmus Darwin was born in Elston, Nottinghamshire, England, as the youngest of seven children, on December 12, 1731. He had his early education at the Chesterfield School and, in 1750, enrolled at St. John's College, Cambridge, to begin his medical studies. He left Cambridge in 1754 without taking a BA degree and moved to Edinburgh Medical School, where he completed his medical training. In 1755, he returned to Cambridge, where he defended a thesis and received a bachelor of medicine degree. In 1756, he was awarded an MD from Edinburgh Medical School and began to practice at Nottingham. After a very brief and unsuccessful experience at generating a medical practice, Darwin moved to Lichfield, where he conducted his practice for twenty-six years. In 1782, he moved his practice to Derbyshire, and maintained an active medical presence until 1797.

Throughout his life, Darwin identified himself primarily as a physician. His medical activities would require him to travel about thirty miles per day or almost ten thousand miles each year. He attended about four thousand patients annually. He cared for the poor without charge and scaled his fees according to the wealth of the patient. Professional generosity was a hallmark of his medical practice. He was an excellent diagnostician and assessor of the patient's prognosis. He zealously condemned the imbibing of alcohol use and minimized the value of herbal remedies and the concoctions of apothecaries, but dispensed opium liberally, at times for inconsequential illnesses. Although Darwin was cognizant of opium addiction and wrote about it, he didn't appreciate the danger of his treatments. Darwin's prescription of a six-month course of opium for Samuel Taylor Coleridge initiated the famous poet's addiction.

In 1760, Darwin published a paper in the *Philosophical Transactions* (of the Royal Society) entitled "An Uncommon Case of an Haemoptysis" (coughing up blood). A year later, he was elected as a fellow of the Royal Society. In time, Darwin became, arguably, the most eminent physician of late-eighteenth-century England. He was consulted regarding patients throughout the country: patients traveled from as far away as London (for over hundreds of miles) to seek his opinion. King George III invited Darwin to become the royal physician, but Darwin refused since he had no desire to move to London. In 1797, Richard Warren, the royal physician at the time, traveled from London to Derby to seek Darwin's opinion regarding his own medical prognosis.

In 1794, the first volume of Darwin's *Zoonomia, or the Laws of Organic Life*, consisting of more than two hundred thousand words, was published. It was his attempt to classify animal life and to develop a theory of diseases. It presents a catalogue of diseases, includes details of how they are manifested, and recommends treatments. His classification was fallacious and based on mistaken premises, but in *Zoonomia* he articulates a process of biological evolution and includes a section on the oxygenation of blood.

Two cotemporary critiques, drawing from a lack of scientific knowledge, opined that *Zoonomia* "bids fair to do for Medicine what Sir Isaac Newton's *Principia* has done for Natural Philosophy" and "it was one of the most important productions of the age." The publication of volume 2 of *Zoonomia*, containing three hundred thousand words, raised Darwin's medical reputation to new heights.

The great diversity of Darwin's "inventions" (none of which was patented) and their forward-looking nature bring into focus the breadth of this polymath, who has been referred to as the English da Vinci. Darwin's writings provide evidence that he appreciated the importance of gases and the important physical laws that explain their composition and behavior. His interest in gases, as a consequence, sparked his interest in improving steam engines and carriages, which, when combined, would produce "a fiery Chariot." He also proposed a steering mechanism for the two front wheels of a carriage that would improve the turning and the stability of the vehicle, a linkage that would be adopted by automobile manufacturers 130 years later.

In 1767, Darwin worked on the development of an efficient steam engine. Two years earlier, his close friend and fellow member of the Lunar Society (to be discussed shortly), James Watt, introduced a separate condenser to improve the steam engine's efficiency, and Darwin made several modifications. In 1768, he began designing a horizontal windmill for another close friend, Josiah Wedgwood, the famous potter and china creator. The windmill was installed in 1779 and continued to grind colors at the Wedgwood factory for thirteen years.

In 1771, Darwin invented a speaking machine, which eventually necessitated the development of a theory of phonetics. By 1776, Darwin was chronicling his ideas and inventions in a commonplace book, each volume consisting of about three hundred pages, and, over the ensuing ten years, he produced about two hundred volumes. His inventions, which are illustrated and detailed in these manuscripts, include a boat lift to allow a vessel to traverse locks of a canal, which is on an incline. Also detailed is an artificial bird with flapping wings; a copier, which duplicates the letters and words as they are written by a quill; and a multi-lens or multi-mirror telescope. Weather was a persistent interest of Darwin, and he continued to consider the development of meteorological instruments.

To satisfy the intellectual companionship that Darwin's fertile mind sought, in 1765, he was one of three founders of the Lunar Society of Birmingham. "Intellectually the most effective provincial group that has ever come together in England," the group constituted a force during the Industrial Revolution in England, and by exchanging ideas they fostered the Enlightenment. In the 1760s, Darwin became a friend of Benjamin Franklin, who was in England at that time, and in the 1770s, Darwin expressed strong sympathy for the American colonists' desire for independence. He was so strongly opposed to slavery that in his work *The Loves of the Planets*, published in the 1780s, he wrote, "E'en now in Afric's groves with hideous yell / Fierce SLAVERY stalks, and slips the dogs of hell" and "Hear him, ye Senates! Hear this truth sublime, / 'HE, WHO ALLOWS OPPRESSION, SHARES THE CRIME.'"

Yet another cause célèbre of Darwin's was women's right to an education. In 1797, he published *A Plan for the Conduct of Female Education in Boarding Schools*, which was a step in the progression of gender equality in education. He proposed that girls should learn modern languages, sciences, shorthand, and should also be devoted to bodily exercise.

Darwin's range of interests was boundless: he analyzed cloud formations, plant nutrition, and photosynthesis, in addition to demonstrating an interest in geology, which, in turn, expanded to include biological evolution. In 1788, he published a significant paper on the formation of clouds without the loss or gain of heat. In Darwin's *Phytologia*, published in 1800 and consisting of 250,000 words of his best prose, he wrote about the sustenance of vegetable life. Describing photosynthesis more completely than had been done previously, he specified that plants require carbon dioxide, water, and sunlight, along with the essential nutrients of nitrogen and phosphorus, which results in the end products of oxygen and sugar.

Darwin's interest in geology can be dated to 1767, when recent excavations revealed fossil shells and bones. He adopted the motto *E conchis Omnia* ("everything from shells") and affixed it to the family crest of three scallop shells. It implied that all animals came from sea creatures with shells. This interest in geology formed a basis for his evolutionary theory, which appears in the first volume of *Zoonomia*. Darwin identifies the changes that occur in animals during their life and the mutations that may be inherited and propagated. He indicates that the three elements that stimulated changes of form are lust, hunger, and security. He concludes, "The final cause of this contest amongst males seems to be, that the strongest and most active animal should propagate the species, which should thence be improved."

He presents examples of anatomical modifications that facilitate the acquisition of food, and the various types of camouflage and mimicry animals use to enhance their security. He writes that all creatures arise from "one living filament," originally derived from microscopic elements in primeval oceans. Thus, he discounts the widely held belief, which had been proposed by Archbishop Usher in the sixteenth century, that the first day of creation was Sunday, October 23, 4004 BCE. The naturalist Jean-Baptist Lamarck doubtless considered Darwin's writings when he synthesized his flawed theory of purposive evolution in 1809. Charles Darwin, who carefully read and annotated Erasmus's *Zoonomia*, wrote beside a paragraph about the beaks of birds, "Lamarck!! Lamarck concisely forestalled by my Grandfather."

Erasmus Darwin demonstrated capability as a poet when he was a twenty-year-old at Cambridge. In 1751, he produced a ninety-two-line poem in memory of Frederick, the Prince of Wales, that was published by the university as part of a memorial volume. Thirty-eight years would pass before another of his poems appeared. At that time, the publication of "The Loves of the Plants" gained Darwin instant fame as a poet, despite the fact that his name does not appear as the author. In 1783, the publication of the poem was preceded by a massive two-volume work entitled *A System of Vegetables*, which was Darwin's translation of *Systema Vegetabilium* by Carolus Linnaeus. "The Loves of the Plants" was compiled and written by Darwin, but he credited it to "a Botanical Society at Lichfield." That work was followed by *The Family of Plants* in 1787, and, in the two publications, Darwin coined the English names of various plants that continue to be used.

"The Loves of the Plants" utilizes humor and imagination to cultivate an interest in botany. Darwin anthropomorphizes vegetables, including intimate details of their sex life, to break down the stodginess of science. He begins an array of descriptions of vegetable sex life with the following couplet:

What Beaux and Beauties crowd the gaudy groves,
And woo and win their vegetable Loves.

And when writing about *Lychnis*, in which the male and female elements are carried on different plants, Darwin describes the mature female as being "In gay undress displays her rival charms, / And calls her wondering lovers to her arms."

The poem immediately evoked appeal from a broad readership. Horace Walpole, a highly regarded contemporary English writer and connoisseur, stated, "You will agree with me that the author is a great poet . . . all is the most lovely poetry," and "Dr. Darwin has destroyed my admiration for any poetry but his own." Anna Seward, the eighteenth-century English romantic poet, known as the Swan of Lichfield, wrote of the poem and its author, "Creative imagination, the high and peculiar province of the genuine Poet, has few more beautiful creations . . . a brilliant little world of Genius and its creations," and "Surely his genius is strong, glowing and original; his numbers grand, rich and harmonious."

"The Loves of the Plants" was incorporated as the second part of Darwin's lengthy poem *The Botanic Garden*, which included "The Economy of Vegetation" as the first part, and appeared in 1791. Darwin was one of the first to popularize science through poetry and, in the 1790s, was one of the most widely read poets in England. He was even under consideration for the position of poet laureate of Great Britain. In 1796, Samuel Taylor Coleridge remarked, "Dr. Darwin possesses, perhaps, a greater range of knowledge than any other man in Europe, and is the most inventive of philosophical men," and "On the whole, I think, he is the first *literary* character in Europe, and the most original-minded man."

The third and last of Darwin's major poems, *The Temple of Nature; or, the Origin of Society*, was published posthumously in 1803. In that work, he presents a pageant of life, as he believed it to be progressing: beginning as microscopic specks in primeval seas, through fish, amphibians, animals, mammals, and including humans. His poetic expressions are prescient of his grandson's *On the Origin of Species*.

> ORGANIC LIFE beneath the shoreless waves
> Was born and nurs'd in Ocean's pearly caves;
> First forms minute, unseen by spheric glass,
> Move on the mud, or pierce the watery mass;
> These, as successive generations bloom,
> More powers acquire, and larger limbs assume;
> Whence countless groups of vegetation spring,
> And breathing realms of fin, feet, and wing.
> THUS the tall Oak, the giant of the wood,
> Which bears Britannia's thunders on the flood;
> The Whale, unmeasured monster of the main,
> The lordly Lion, monarch of the plain,
> The Eagle soaring in the realms of air,
> Whose eye endazzled drinks the solar glare,
> Imperial man, who rules the bestial crowd,
> Of language, reason, and reflection proud,
> With brow erect, who scorns the earthly sod,
> And styles himself in the image of God;
> Arose from the rudiments of form and sense,
> An embryon point or microscopic ens!

He also presents in rhyme how the evolutionary progress from life in water to life on land is manifest in the development of the human embryo:

Thus in the womb the nascent infant laves
Its natant form in the circumfluent waves . . .
With gills placental seeks the arterial flood,
And drinks pure ether from its Mother's blood.

The esteem in which Darwin was held in the realm of poetry during the last decade of the eighteenth century rapidly waned after he died. One of his successors, Sir Walter Scott, gave Darwin a ranking among "British poets of the highest class." But Coleridge, while impressed by Darwin's range of knowledge, had little regard for the poetry and wrote, "I absolutely nauseate Darwin's poem." William Wordsworth indicated that he had been under an injurious influence of Darwin and deliberately developed a different style. He attacked Darwin in print "for his gaudiness and inane phraseology."

Erasmus Darwin's role in the development of and the appreciation for evolution is difficult to define. His famous grandson, Charles, who is credited with the theory of evolution, gave Erasmus no credit and did not mention Erasmus in *On the Origin of Species*. In a later edition, Charles Darwin added in a footnote, "It is curious how large my grandfather, Dr. Erasmus Darwin, anticipated the views and erroneous opinion of Lamarck in his *Zoonomia*." In Charles's *Life of Erasmus Darwin*, there is no mention of the latter's evolutionary views.

In 1994, the Erasmus Darwin Foundation was established, and, in 1999, the Erasmus Darwin House was opened in Lichfield. These memorials pay homage to a highly esteemed physician and a notable literary figure of the eighteenth century, a man whose biographer Desmond King-Hele deemed to be the greatest Englishman of that century, unmatched for his numerous and significant accomplishments.

SOURCES

Dictionary of National Biography (1993), s.v. "Darwin, Erasmus."
King-Hele, Desmond. *Doctor of Revolution: The Life and Genius of Erasmus Darwin.* London: Faber & Faber, 1977.

12

GEORGE CRABBE

Part Medicine, Part Ministry, but Persistent Poetry

It is convenient that, on a chronological roster of notable contributors to literature who can also be identified with a medical practice or education, George Crabbe closely follows Oliver Goldsmith. In the realm of medicine, both had a presence that was ephemeral and without distinction. Goldsmith's poem "The Deserted Village," which was published in 1770, and Crabbe's *The Village*, which came thirteen years after, have often been compared.

Robert Southey, eighteenth-century English poet laureate, referred to Crabbe as the "antithisizer" of Goldsmith. Whereas Goldsmith's portrait of a rural English village was sublime, emphasizing

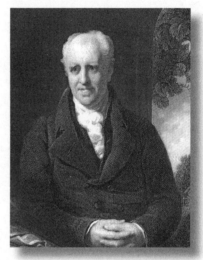

Portrait by Thomas Phillips, RA, and engraved by E. Findon.

intrinsic loveliness, ideality, innocence, and joy even with humanity's vices invading it, Crabbe presents a picture of gloom and pity for rural sins and a sense of sorrow that emanates from within. A comparison of the two contributors to English literature concludes with the ultimate measure of their respective impact: Goldsmith is still remembered while Crabbe is all but forgotten.

George Crabbe was born on Christmas Eve 1754 in Aldeburgh, Suffolk, England. At the time of his birth, the seacoast town, which took its name from the Ald River, was a poor and squalid fishing community. Crabbe's father, who had been a teacher, held the position of collector of salt duties and owned a partnership in a fishing boat. Crabbe spent the early years of his life in the area, where his education was, at best, modest. He was sent to two local boarding schools to study Latin and the classics, and his father read poetry to him. The family subscribed to the periodical *Poet's Corner*.

At age fourteen, Crabbe was apprenticed to a surgeon at Wickhambrook, a village in Suffolk, where he spent three years mainly performing farm chores for his mentor. Crabbe then moved on to Woodbridge, where he was a pupil of the surgeon Mr. Page from 1771 to 1775. While there, Crabbe won a prize for a poem that he titled "Hope," which he had submitted to a lady's magazine. In 1775, he paid to have small pamphlets of his poems published. After a brief stay in London to explore the potential of earning a living there, he returned to Aldeburgh, where he became apprenticed to an apothecary and tended to a few poor patients. During that period, Crabbe developed a lifelong interest in botany.

In April 1780, Crabbe sailed for London with his surgical instruments and a mere three pounds in cash, planning to establish himself in the city. He lived in poverty and pawned the instruments, which he referred to as "some of my more useless articles." He submitted several poems for publication, but none were accepted. In the hope of becoming recognized, Crabbe had a publisher print, at his expense, an article titled "The Candidate—a Poetical Epistle to the Authors of the *Monthly Review*." The *Monthly Review* journal was the main vehicle of literary criticism, and the article was Crabbe's attempt to gain the recognition of the critics, but instead they responded negatively.

In desperate financial straits, Crabbe submitted a letter to Edmund Burke in early 1781. The English statesman was known to have previously endorsed and supported literary efforts. Burke responded by providing Crabbe with financial support and an apartment supplied with books. He even introduced him to Sir Joshua Reynolds, Samuel Johnson, and their circle of artistic associates. In June 1781, Burke arranged for the publication of Crabbe's four-hundred-line poem "The Library," which praised libraries and books. Burke suggested to Crabbe that, based on his tastes, gifts, and religiosity, Crabbe was more suited to the ministry. Crabbe concurred, and the bishop of Norwich ordained him in December 1781. He was assigned to the curacy of his native town, Aldeburgh, and moved there.

Initially, Crabbe was not accepted by his fellow townspeople, but due to Burke's influence, he assumed the position of domestic chaplain for the family of the Duke of Rutland at Belvoir Castle, in Leicestershire, overlooking the

Vale of Belvoir. At the same time, he held small religious posts in Dorsetshire, Frome St. Quintin, and Evershot.

In May 1783, Crabbe published his first significant work, *The Village*, which he had begun before ever meeting Burke. The consequence of this long poem was that Crabbe was anointed "the first great realist in verse." His detailed descriptions of the natural scenes were deemed to be perfect reproductions, and were ascribed, in part, to his knowledge of botany. He introduced pity into the poetry of this naturalist poem, which was considered to be unique for its day. The bold realism of village life, as described in the poem, was assessed by Samuel Johnson, who wrote, "It is original, vigorous and elegant." The metric structure is that of "heroic couplets," which characterized Crabbe's works.

> What form, the real picture of the poor.
> Demand a song—the Muse can give no more.

The poem was well received and initially became part of popular literature. In writing to Crabbe in 1809, Sir Walter Scott stated that, as an eighteen-year-old in 1789, he read the poem and committed it to memory.

In 1784, the Duke of Rutland became the lord lieutenant of Ireland, and it was decided that Crabbe would not accompany him. Crabbe, who had married the year before, moved four miles from the castle to a curacy in the village of Stathern. There, he not only served as a minister but attended to the medical needs of the poor. In 1785, Crabbe's work *The Newspaper* was published. It is both didactic and satirical and added little to Crabbe's reputation as a poet. It was regarded as having little literary consequence by the critics. For twenty-two years, although Crabbe wrote thirty lines of heroic couplets as part of his daily routine, he published nothing more.

In 1789, Crabbe and his family moved to the rectory house in the village of Muston, Leicestershire, where he was compensated for ministerial duties in that village and in Allington, Lincolnshire. He maintained that position for twenty-five years, thirteen of which he was in absentia. For the thirteen years between 1792 and 1805, the Crabbe family resided at Parham Hall in Suffolk. The master of Parham Hall, the uncle of Crabbe's wife, died, and Crabbe's family was invited to reside in the more ample and comfortable surroundings that the venue would provide. Shortly thereafter, Crabbe accepted the office of curate in charge at Sweffling and later added Glemham, which were in the same vicinity and allowed him to maintain a residence at Parham Hall.

Crabbe continued to write, and for a brief period he turned to prose. He completed three novels, though none of them were ever published. While in Suffolk, he began writing a very different type of poetry, which was presented in an 1807 volume titled *The Hall of Justice*. The title work is a drama in monologue of Aaron the gypsy, but the most significant segment is the poem "Sir Eustace Grey," in which a patient in a madhouse tells his physician and a visitor about his downfall and madness. Edward FitzGerald, the translator of Omar Khayyam, indicated that Crabbe had taken opium in 1790 for an intestinal ailment and became addicted. The addiction, FitzGerald contended, caused the dreams that formed the basis of Crabbe's descriptions in "Sir Eustace Grey" and in another poem, "The World of Dreams," which was published after Crabbe's death.

In 1805, Crabbe returned to his parish at Muston, where he was appreciated by the parishioners as a dedicated minister. After Crabbe's publishing hiatus of twenty-two years, a new publication of his works appeared. It included *The Library*, *The Newspaper*, *The Village*, "Sir Eustace Grey," and *The Hall of Justice*. The principal new poem was "The Parish Register," in which Crabbe returns to the theme of *The Village* but on a larger scale. A village clergyman narrates to his audience the characters and incidents that are brought to mind, and the registers of baptisms, marriages, and deaths are perused. The work repudiates the idyllic imagery of Goldsmith's "The Deserted Village."

Is there a place, save one the poet sees,
A land of love, of liberty, and ease;
Where labor wearies not, nor cares suppress
Th' eternal flow of rustic happiness:
Where no proud mansion frowns in awful state,
Or keeps sunshine from the cottage gate;
Where young and old, intent on pleasure, throng,
And half man's life is holiday and song?
Vain search for scenes like these! No view appears,
By sighs unruffled, or unstain'd by tears;
Since vice the world subdued, and waters drown'd,
Auburn and Eden can no more be found.

Crabbe mixes tragic incidents of village life with some more pleasant and humorous vignettes. The poem was a success as a consequence of the stories it told, and the unique realism and pity that it embodied.

FROM MEDICINE TO MANUSCRIPT

Crabbe's magnum opus, *The Borough*, was published in 1810. He began the composition in 1801, continued his writing after he returned to Muston, and completed the poem during a long visit to Aldeburgh in 1809. The result is more than ten thousand lines of verse made up of couplets. The theme is an extension of the topics covered in *The Village* and "The Parish Register." The narrator extends his observations and interpretations concerning a rural village, its scenery, institutions, and personalities.

The work is written as a series of letters, divided into twenty-four cantos, to a correspondent who had requested a description of the borough, which is undisguisedly Aldeburgh. The almshouse, hospital, prisons, and inns are described. The descriptions include detailed stories of the persons associated with the structures. Letter XXII from "Peter Grimes" in *The Borough* formed the basis for a Benjamin Britten opera of the same name that opened in London in 1945.

Characteristically, Crabbe's description of the natural scenery is detailed and precise rather than panoramic. He was an artist who painted with a fine-tipped brush. Following the pattern of his previous publications, he brings forth the misery, loneliness, and unattractive aspects of the personalities. The work was an immediate success, and, over the ensuing six years, six editions were published.

Crabbe's next publication, *Tales*, appeared in 1812. The work consists of twenty-one episodes, often evolving from events that occurred in his family. The stories that represent fiction in verse are generally sad and evoke pathos. But there are occasional comedies interspersed throughout. The reviews by literary critics were warm and positive. Five editions were published within the first two years of its appearance.

Crabbe's final move, from Muston to Trowbridge in Wiltshire, where he held the position of rector for the remainder of his life, took place in 1814. The last of his literary contributions was *Tales of the Hall*, which was published in 1819. The "Hall" is the home of an elderly, financially successful bachelor who is visited by a half brother whom the host had previously scarcely met. The two brothers, at times joined by a parish clergyman, relate their experiences to one another. These constitute the "Tales." Crabbe died on February 3, 1832. Two years later, several of his poems, which had not appeared in print, were published as *Posthumous Poems*.

Crabbe's writing was uneven and ranged from exceptional excellence to amateurish exposition. Among the band of his admirers was Edward

FitzGerald, who had a long-term association with Crabbe's son, George, who became a rector at Merton in Norfolk. In FitzGerald's *Letters*, he repeatedly recommends Crabbe and quotes from him. FitzGerald selected some of Crabbe's later works, added his own personal prose annotations, and had a volume published in 1882. In the preface, FitzGerald wrote, "Miss [Jane] Austen, who is now so great an authority in the representation of gentle humanity, so unaccountably smitten with Crabbe in his worsted hose that she is said to have pleasantly declared he was the only man whom she would care to marry."

Joining Austen, FitzGerald, Sir Walter Scott, and Samuel Johnson as admirers of Crabbe's literary contributions were William Wordsworth, Alfred Lord Tennyson, and Lord Byron, who in a eulogy for Crabbe referred to him as "Nature's sternest painter, yet the best." Byron opined that poetry had steadily declined since the presence of Alexander Pope, and he regarded Crabbe as the last remaining hope. Wordsworth wrote that Crabbe's poetry would last "as long as anything that has been expressed in verse since it first made its appearance." Wordsworth erred; Crabbe's work has persistently declined in favor, and it now attracts little attention.

SOURCES

Ainger, Alfred. *Crabbe*. New York: Macmillan, 1903.
Dictionary of National Biography (1993), s.v. "Crabbe, George."

13

JOHANN CHRISTOPH FRIEDRICH von SCHILLER

Literary Largess of an AWOL Regimental Doctor

Escape from a brief and thoroughly dissatisfying medical career provided the opportunity for the creative evolution of one of the greatest contributors to the literary arts. Spanning the fields of history, philosophy, drama, and poetry, Johann Christoph Friedrich von Schiller's productivity is unmatched when the sheer number and diversity of projects are taken into account. Schiller wrote meaningful histories, significant philosophical papers on ethics and aesthetics, ten successful dramas, six ballads, and many poems. His prose and poetry were the stimulus for several musical masterpieces.

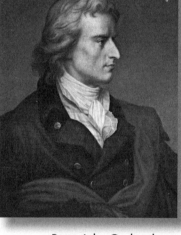

Portrait by Gerhard von Kügelgen.

Schiller was born on November 10, 1759, in the small town of Marbach, about twenty miles from Stuttgart in the Duchy of Württemberg. His father had served in the Seven Years' War (1756–1763), first as a noncommissioned military surgeon and eventually as a combat officer with the rank of captain. Schiller's father's service to Duke Karl Eugen provided the opportunity for the son of a military officer to enter the duke's newly founded educational establishment.

Schiller previously attended the Latin school at Ludwigsburg, twelve miles from Stuttgart, between 1768 and 1772. At the age of thirteen, he entered the ducal school at Solitude Palace, in the forest about two miles west of Stuttgart. Initially intending to study law, Schiller concentrated on Latin, Greek, history, mathematics, philosophy, poetry, and jurisprudence. The atmosphere of the school was restrictive and dominated by regulations, which had to be adhered to throughout the day and night. He found the experience repugnant, and when a medical faculty was added to the academy, Schiller immediately transferred to that discipline. Although he preferred drama and poetry, medicine offered better prospects for supporting himself financially when he completed his studies.

There were only nine medical students in the first class, and Schiller had to replace his Greek, Latin, and French studies with anatomy, chemistry, botany, pathology, and semiotics. One of the textbooks that he used was Albrecht von Haller's *First Lines of Physiology*. Haller (see chapter 8), who combined medical practice and scientific productivity with highly regarded poetry and prose, served as a role model for Schiller, who was diligent in his medical studies and was permitted to submit his mandatory final dissertation in 1779.

Schiller's dissertation, "Philosophy of Physiology," considered the relationship between humans' physical being and their soul, and also the nature of perception. The work was reviewed by Schiller's favorite teacher (Professor Consbruch), by the court physician, and by Surgeon-Major Klein. The professor indicated that "his argument is in many cases too contrived and in an essay where language should be distinct and clearly defined I should have desired a less flowery style." The court physician rejected the essay, while Surgeon-Major Klein stated, "This laboriously completed essay is exaggerated and also based on many false premises. . . . He is belligerent against everything that does not suit his new theories. Otherwise his vivid presentation of an entirely novel scheme is unmistakable evidence of the author's excellent and striking intellectual powers, and his ever exploring mind gives promise of a really diligent and useful man of learning once the ferment of youth has passed away."

A year later, to improve his chance of success, Schiller presented two dissertations—the essay "On the Difference between Inflammatory and Putrid Fevers," and "Essay on the Connection between the Animal and Spiritual Nature of Man." The essay on fevers was rejected, but the second essay was accepted, allowing Schiller to graduate after five years of medical study. Because Schiller qualified one year before the academy was granted a university charter, enabling it to grant doctorates and licentiates in medicine, he was precluded from establishing a civilian practice. Therefore, he accepted an appointment as a regimental doctor for Duke Karl Eugen's troops.

FROM MEDICINE TO MANUSCRIPT

In early 1781, Schiller wrote a friend, "I feel that my future and vocation lie in a post in which I can continue to study and make use of my physiology and philosophy . . . if ever I should write outside, it would be in this line. Compositions in the field of poetry, tragedy, etc. would rather disturb than promote my project to become a professor of physiology and medicine."

Schiller probably began writing his play *Die Räuber* (*The Robbers*) in 1777, while a student at the academy. In 1781, amid increasing dissatisfaction with his medical assignment as a regimental doctor, he revised the work. Because he was unable to arrange for immediate staging, he elected to adapt the play for publication, which was carried out at his own expense. In January 1782, *Die Räuber*, which centered around a conflict between two aristocratic brothers with different personalities, was performed at an auditorium in the city of Mannheim and was a great success. The audience was emotionally affected and responded with loud applause. As Schiller started working on his second play, *Fiasco's Conspiracy at Genoa*, *Die Räuber* was receiving acclaim from audiences in Hamburg, Leipzig, and Berlin.

While attached to his regiment, Schiller was sentenced to two weeks of detention for two absences without leave, on which occasions he had gone to Mannheim to see a performance of his play. Later, Schiller petitioned Karl Eugen to be allowed to engage in literary works and to communicate with foreigners. The duke rejected the request and issued the instruction that Schiller should be arrested if he was found writing on any subject other than medicine. On the night of September 22, 1782, a frustrated Schiller deserted his regimental post at Stuttgart and traveled under the alias of "Dr. Ritter" to Mannheim. Although his subsequent correspondence expressed the hope of returning to medicine, this never took place. The sole significance of Schiller's medical training was that it introduced him to psychological and philosophical thinking, which found expression in his prose, poems, and plays.

Schiller's first published poem, "Der Abend" ("The Evening"), appeared in *Schwäbische Magazin* in 1776, one year after he began his medical studies. His first significant collection of poetry appeared in *Anthologie für das Juahr 1782* (*Anthology for the Year 1792*). His range of poems was wide, but many focused on the disparity between the joy of life and the negativity of death. "Laura am Klavier" ("Laura at the Piano") and "Triumph der Libe" ("Triumph of Love") espouse the sentiment that love can conquer all adversity. "Die Freundschaft" ("Friendship") is considered as a powerful driving force in human relations.

"An die Freude" ("Ode to Joy"), which became the basis for the fourth and climactic movement of Beethoven's Ninth Symphony, was published three years later in 1785. Other examples of Schiller's works stimulating musical composition were "Die Bürgschaft"("The Hostage"), which Franz Schubert set to music twice, once as a song and then as an opera, and "Nänie." Nänie was the Greek goddess of funerary lamentation who formed the centerpiece for Schiller's treatment of lamentation. Brahms used the poem to structure his Opus 82, a lamentation of his friend's death.

In the spring and winter of 1783, Schiller wrote the play *Luise Millerin*, or *Kabale und Liebe(Intrigue and Love)*, and began *Don Karlos, Infant von Spanien (Spanish Infant)*, which would take four years to complete. His second drama, *Fiesco (Die Verschwörung des Fiesco zu Genua*, or *The Conspiracy of Fiesco at Genoa)*, premiered in Bonn in January 1783, and was performed in Mannheim six weeks later. In August of that year, Schiller was appointed theater dramatist at Mannheim, a position that he held for only one year, when his contract was not renewed.

In 1787, Schiller met Charlotte von Lengerfeld, whom he married in February 1790. The couple had two sons and two daughters. In 1788, he completed his history of the fall of the Spanish Netherlands, *Geschischte des Abfalls der vereinigten Niederlande von der spanischen Regierung (The Revolt of the Netherlands from Spanish Rule)*, a work that grew out of research he conducted while writing *Don Carlos*, the latter of which premiered in Hamburg in 1787.

In 1789, after his name had been put forward by noted writer Johann Wolfgang von Goethe, Schiller was appointed professor of history and philosophy at the University of Jena in Thüringia near Weimar. Schiller remained at the university, which has been renamed Friedrich Schiller University of Jena, for ten years. While in his professorial post, Schiller initially devoted his efforts to history, philosophy, and aesthetics. The two histories that he published in 1790 and 1793 were *Geschichte de dreißigjähren Kriegs (A History of the Thirty Years' War)* and *Über Völkerwanderung, Kreuzzüge und Mittelalter (On the Barbarian Invasions, Crusaders and Middle Age)*.

As part of his academic interests, Schiller embarked on an intense study of philosopher Immanuel Kant's (1724–1804) critical philosophy, for which Schiller received a three-year grant. Kant focused on resolving the dispute between empiricists, who posited that all knowledge comes from experience, and rationalists, who opined that reason and innate ideas preempted experience. Kant espoused the concept that cause and effect were integral to all human experience.

Schiller's interest in aesthetics found expression in *Über Anmut unt Würde (On Grace and Dignity)*, published in 1793, and *Briefe über die ästhetische Erziehung*

(*Letters of Aesthetic Education*), published in 1794. The former presents a theory of tragedy, while the latter is a theory of art based on aesthetic experience, which contributes to social and political consequences.

In 1792, the First French Republic granted Schiller citizenship in the republic, in part as a reward for the presentation of a French translation of *Die Räuber* in Paris the previous year. The same honor was bestowed on George Washington. In 1794, Schiller and Goethe met at a meeting of the Society for Natural Research in Jena and firmly cemented their intellectual relationship. Their association has been referred to as "the most significant intellectual friendship in the history of German literature." Their names are joined as developers of what has been termed "Weimar Classicism." The name referred to a new humanism that was a synthesis of Romantic, classical, and Enlightenment ideas.

In 1795, Schiller resumed writing poetry and dramas. Among the poems he wrote during the early period of his transition were "Der Spaziergang" ("The Walk") and "Das Ideal und das Leben" ("The Ideal and the Actual Life"). The year 1797 was named by Schiller as "Balladenjahr" ("The Year of the Ballad"). That year, Goethe and Schiller were energized by a friendly competition. Goethe composed five ballads, and Schiller countered with six, including "Der Taucher" ("The Diver"), "Der Handschuh" ("The Glove"), "Der Ring des Polykrates" ("Polycrates' Ring"), "DasLied von der Glocke" ("Song of the Bell"), and "Die Kraniche des Ibykus" ("The Cranes of Ibykus").

On October 12, 1798, the first installment of Schiller's masterpiece dramatic trilogy, *Wallenstein*, premiered and celebrated the opening of the new theater in Weimar. The next year, Schiller and his family moved to Weimar, where he spent productive time as a dramatist, clearly a vocation that was the most notable aspect of his career. According to author Charles E. Passage, Schiller is considered to have been "the greatest writer of serious drama between the death of Racine in 1699 and the emergence of Ibsen as a master of the European theater around 1880." When polled, a twenty-first-century French television audience placed Schiller second only to William Shakespeare as a dramatist.

It is important to take a closer look at the recognition Schiller received as a dramatist. *Die Räuber*, written when Schiller was about twenty-one, was expressive of the Sturm und Drang ("storm and urge") overt emotionalism and violence, and made him an overnight sensation. The drama concerns the conflict between two sons of an elderly and infirm count. The older brother leads a revolutionary group in the forest, while the villainous younger brother plots to gain his older brother's inheritance. The play is referred to in Dostoyevsky's book *The Brothers Karamazov* and Charlotte Brontë's work *Jane Eyre*, and was adapted for composer Giuseppe Verdi's opera *I masnadieri* (*The Bandits*).

Fiesco was based on a historical event that took place in the mid-sixteenth century. It revolved around a conspiracy in which a young count was involved in an attempt to depose the eighty-year-old Doge of Genoa, Andrea Doria. Three subplots added to the substance of the play, which, although more mature in style than *Die Räuber*, was not as well received.

Kabale und Liebe was first performed in 1784, initially in Frankfurt am Main and then two days later in Mannheim with Schiller present. Both productions evoked great applause. The work depicts the contemporary differences between the German social classes. Intrigue and manipulations are employed to destroy the love between a nobleman's son and the daughter of a middle-class musician. Giuseppe Verdi's opera *Luisa Miller* was based on the play, which Schiller had originally entitled *Luise Millerin*.

Don Karlos, Infant von Spanien is a historical tragedy that Schiller worked on between 1783 and 1787, when it was premiered in Hamburg. The drama had as its focal point Don Carlos, the notorious son of King Philip II of Spain, but bore little resemblance to the historical facts or Don Carlos's aberrant personality. The first act was initially published as prose in a literary magazine in 1785. Additional installments were also published in magazines. Eventually the completed drama was transformed from prose into blank verse. Schiller's drama formed the basis for Verdi's opera *Don Carlos*, which was composed when the maestro was at his zenith and premiered in 1867.

Wallenstein was a trilogy built around the life of Albrecht von Wallenstein, the general of the Imperial and Catholic army during the Thirty Years' War, who was later assassinated in 1634. The dramas are regarded as Schiller's greatest work and the centerpiece of his literary career. The three plays—*Wallensteins Lager* (*Wallenstein's Camp*), *Die Piccolomini* (*The Piccolomini*, the name of an Italian family that produced Pope Pius II), and *Wallensteins Tod* (*Wallenstein's Death*). The first play premiered at the reopening of the Weimar Theater in 1798, the second opened in early 1799 at the same venue, and the third play was presented three months later.

Schiller's remaining four dramas were written after he moved to Weimar. *Maria Stuart*, a drama depicting the final days of the claimant to the English throne, premiered at the Weimar Theater in June 1800. The play formed the basis for Gaetano Donizetti's 1835 opera, *Maria Sruarda*. Drawing from the heroic and tragic life of Joan of Arc, Schiller's *Die Jungfrau von Orleans* (*The Maid of Orleans*) reached the Weimar stage in April 1803. The printed text had been selling well for over a year previously. The drama outstripped both the *Wallenstein* trilogy and *Maria Stuart* in popularity for over two generations after it first appeared.

Die Braut von Messina, oder Die feindlichen Brüder (*The Bride of Messina, or the Hostile Brothers*) premiered in March 1803 in Weimar. The play is about two brothers who quarrel over a woman, who is later revealed to be their sister, although neither she nor her brothers are aware of the relationship. The play is a unique effort by Schiller to combine elements of Greek tragedy with modern theater. The drama ends with one of Schiller's memorable lines: "The worst of evils is, however, guilt." The work was adapted for two operas, *La sposa di Messina* by Nicola Vaccai and *Nevěsta messiniká* by Zdeněk Fibich.

Schiller's last complete play, *Wilhelm Tell*, based on folklore, was his most popular. It premiered at the Weimar Theater in March 1804. The tale of the legendary Swiss bowman's role in the Swiss attempt to gain independence from the Habsburg Empire in the fourteenth century has had many adaptations, most notably the opera by Gioachino Rossini.

Schiller died in Weimar on May 1805, at the age of forty-five. He is memorialized in Europe and the United States. Among his oft-quoted lines are "The voice of the majority is no proof of justice"; "It is not flesh and blood, but heart which makes us fathers and sons"; and "Truth exists for the wise, beauty for the feeling heart."

The earliest monument for Schiller was built in Stuttgart in 1839. The Weimar Goethe-Schiller bronze statue, which was erected in 1857, is the most notable and most imitated. Copies can be viewed in San Francisco, Cleveland, Milwaukee, and Syracuse. A grand statue of Schiller stands in Berlin in front of a concert hall, the former Royal Theater. Seated around the pedestal are the allegorical figures of history, lyrical poetry, philosophy, and tragedy, the four literary areas to which Schiller contributed. A replica of that representation resides in Lincoln Park in Chicago.

SOURCES

Newhurst, Kenneth, and Nigel Reeves. *Friedrich Schiller: Medicine, Psychology, and Literature*. Berkley: University of California Press, 1978.

Passage, Charles E. *Friedrich Schiller*. New York: Frederick Ungar, 1975.

Reed, T. J. *Schiller*. Oxford: Oxford University Press, 1991.

14

JOHN KEATS

A Bard Who Shed the Bard Parker

For almost a century, modern surgeons have used Bard Parker knives and blades to incise or excise. About three centuries have passed since a young surgeon put away his sharp knife and left the profession in which he had been licensed. During his brief remaining life, he produced poems and letters that would gain him recognition as one of the great Romantic English literary figures, assuming a position alongside William Wordsworth, Lord Byron, and Percy Bysshe Shelley.

The Romantic poet John Keats was born in Moorgate, London, on October 31, 1795. His father worked at the Swan and Hoop Inn, first as a hostler tending patrons' horses and later as the manager

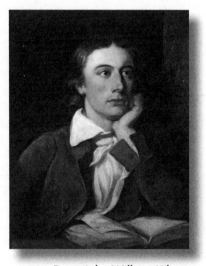

Portrait by William Hilton.

of the establishment. Keats's father died in a riding accident when Keats was eight, and his mother died of tuberculosis after young Keats had dedicated himself to caring for her. The fourteen-year-old orphan was left to the custody of his grandmother. At that time, Keats, who had received his early education at a small boarding school, was apprenticed to Thomas Hammond, a surgeon and apothecary with whom Keats lodged.

In Keats's time, the English medical scene consisted of a clear divide between socially elite university-educated physicians acceptable to the Royal College of Physicians or Surgeons and those who embarked on a career in surgery or as an apothecary after an appropriate apprenticeship. The apothecaries had been given the right to practice medicine early in the eighteenth century under the Apothecaries Act of 1815, which granted the society of apothecaries the power to license and regulate medical practitioners.

During his apprenticeship, Keats would have learned how to make the common drugs from herbs, plants, and berries, using the mortar and pestle, and he would have acquired basic surgical skills, such as setting bones, pulling teeth, cupping (suction therapy), bleeding, and applying leeches. He would have studied anatomy and physiology texts, and he would have gained clinical experience as he attended patients with the physician to whom he was apprenticed.

After Keats completed his apprenticeship, as was mandated for licensure, he went to the United Hospitals of Guy's and St. Thomas, where he studied during sessions of 1814–15 and 1815–16. He became a surgical dresser at Guy's, where he attracted the attention of one of the most famous of British surgeons, Sir Astley Cooper. During his training, Keats would have performed minor surgical procedures before he was allowed to take the licensure examination, which he passed, at Apothecaries' Hall in 1816.

Keats's surviving "Anatomical and Physiological Notebook" testifies to his conscientious application to medicine and his dedication to relieving human suffering. But the attainment of a license failed to detract Keats from his goal of becoming a notable poet.

Keats was poised to study for the examinations that would gain him membership in the Royal College of Surgeons, but he shifted his attention to his literary career. In 1816, shortly after Keats received his apothecary's license, which allowed him to practice as a physician and surgeon, he severed his ties with medicine and announced that he would devote himself to poetry. On a few occasions, however, his thoughts returned to medicine.

In 1818, Keats wrote this to a friend: "Were I to study physic, or rather medicine, again, I feel it would not make the least difference in my poetry." In a letter to his brother George a year later, he wrote, "I have been at different times turning it in my head whether I should go to Edinburgh and study for a physician; I am afraid I should not take kindly to it; I am not sure I could take fees—and yet I should like to do so." After a bout of hemoptysis in 1820, he wrote, "I have my choice of three things—or at least two—South America or surgeon to an Indiaman."

Poetry began to take over Keats's life while he was actively training to become a physician. He composed his earliest extant poem, "An Imitation to Spenser," in 1814, as a student at Guy's.

During the week of October 13, 1816, Keats, with the manuscripts of several poems in hand, presented himself at the home of Leigh Hunt (James Henry) at Hampstead Hill on the outskirts of London. Hunt, whose home had become a gathering place of literary endeavor, was viewed as a hero by Keats. Hunt was an essayist, poet, and critic who edited the *Examiner*, a radical reformist newspaper, which published the leading writers of the day, including Byron, Shelley, and William Hazlitt, to which Keats's name would be added.

In 1816, the first publication of one of Keats's poems, the sonnet "O Solitude," appeared in the *Examiner*. Hunt wrote in that periodical an essay titled "Young Poets," in which he referred to Shelley, John Henry Reynolds, and Keats. About Keats, Hunt wrote, "He has not yet published anything except in a newspaper, but a set of his manuscripts was handed us the other day, and fairly surprised us with the truth of their ambition, and ardent grappling with nature."

Perhaps, as a consequence of his medical experience, Keats singled out Apollo as a personal deity. Apollo, who, according to Greek mythology, was the son of Zeus and the Titan Leto, was the god of medicine and, also, the fine arts, including poetry. As is pointed out by Stephen Coote in his *John Keats: A Life*, "the sense of service to humanity, the devotion of the divinely inspired poet to the well-being of the world, is central to Keats' poetry."

In 1817, the first of three volumes of Keats's works was published with the banal title of *Poems*. Sir William Osler regarded the sonnet "On First Looking into Chapman's Homer" to be the most remarkable poem in the collection. The book was poorly received by the public and the critics.

In 1818, *Endymion*, based on the Greek myth of the shepherd beloved by the moon goddess, was greeted with similar derision by the critics. That poetic romance of 993 lines begins with the following:

> A thing of beauty is a joy forever;
> Its loveliness increases; it will never
> Pass into nothingness.

Also included are these lines:

> Pleasure is oft visitant; but pain
> Clings cruelly to us.

and

> Time, that aged nurse,
> Rock'd me to patience.

The work evoked general negative comments, though, at times, these were tempered by the critics. The *Quarterly Review*, which had a strong political bias against those with whom Keats was associated, referred to the poem as "the most incongruous ideas in the most uncouth language." Keats accepted the criticism. He wrote, "Praise or blame has but a momentary effect on the man whose love of beauty in the abstract makes him a severe critic in his own works."

Keats was introduced to the lawyer Richard Woodhouse, who befriended him and became one of his most strident supporters. The first publication of Keats's poetry convinced Woodhouse of the poet's genius, and he regarded Keats as one of England's greatest writers. Woodhouse began collecting material by and about Keats as the poet's work evolved. The collection continued during and after Keats's life, thereby constituting one of the most significant Keatsiana archives.

During the five years in which John Keats had shed his medical mantle and devoted himself to poetry, some of the most beautiful and lasting verses in the English language evolved. An edition of his complete poems includes 150 titles, almost fifteen thousand lines of verse. In June 1818, Keats embarked on a walking tour of Scotland, Ireland, and the Lake District of England. On his return he cared for his youngest brother, Tom, who died of tuberculosis on December 1, 1818. In the period between September 21, 1818, and September 21, 1819, Keats had his most prodigious outpouring of poetry.

Two long, unfinished poems, *Hyperion* and *The Fall of Hyperion*, mark the opening and close of this period. During those twelve months, Keats met Fanny Brawne and established a relationship that generated a memorable correspondence. "The Eve of St. Agnes," a poem that has been compared to Shakespeare's *Romeo and Juliet* because of the comparable plot, was written during the stated period. It begins, "St. Agnes' Eve—Ah, bitter chill it was! / The owl, for all his feathers, was a-cold," and includes, "Asleep in lap of legends old" and "As though a rose should shut, and be a bud again."

The ballad "La Belle Dame Sans Merci" was also penned by Keats at this time as were several sonnets and the three great odes "Ode to Psyche," "Ode to a Nightingale," and "Ode on a Grecian Urn."

"Ode to a Nightingale" includes this line: "I have been half in love with easeful Death, / Call'd him soft names in many a mused rhyme." "Ode on a Grecian Urn" contains the lines "Heard melodies are sweet, but those unheard / Are sweeter," and "Beauty is truth, truth beauty,—that is all / Ye know on earth, and all ye need / to know." Other odes followed, including "Ode on Melancholy" and "Ode on

Indolence." The narrative poem "Lamia," which drew from mythology, was also composed during this energetic period of Keats's productivity.

Tuberculosis pervaded the Keats family. In addition to his mother and youngest brother, Tom, another brother, George, who immigrated to America in 1819, died of the disease in 1841. Ultimately, Keats himself was affected with tuberculosis. Symptoms became more apparent in 1820, and he traveled to Rome in the hope that a warmer climate would improve his status. He had written to Fanny Brawne that "there is a great difference between going off in warm blood like Romeo, and making one's exit like a frog in a frost." Keats died in Rome on February 23, 1821, at the age of twenty-five, and was buried in a Protestant cemetery there. Several weeks after the funeral, Shelley wrote the elegy "Adonais" honoring his friend and colleague. Keats is memorialized in the Poets' Corner of Westminster Abbey along with contemporaries Wordsworth, Byron, and Shelley.

Among the many oft-quoted lines of John Keats, it is difficult to find any that utilize his exposure to medicine. A faint suggestion appears in "Ode to a Nightingale":

My heart aches, and a drowsy numbness pains
My sense, as though of hemlock I had drunk,
Or emptied some dull opiate to the drains
One minute past, and Lethe-wards had sunk.

SOURCES

Coote, Stephen. *John Keats: A Life*. London: Hodder & Stoughton, 1995.

Gitting, Robert. *John Keats: The Living Year*. Cambridge, MA: Harvard University Press, 1954.

Osler, William. *An Alabama Student and Other Biographical Essays*. New York: Oxford University Press, American Branch, 1908.

Stillinger, Jack. *John Keats Complete Poems*. Cambridge, MA: Belknap Press of Harvard University Press, 1982.

15

MARIE-JOSEPH EUGÈNE SUE

From Surgery at Sea to Successful Serials

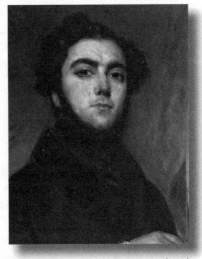

Marie-Joseph Eugène Sue, who wrote under the name of Eugène Sue, was born at the beginning of the First French Empire under Napoleon I (1804–1814/1815). During the Bourbon Restoration under Louis XVIII and Charles X (1814/1815–1830), he served as an auxiliary surgeon in Spain and in the French navy. During the July Monarchy under Louis Philippe d'Orléans (1830–1848), he became one of the most widely read literary figures in France. In France's Second Republic (1848–1852), he was elected, as a Socialist, to the Legislative Assembly from the Paris-Seine constituency. Later, in the Second Empire

Portrait by François Gabriel Guillaume Lépaulle.

under Napoleon III (1852–1870), he was exiled to Savoy, where he continued his literary career until his death. His volatile and varied life, which included a significant political and personality transformation, was so unusual that it could have been the subject of a work of fiction.

Marie-Joseph Eugène Sue was born into an affluent and distinguished family in Paris on January 26, 1804. His father had been the physician in chief of the Guard of the Consuls in the administration that preceded the First French Empire. His father, a favorite of Napoleon, was called to accompany the emperor on the Russian campaign of 1812, but took ill in Germany and returned home. He witnessed the birth certificate of Eugène de Beauharnais, the only son of Alexandre de Beauharnais and Joséphine Tascher de la Pagerie, the future wife of Napoleon I. Joséphine was Eugène Sue's godmother.

Sue began his schooling in France at the prestigious Collège Bourbon and showed signs of high intelligence, but also demonstrated resistance to his father's authority. As a seventeen-year-old, he surrendered to parental pressure and joined the staff at his father's hospital as a surgeon in training. In 1823, he ended his training and assumed the position of an auxiliary surgeon, initially with the French army and subsequently with the French navy. He participated in an expedition to the Spanish border to apply sanitary measures to combat yellow fever. He lived for a brief period in Madrid.

In October 1827, he served aboard the *Breslaw* during the decisive naval Battle of Navarino in the Ionian Sea as part of the Greek war for independence from Turkey. Sue's military service was not particularly praiseworthy. When he was found asleep on watch, an uncomfortable chair was designed for him so he would not doze off again. It was named the "Eugene Sue chair." As for his medical duties aboard the ship, he performed any needed amputations, which prompted the following comment: "This young surgeon did the amputations with the clumsiness of a novice combined with the composure of an old surgeon." His naval experience would eventually play a role in his early literary works.

Sue resigned his naval commission in 1829 and returned to Paris, where his medical career came to a permanent end. He began writing, but he hoped to become a painter. A year later, his father's death brought him a considerable inheritance, which altered his lifestyle. Self-impressed and favored with good looks, he patterned himself after Lord Byron: adopting the presentment of a dandy, living in luxurious surroundings, and changing his attire three times daily, often in the presence of an invited audience. Within seven years, he squandered the sizeable inheritance.

In order to pay off his debts, Sue worked as a reporter for the Paris *Herald* and wrote at an accelerated pace. The earliest of Sue's literary attempts can be dated January 23, 1826, when, still in the navy, he wrote a series of letters describing the adventure of a spy. Sue's first publications, after resigning his commission, *Kernock le pirate* (*Kernock the Pirate*) and *El Gitano* (*The Gypsy*), appeared in 1830. These two novellas, dealing with piracy and smuggling, were of little literary consequence. The following year, two more novellas, *Plick and Plock* (the name of two gnomes) and *Atar-Gull* (the name of the slave ship), were published in magazines. The latter told the story of the revenge of a slave directed against the family of a master, who had hung the slave's father.

Le Salamandre (*The Salamander*), a novel in two volumes, was the first of Sue's large works. The title took its name from a French corvette and tells of a naval lieutenant, on trial for rebellion, who sacrifices himself for his captain. The early Sue novels ridicule virtue, and their plots have evil triumphing over good. He presents scenarios emphasizing that wealth does not necessarily equate with happiness.

Initially, most of Sue's works appeared in serialized forms in *feuilletons*, which were detachable portions of French newspapers. This form of publication allowed for expansion of the readership because, at the time, books were very expensive and beyond the means of most people. The works of Sue gained the attention of the English publication *Foreign Quarterly Review*, which neglected other French writers, such as Stendhal, Alfred de Vigny, and George Sand. Sue was referred to as a French writer of interest.

In 1837, Sue's five-volume *Histoire de la marine François 1835–1837* (*History of the French Navy 1835–1837*) was published. It was a popular success, but the author was criticized for taking liberties and reporting inaccuracies. The same year, *Lautréamont*, a gothic novel set in the time of Louis XIV, was published. *Arthur* and *Mathilde* were two of Sue's early novels, which depicted the indolence of the high life of socialites. In 1841, his writing changed focus and concentrated on the disadvantaged common people and the social ills they confronted.

Sue's writings reflected the concurrent transition in his personal life. He had become an outspoken Socialist who used his literary talents to bring attention to the social ills and the adverse consequences of capitalism and the Catholic Church. His two best-known novels, *Les Mystères de Paris* (*The Mysteries of Paris*, 1842–43) and *Le Juif errant* (*The Wandering Jew*, 1844–45), were published in installments in the periodical *Le Constitutionnel* (*The Constitutional*). The two monumental works made Sue one of the wealthiest and most widely read writers in France, rivaling Alexandre Dumas père, and Victor Hugo, who was influenced by *Les Mystères de Paris* in his writing of *Les Miserables*.

The earlier of Sue's two novels had its origins in a cholera epidemic that spread throughout the poor people of Paris, and was the first work to express Sue's socialistic conviction. The novel, in which the protagonist is a nobleman from a fictional German kingdom and is disguised as a Parisian laborer, explores the various levels of society. Sue emphasizes the inhumane conditions that the lower classes endure, and how the lower strata of society are victimized by the upper classes. The melodrama, which was contained in over one thousand printed pages, pits good against evil in multiple engagements.

In 1845, Karl Marx included an extensive criticism of the work in his publication *The Holy Family*. Edgar Allan Poe wrote an essay about Sue's novel, referring to the work as "a paradox of childish folly and consummate skill." Shortly after the publications of *Les Mystères de Paris* and other novels by Sue and Dumas, they were translated by the English author Henry William Herbert. The books were popular in England.

The most widely read of Sue's novels was *Le Juif errant*, which took its name from a legend that first appeared in a German pamphlet in 1602. The legend told of a Jewish shoemaker who taunted Jesus on the road to Calvary, and was told to wander on forever until the Second Coming. The 1,400-page novel, which is distinctly anti-Catholic, particularly regarding the Jesuits, is a multifaceted melodrama and is included in *Horror: The 100 Best Books*, edited by Stephen Jones and Kim Newman and published in 1988. *Le Juif errant* was the basis of an opera by Fromental Halévy and several motion pictures.

In 1847, Sue published an eight-volume novel titled *Martin, l'enfant trouvé, ou Les Mémoires d'un valet de chamber* (*Martin, the Foundling, or Memoirs of a Valet*). This was followed by *Les Sept péchés capitaux* (*The Seven Cardinal Sins*). In 1848, Sue began his role as a Socialist deputy to the National Assembly, a post he retained until he was exiled to Savoy in 1851, following Louis Napoleon's coup d'état.

While in exile, he continued to publish at a rapid rate and became one of the highest-paid authors in France, second only to Alexandre Dumas. In Savoy, Sue wrote about two dozen novels, all of which continued to stress the evils and persecution encountered by the lower classes and projecting horror. *Les Mystères du peuple, ou Histoire d'une famille de prolétaires à travers les âges* (*The Mysteries of the People, or History of a Proletarian Family across the Ages*, in nineteen volumes), which appeared in serial form between 1849 and 1857, was suppressed by the French government.

In his later years, Sue acquired several printing houses that continued to publish his works and added to his wealth. He died in Annecy, Savoy, on August 3, 1857. His name appears on a street sign near Montmartre and the Sacré Coeur Basilica in the eighteenth arrondissement of Paris. Sue is referred to in a chronicle about French authors as "un remarquable feuilletoniste," or "a remarkable serialist."

SOURCES

Bory, Jean-Louis. *Eugène Sue*. Paris: Hachette Littérature, 1962.

16

CHARLES JAMES LEVER
Fiction Focuses on the Irish from Afar

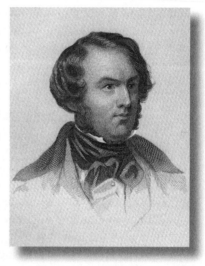

The biographers of Dr. Charles Lever have referred to him as "Dr. Quicksilver" and "the Lost Victorian." The first name was given when he was a young physician because of his mercurial personality. The second name refers to the fact that, although he was a most prolific novelist who wrote more about the Irish people and life on the European continent than any other British author during the reign of Queen Victoria, he has lapsed into obscurity. George Bernard Shaw wished to be affiliated with Lever "as a countryman and immediate forerunner."

Charles James Lever was born in Dublin on August 31, 1806, into a comfortable Protestant family. His youth was marked by the establishment of a reputation as a storyteller and for a love of reading that was offset by a propensity for mischief. At the age of sixteen, he enrolled at Trinity College, where his activities and pranks would attain legendary status. Indeed, seventy-five years later, they would be invoked in comparison with the behavior of noted prankster Oliver St. John Gogarty (see chapter 31). Lever's undergraduate education was extended to five years, after which he received a BA in 1827.

A year before his graduation, Lever's earliest publication, an essay titled "Recollections of the Night," which related to his experimentation with opium, was published in an obscure magazine. After graduation, unable to determine his ultimate goal, Lever left on a ship for Canada, with the temporary appointment as a "doctor." After a short stay in Quebec, he traveled through Indian lands and upper New York State and in the vicinity of Lake Erie. He returned to Ireland with a canoe and soon thereafter extended his travels to Europe. He studied for a brief period at the universities in Göttingen and Heidelberg, and traveled to Weimer, where he joined an audience listening to Johann Wolfgang von Goethe.

He returned to Dublin and to the study of medicine at Trinity in 1829. His medical studies did not preclude his literary contributions. In 1830, the second edition of a newly launched magazine, the *Dublin Literary Gazette*, contained an essay by Lever titled "News from the Log-Book of a Rambler," based on his various travels. Lever failed his examination for licensure from the Royal College of Surgeons, but, in 1831, he received a bachelor of medicine degree from Trinity, entitling him to practice medicine independently, but not surgery.

In 1832, Lever accepted an assignment by the local board of health to serve the impoverished districts of Kilrush and Kilkee in County Clare. He spent most of the time treating cholera-stricken patients, who were impressed by his kindness and cheerfulness. He married a year later and eventually moved on to fill a vacant position at Portstewart in County Derry. During his stay at Portstewart, his extra-medical antics resulted in his being assigned the nickname "Dr. Quicksilver."

In 1836, three years after the *Dublin University Magazine* was established, Lever had his first short story, "The Black Mask," published in that periodical. Within a year, the initial installment of his first novel, *The Confessions of Harry Lorrequer*, also appeared in that magazine, and was met with enthusiastic popularity. The entire novel was published as a book in 1839. By that time, Lever had agreed to serve as a doctor in the English colony in Belgium.

Lever's reputation is generally related to his first two extremely popular novels. *The Confessions of Harry Lorrequer* already established him as one of Great Britain's most sought-after writers. He was even compared with his main rival, Charles Dickens. According to author Stephen Haddelsey, when comparing Lever to Dickens, it was stated that "the author of *Lorrequer* is a person of equal buoyancy of spirits, of more extended observation, and not inferior in vigour of fancy and description."

The Confessions of Harry Lorrequer consists of a series of linked stories that are both humorous and picaresque, in which the focus lies in the eponymous narrator rather than a sustained plot. The hero moves almost uninterruptedly from duel to duel and one romantic encounter to the next. In a conscious appeal to a predominantly English readership, the Irish peasantry is presented merely as quaint, and the English policy toward them is not analyzed or criticized. Lever responded to the readership's applause: "If this sort of thing amuses, thought I, I can go on forever," and thereafter committed himself to the profession of a novelist.

Charles O'Malley, the Irish Dragoon, Lever's second novel, is usually paired with *The Confessions of Harry Lorrequer* when considering the author's corpus. *Charles O'Malley, the Irish Dragoon* represents a significant advance of Lever's authorial skills. Although it is a comedy and the protagonist evidences similarities with Shakespeare's Falstaff's rascality, it is a serious work about an idealistic young man and incorporates several well-developed comic characters. It combines hilarious events with exciting adventures and dynamic descriptions of battles that take place in the campaign against Napoleon. The fictional descriptions of battles are among the best published during the nineteenth century. The opening scenes of the novel, which occur at Trinity, were taken directly from the author's experiences, and many of the characters were derived from Lever's personal associations. The novel cemented his reputation as one of Great Britain's most popular writers. Forty-one editions of *Charles O'Malley, the Irish Dragoon* were published during the nineteenth century and an additional fifteen in the twentieth century.

In George Saintsbury's review of nineteenth-century English literature, the book is referred to as Lever's masterpiece. By contrast, contemporary Irish critics, favoring Irish nationalism, denounced the author's treatment of the peasantry and the choice of aristocratic landholders as heroes.

In 1842, at a time when Lever was financially stressed, he made a deliberate change in the direction of his life. He permanently ended his medical activities, which had consumed his daytime hours and required that he work late at night on his writing. He chose to dedicate the remainder of his life to literature, moving back to Ireland and assuming the editorship of the *Dublin University Magazine*.

He soon began to anonymously contribute essays to the magazine. Between January 1842 and May 1844, a series of papers titled "Nuts and Nutcrackers" appeared and were incorporated as a book by the same title published in 1845. Most of the essays were specifically related to current events and lost their relevance with the passage of time. As a Tory, Lever targeted Whigs and the Repeal Movement, by which the 1800 Act of Union between Great Britain and Ireland would be negated.

Lever produced five volumes of essays. In the same year *Nuts and Nut-*

crackers appeared, *Arthur O'Leary: His Wanderings and Ponderings in Many Lands* was also published. In that work, Lever revived a character from *Charles O'Malley, the Irish Dragoon* to present a series of sketches about continental travel.

Early in 1845, Lever left his position at the magazine and moved back to Europe. As pointed out by Stephen Haddelsey, the year 1845 represented a watershed time for Lever as a novelist. The two novels published that year, *The O'Donoghue* and *St. Patrick's Eve* ushered in an author with serious intent and with a concern for the political and social status of Ireland. He wrote for an English audience and attempted to erase their prevalent misconceptions of the Irish. The story told in *The O'Donoghue* takes place at the end of the eighteenth century, during the time of an abortive attempt by the French to land in Ireland to aid the rebels. It focuses on the interplay between the inept English landlord and the shrewd, pragmatic Irish tenants, who previously possessed the land.

St. Patrick's Eve was modeled after the contemporary Christmas books by Charles Dickens. It describes the horrors of poverty and draws from Lever's experience with cholera patients at Portstewart. In that work, Lever provides evidence for an admiration of Irish peasants, contradicting some of the criticism that had been directed against him, namely, that he was not sympathetic to their plight.

Lever's next novel, *The Knight of Gwynne*, was produced while he and his family led an itinerant life in Europe. It was the first of his novels to have a well-structured and cohesive plot. Some of the action derives from his experiences at Portstewart. Politically, he describes how the Irish aristocracy, whose members were opposed to the Act of Union, was circumvented by selfish opportunists. But, it is the knight, as a character in that tale, who generates the novel's greatest appeal. That work was followed by *The Confessions of Con Cregan: The Irish Gil Blas*, which was well received. Lever wrote in relation to that novel, "My notion was that the hero, once created, would not fail to find adventures. The vicissitudes of daily poverty would beget shifts and contrivances; with his successes would come ambition and daring." A large geographical range, which includes Ireland, France, Canada, Texas, and Mexico, is covered in the novel.

During the decade of the 1850s, Lever published ten more novels, the most significant of which were *The Dodd Family Abroad* (1854) and *The Martins of Cro' Martin* (1856). *The Dodd Family Abroad* is an epistolary novel, which describes hilarious situations of the Dodds during their travels to indicate how the English and Irish could better understand Europeans.

FROM MEDICINE TO MANUSCRIPT

The comical nature of *The Dodd Family Abroad* is contrasted with *The Martins of Cro' Martin*, which is characterized by pessimism, gloom, and tragedy resulting from the ineptness and irresponsibility of the Protestant aristocracy and an English landlord as it affects the Irish peasant tenant. Once again Lever includes descriptions of pestilent-ridden hovels and a cholera epidemic in his narrative. Modern critics consider the latter book to be one of Lever's best novels.

In 1859, to help resolve his persistent financial problems, Lever assumed the position of vice council of Spezia, a sinecure with little administrative responsibility, which allowed him to maintain his home in Florence. Prior to the move, Charles Dickens began representing Lever in negotiations with Lever's publishers. Lever's appreciation for this help and his friendship with Dickens is expressed in the published dedication of his 1863 novel, *Barrington*. While serving as vice council, Lever continued to produce novels at an exhausting pace to offset his own debts, which were compounded by those of his son.

A Day's Ride, a novel published in 1863, initially in serial form in Dickens's magazine *All the Year Round*, was so unpopular that it caused sales to plummet and accelerated Dickens's publication of *Great Expectations* to stabilize his own financial status. George Bernard Shaw referred to *A Day's Ride* as a work that had a profound influence on him. Shaw compared the novel's protagonist to Hamlet as an original contribution to the study of character.

In 1867, Lever received a political promotion when he was appointed as council at the northeastern Italian seaport of Trieste. He abhorred the place, which made him intensely despondent. This may have contributed to the fact the *That Boy of Norcott's*, published in 1869, was deemed to be Lever's worst novel. But, in 1872, this setback was compensated for by the publication of *Lord Kilgobbin*, his last and, arguably, best novel.

The modern Irish literary scholar A. Norman Jeffares wrote that *Lord Kilgobbin* is "the novel by which Lever should be judged. It is a despairing picture, of a decaying and discontented Anglo-Irish Ascendancy at the mercy of political unrest, angry terrorism and that English ineptitude, swinging between repression and appeasement, which he could not venerate." This, the most political of Lever's novels, was dedicated to his wife, who had died two years previously. In 1872, Lever received an honorary degree of LLD (or doctorate of laws) from Trinity College. A few months later, on June 11, 1872, he died in Trieste. Noted British author Anthony Trollope, who maintained a friendship with Lever that extended over more than fifteen years, wrote of him in his *An Autobiography*: "Surely never did a sense of vitality come so constantly from a man's pen, nor from a man's voice, as from his." But, Charles Lever, the prolific author who wrote of Ireland and the Irish people during trying times from several European venues, producing thirty novels and five volumes of essays, has lapsed into virtual obscurity.

SOURCES

Dictionary of National Biography (1893), s.v. "Lever, Charles James."

Haddelsey, Stephen. *Charles Lever: The Lost Victorian*. Buckinghamshire: Colin Smythe, Gerrards Cross, 2000.

Stevenson, Lionel. *Dr. Quicksilver: The Life of Charles Lever*. London: Chapman & Hall, 1939.

17

OLIVER WENDELL HOLMES

A Most Successful Combination

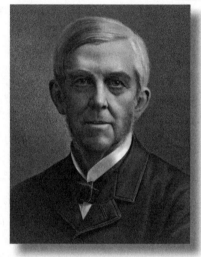

In 1907, Sir William Osler (see chapter 20) referred to Oliver Wendell Holmes as "the most successful combination which the world has ever seen of the physician and the man of letters." Holmes was often referred to as the American Oliver Goldsmith, in that both could write prose and poetry equally well. Holmes was unique, in that his poetry contributed to saving an iconic ship, while his prose led to the salvation of a multitude of newborns and the women who bore them.

Holmes had poetry in his genes. He was born in Cambridge, Massachusetts, on August 29, 1809, the first son of Abiel Holmes, a minister, and Sarah Wendell, who was a descendent of Thomas Dudley, the first published American poet. As a child, Holmes had the distinction of receiving a cowpox vaccination from Dr. Benjamin Waterhouse, who was the first to employ the method in the United States.

Holmes began his schooling near his home. When he was fifteen, he was sent for one year to Phillips Academy in Andover, Massachusetts, to prepare him for Harvard College, which he entered in 1825. During his four years at Harvard, his sociability and prowess as a poet offset his less than impressive physical presence, a height of five feet three inches. As an undergraduate, he distinguished himself academically, socially, and as a literary personality. He was elected to the Phi Beta Kappa honor society based on academic achievement. As a junior, he became a member of the Hasty Pudding Club, which provided a venue for his celebratory poems and public recitations. As poet laureate of the class of 1829, he presented a poem at the valedictory exercises. The reporter for the *New England Palladium* chronicled Holmes's performance in this way: "Though of a light and sarcastic character [it] was received with much applause."

Holmes ruled out the possibility of "the trade of authorship," and, after vacillating between the law and medicine, elected the law. He began studying law but was almost immediately disheartened, choosing to distract himself by writing poems for anonymous publication in periodicals initiated by Harvard undergraduates. In response to his learning that the secretary of the navy was considering dismantling the frigate *Constitution*, one of the original six frigates of the US Navy, Holmes wrote the three stanzas of "Old Ironsides," which appeared on September 16, 1830, in the *Advertiser* with the author listed as "H." The poem was widely circulated and might have played a role in saving the ship. The same year, Holmes wrote "The Last Leaf," which Edgar Allan Poe called one of the finest works in the English language, and was one of Abraham Lincoln's oft-recited favorites. The poem was published on March 26, 1831, in the *Amateur*, signed "O.W.H."

After Holmes had ruled out law as a career, he directed himself to the study of medicine. The curriculum, at the time Holmes prepared for a medical career, was limited, and the number of faculty to whom a student was exposed was small. Holmes studied at Harvard Medical School (then called Massachusetts Medical School) and at a private school (run by five local respected physicians), where he received clinical training. While conducting his studies, Holmes found time to continue writing. During that period he wrote essays that appeared in the *New England Magazine*.

From the spring of 1833 until Christmas 1835, Holmes lived in Europe, mainly enhancing his medical knowledge in Paris. At the time, there was general agreement that a French medical education was most prestigious. Historian David McCullough's recent work, *The Greater Journey: Americans in Paris*, chronicled the attraction that Paris had for Americans, including those aspiring to medical careers. No degree was required, and there was no tuition for foreigners who attended lectures.

Although Holmes attended lectures by most of the notable Parisian physicians, anatomists, pathologists, and surgeons, the one to whom he ascribed the most significant influence on his own thinking was Charles Pierre Alexandre Louis, pathologist at the Pitié-Salpétriere ("small hospital"). Louis taught that a physician should be skeptical and not rely on dogma or haphazard experience. The liberal use of drugs and method of bleeding were considered to be inappropriate. The lessons that Holmes learned from Louis found expression in 1860 when Holmes suggested that "the whole of material medica with a few exceptions might be tossed to the fishes with no harm done, except possibly to the fishes."

A memorable acquisition by Holmes during his stay in Paris was a first edition in Greek of *The Aphorisms of Hippocrates*, published in 1532 and edited by François Rabelais (see chapter 3). Holmes returned home to Cambridge, Massachusetts, for Christmas in 1834, and the following January, Holmes, who had not completed his medical degree before he left for Paris, presented a required thesis, successfully completed final examinations, and was awarded the medical degree on February 11, 1835. On May 22, he became a member of the Massachusetts Medical Society.

Although Holmes had not written a stanza of poetry while he was abroad, shortly after his return to Cambridge, he contributed "An Evening Thought" and "The Last Reader" to the *American Monthly Magazine*. He became the Phi Beta Kappa poet at Harvard and prepared and presented verses for the Harvard centennial. In 1836, a volume of his *Poems* was published.

Holmes continued to concentrate on his medical career. He hung out a shingle to attract patients and won the Boylston Medical Prize for his dissertation on "Direct Exploration." The work concerned the diagnosis of internal conditions by external means, and focused on listening to the sounds of the body usually by means of the stethoscope, which had been introduced by French physician René Laennec in 1815. In the fall of 1836, Holmes began the post of visiting physician at the Boston Dispensary, a charitable facility. In response to another call by the Massachusetts Medical Society for a Boylston Medical Prize contribution, Holmes submitted an essay on malaria in New England and another on neuralgia. Both essays won prizes, and his three essays were published in January 1838 by the *Boston Medical and Surgical Journal* (the forerunner of the *New England Journal of Medicine*). The essay on malaria received praise a century later as the best regional history of the disease.

Holmes's visibility throughout the Boston community was enhanced when, on December 7, 1837, he gave his first lecture at the civic association known as the Boston Lyceum. He presented his work there irregularly until the 1850s, when he started appearing more frequently. He would receive ten or fifteen dollars for each lecture (the equivalent of three hundred to four hundred dollars currently).

Holmes began his role as a medical educator in 1838, when he joined several Boston physicians to form the Tremont Medical School, which eventually merged with the Harvard Medical School. Holmes taught physiology and pathology, and assisted in anatomy. In July 1838, Holmes was appointed professor of anatomy and physiology at Dartmouth College. He had a year to prepare for the position, which required fourteen weeks away from Boston. Holmes would maintain that position for two years. In Holmes's introductory lecture at Dartmouth, he stressed the interrelationship between the disciplines of anatomy and physiology, stating, "One shows us the wheels and levers of the machine which we are to study; the other sets them all in operation." One hundred fifty years would pass before medical schools would routinely teach structure and function and entwine interdependent elements, a "double helix."

In 1840, Holmes married the daughter of a distinguished Massachusetts Supreme Court justice. She was also the niece of James Jackson, the physician with whom Holmes studied. In the early 1840s, Holmes's practice increased, and his experience with patients seeking strange cures or needing relief from such "cures" found him using his Lyceum lectures as a platform to denounce the quackeries of hydropaths, vegetarians, and, most particularly, homeopathy. In 1842, he published a volume titled "Homeopathy and Its Kindred Delusions" based on two lectures he had given.

In 1843, Holmes published an essay, based on a paper, which he had read at the Boston Society for Medical Improvement. The essay, "The Contagiousness of Puerperal Fever," appeared in the April issue of the only volume of the *New England Quarterly Journal of Medicine and Surgery*. An abstract of the essay appeared three months later in the *American Journal of Medical Sciences*. Holmes, based on his personally conducted survey of the literature and the records of individual physicians, concluded that puerperal fever (postpartum infection or childbed fever) was contagious and that it was spread from one patient to another by physicians and other attendants of those patients. In 1852, Hugh L. Hodge, professor of obstetrics at the University of Pennsylvania and, two years later, Charles D. Meigs, professor of midwifery and the diseases of women and children at Jefferson Medical College, attacked the concept of contagion and assailed Holmes's essay. In 1855, Holmes, as a rebuttal, republished his essay under the title of "Puerperal Fever as a Private Pestilence."

In 1846, Holmes placed his imprimatur of what has been referred to as "America's greatest contribution to surgery." On October 16, at the Massachusetts General Hospital, the first successful use of inhaled sulfuric ether, administered by the dentist W. T. G. Morton, to relieve pain during a surgical procedure took place. On November 21, Holmes wrote Morton, "Everybody wishes to have a hand in a great discovery. . . . The state should I think be called 'Anaesthesia.' This signifies insensibility . . . . The adjective will be 'Anaesthetic.'" It is to be noted that the word "anaesthesia" was widely used at the time and dates to the first century when Dioscorides, a celebrated Greek physician, introduced it.

In 1847, Holmes was appointed the Parkman Professor of Anatomy and Physiology at Harvard Medical School, a position named in recognition of Dr. George Parkman, who had gifted land on which a new medical school building was erected. It was the first time that physiology was recognized as a subject by Harvard. Within months, Holmes also assumed the post of dean of the Harvard Medical School faculty, a position he would hold for six years. Shortly after this appointment as dean, Holmes was criticized for considering the admission of a woman as a student (she was asked to withdraw her application). Ninety-eight years would elapse before the first woman would be accepted to Harvard Medical School. In 1850, Holmes admitted three African Americans to the school, but pressure from their classmates, faculty, and overseers allowed them to complete only one semester before they were dismissed. At that time, the medical school functioned almost completely independent of the college. Holmes was responsible for developing the curriculum, including the introduction of microscopy, and served as an intermediary between the faculty and the college.

In January 1849, Holmes notified his patients that he would no longer be conducting a private practice. He then resigned from the staff of the Massachusetts General Hospital, intending to devote himself to teaching and becoming a public lecturer, speaking to audiences on a circuit that included small towns and large cities mainly in the northeastern states. Between 1851 and 1856, Holmes maintained an exhausting schedule: his days were spent teaching medical students anatomy while at night Holmes traveled away from Boston to provide audiences with medical, scientific, and literary knowledge coupled with amusing anecdotes.

Attending public lectures had become a popular form of entertainment, and lecturing turned into quite a marketable commodity. Between November 1851 and April 1852, Holmes gave around sixty lectures in about fifty different cities in Massachusetts, New Hampshire, Vermont, Connecticut, Rhode Island, Maine, and New York. His repertoire included three or four lectures. The titles included "History of Medicine," "Love of Nature," and "Lectures and Lecturing." In 1853, he gave a series of twelve lectures on poets as part of the popular Lowell Institute Lectures.

The first issue of the *Atlantic Monthly*, which Holmes had named during the organizational meetings, appeared in November 1857. It included an unsigned contribution by Holmes that bore the title "The Autocrat of the Breakfast-Table." The autocrat articles, consisting of fictional table talk, as they appeared in ensuing issues of the periodical, were extremely popular and gave evidence of Holmes's humor and prowess as a poet. One of the most notable inclusions was "The Deacon's Masterpiece," better known as "the wonderful one-hoss shay."

A collection of his articles was published in 1858 as a book titled *The Autocrat of the Breakfast-Table*, which was well received, selling ten thousand copies in three days. A sequel, *The Professor at the Breakfast-Table*, which took over from the previous collection as serial installments in the *Atlantic Monthly*, was published in book form in 1860. That year, Holmes presented his lecture "Currents and Counter-Currents in Medical Science" to the Massachusetts Medical Society. He decried the liberal use of unproven drugs and stressed that the main duties of a physician were to prevent disease and make patients comfortable. He criticized patent medicines and homeopathy and indicated that more time should be spent on the determination of the cause of disease.

When the Civil War broke out, Holmes became a strident voice for the North. His lectures and poems provided expression of his sentiments regarding the preservation of the Union. Holmes's oldest child, Oliver Wendell Holmes Jr., who became known as the "Great Dissenter," during his long tenure on the US Supreme Court, left Harvard prematurely to join the Union forces and was injured three times. At the beginning of the war, *Elsie Venner*, the first of Holmes's three novels, which began as a serialization in the *Atlantic Monthly*, was published. It was followed by *The Guardian Angel* in 1867 and *A Morbid Antipathy* in 1885. Holmes's medical background finds expression in *Elsie Venner*, the tale of a complex and disturbed young lady, whose mother was bitten by a rattlesnake while pregnant. In that work, the term "Boston Brahmin" was introduced. In *The Guardian Angel*, Holmes presents the limits of the human will and how inborn, inherited elements can alter that will. *A Morbid Antipathy* concerns a character whose phobias are related to psychic trauma. Holmes's novels never reached the level of appeal that his poetry enjoyed.

The last of the Breakfast-Table series, *The Poet at the Breakfast-Table*, was published as a book in 1872. It gives voice to the circumstance of no longer being an active participant in life but rather reflecting on the past. In that work, the father-son relationship is considered, as are the modern theories of evolution and physics. The publication coincided with the transformation of the Harvard Medical School and Harvard College by Charles William Elliot, its twenty-first president. The medical school became part of the university, and physiology became a separate department, which allowed Holmes to dedicate all of his teaching to the subject of anatomy.

In 1876, Holmes's work titled *John Lothrop Motley: A Memoir* was published. It chronicled the life of one of his friends, a Harvard graduate, historian, novelist, and diplomat, who served as US minister to the Austrian Empire in 1861 and ambassador to the United Kingdom from 1860 to 1870. Toward the end of 1882, Holmes resigned from his position at the Harvard Medical School. In April of the following year, some two hundred New York State physicians feted Holmes at a banquet, during which he was referred to as "the most versatile member of their profession."

In1884, Holmes published another biography, *Ralph Waldo Emerson*. Although the book is deemed to be of little value for a modern student of Emerson and transcendentalism, the section on Emerson's poetry provides insight and enthusiastic appreciation on Holmes's part. A year later, during a vacation with his daughter in England, Scotland, and France, he received an honorary doctor of letters (DLitt) degree from both Oxford and Cambridge, a rare circumstance that would be matched by the noted surgeon Sir Geoffrey Keynes a century later. Holmes's book *Our One Hundred Days in Europe* chronicled his trip.

In 1891, he published *Over the Teacups*, the last of his Breakfast-Table books. On October 7, 1894, he died at home. A memorial tablet in King's Chapel in Boston where Holmes worshiped reads, "Teacher of Anatomy, Essayist and Poet," followed by a quote from Horace that translates as "He mingled the useful with the pleasant."

SOURCES

Leslie, Stephen. "Oliver Wendell Holmes." In *Studies of a Biographer*. London: Duckworth, 1898.

McCullough, David. *The Greater Journey*. New York: Simon & Schuster, 2011.

Tilton, Eleanor M. *Amiable Autocrat: A Biography of Oliver Wendell Holmes*. New York: Henry Schuman, 1947.

18

SILAS WEIR MITCHELL
Neurology and Nineteen Novels

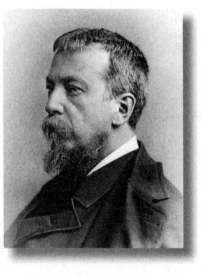

Silas Weir Mitchell or, as he preferred to be called, S. Weir Mitchell is credited with fathering American neurology and pioneering scientific medicine in the United States. A native of Philadelphia, Pennsylvania, where he spent almost his entire academic career, he was proud of a medical heritage that extended over three generations. All five of his great-grandparents' sons, who were born in Scotland, studied medicine. S. Weir Mitchell's grandfather studied medicine at Edinburgh and immigrated to Shepherdstown, Virginia, where S. Weir's father, John Kearsley Mitchell, was born in 1793.

John Kearsley graduated from the University of Pennsylvania Medical School in 1819, and was appointed professor of the practice of medicine at Jefferson Medical College in Philadelphia in 1839. He held the position while S. Weir Mitchell was a medical student at that school, and remained a highly regarded member of Philadelphia's medical community until his death in 1858.

The third oldest of nine children, S. Weir Mitchell was born in 1829. At age fifteen, he entered the University of Pennsylvania, where he studied the classics, philosophy, literature, rhetoric, mathematics, chemistry, and physics. In 1848, he proceeded to Jefferson Medical College in Philadelphia and graduated two years later as one of 210 graduates, all of whom were taught by a faculty that consisted of seven professors, including his father. Shortly after his graduation, he sailed for Europe, where he met several eminent physicians in London. He subsequently attended physiology lectures given by Claude Bernard and histology lectures by Charles-Phillipe Robin in Paris.

When Mitchell returned to Philadelphia, he declared to his associates that he would direct his attention to becoming a physician who would devote time to laboratory research. This goal was contrary to his father's strong desire that he become a surgeon. During the next decade, prior to his participation in the Civil War, Mitchell divided his time between the practice of medicine accompanied by clinical research and laboratory studies, particularly in toxicology. He presented and published over a dozen papers on widely diverse subjects after conducting experiments on opossums, muskrats, pigeons, frogs, turtles, dogs, ducks, and chickens. In 1860, Mitchell published his first major work, a 145-page monograph titled *Researches upon the Venom of the Rattlesnake, with an Investigation of the Anatomy and Physiology of the Organs Concerned.*

Simultaneously, Mitchell practiced medicine as a partner in his father's successful practice until his father died, at which time he took over the practice. Mitchell intermittently continued his research on venomous snakes for forty years. The 1861 paper titled "On Treatment of Rattlesnake Bites with Experimental Criticism upon the Various Remedies Now in Use" was among his many publications on the subject.

At the onset of the Civil War in 1861, Mitchell's medical reputation had already been established. The famous European physiologist Charles Edouard Brown Séquard wrote Mitchell a letter, in which he stated, "You and your friend and scientific partner, Dr. [William A.] Hammond, are the most original Physiologists of the United States."

The period of the Civil War represented an important time in Mitchell's medical career. In 1862, he was elected a member of the American Philosophical Society. Also that year, he received his first hospital appointment related to the war effort. He contracted with the Union Army at the Filbert Street Hospital in Philadelphia. By his own account, "There I became interested in cases of nervous disease and wounds of nerves, about which little was then known."

Surgeon General of the Union Army William A. Hammond, who had been Mitchell's former collaborator, had created a small hospital for nervous diseases at the Christian Street Hospital, which grew into the four-hundred-bed Turner's Lane Military Hospital. Mitchell joined the staff while, at the same time, increasing his own general practice. Mitchell's efforts at that facility resulted in a series of significant papers and a book, *Gunshot Wounds and Other Injuries of Nerves*, coauthored by S. Weir Mitchell, George Morehouse, and William K. Keen, which revolutionized knowledge about wounds of the nerves and became a medical classic. In that work, a description of "burning pain," which Mitchell would later name "causalgia," first appeared. In 1864, Mitchell resigned his position in the army and concentrated on his private practice, which transitioned from general medicine to consultations related to neurological disorders.

Mitchell's scientific contributions were given recognition when he was elected to the National Academy of Sciences in 1865. He next expanded his medical reach by embarking on research concerning the physiology of the cerebellum, a part of the hindbrain. In spite of his productivity, on three occasions, he was unable to obtain professorships in physiology that he sought at Jefferson Medical College and the University of Pennsylvania.

In the early 1870s, Mitchell was appointed to the staff of the Orthopaedic Hospital in Philadelphia, the name of which was expanded to become the Orthopaedic Hospital and Infirmary for Nervous Diseases. It was there that his reputation grew substantially as he concentrated intensely on the treatment of neurological disorders. At the same time, Mitchell championed a theme that had been espoused by physiologist and literary figure Albrecht von Haller whose life and work we have already discussed (see chapter 8). Like Haller, Mitchell believed that rural areas of the country were more healthful than the urban areas.

In 1872, Mitchell published his work on neurological conditions, *Injuries of Nerves and Their Consequences*, which underwent many editions and translations. In 1875, members of the American Neurological Association wanted to nominate him for the first presidency of the organization, but he declined. He would later assume the organization's presidency in 1909 at the age of eighty.

Mitchell expanded his research interests to include disorders of sleep, along with conducting research on tendon reflexes. But his reputation as the most prominent neurologist in America was, in large part, based on his management of hysteria and the application of rest as the major therapy. In 1877, he published the first definitive description of the rest treatment in *Fat and Blood: And How to Make Them*, with the subtitle *An Essay of the Treatment of Certain Forms of Neurasthenia and Hysteria*. The five therapeutic elements that constitute his regimen are seclusion, bed rest, diet, massage, and electricity with an induction current.

In 1877, on the occasion of the centennial of the College of Physicians of Philadelphia, Mitchell was elected its president. Six years later, he would finally meet William Osler, with whom he maintained a long friendship based on mutual respect. Then in 1883, Mitchell met with Osler while both were in Europe. He hoped to negotiate with Osler to fill the position of professor of clinical medicine at the University of Pennsylvania and succeeded.

In 1886, at Harvard's 250th anniversary, Mitchell received an honorary doctor of letters degree, and two years later, at the 800th anniversary of the University of Bologna medical school, he received an honorary doctor of medicine degree. A year later, the American Physiological Society was formed as a direct result of a suggestion by Mitchell.

In 1897, Mitchell's *Clinical Lessons on Nervous Diseases* was published, offering a profile of his breadth of knowledge, experience, and expertise. That work includes a full description of the eponymous "Mitchell's disease" or erythromelalgia, a rare disease involving smaller blood vessels, a disorder characterized by pain in the extremities associated with redness and warmth of the skin. Between 1898 and Mitchell's death on January 4, 1914, forty-three of his medically related publications appeared, bringing the total to 285. The last four were focused on the medical department in the Civil War and the contributions of John Shaw Billings, an old friend who had been integral to the development of the surgeon general's office. When Harvey Cushing (see chapter 28) met Mitchell for the first time in 1902, he wrote, "He [Mitchell] was probably the most picturesque and many-sided physician of his time— and knew it." Mitchell's medical publications were characterized by lucid and appealing prose.

His literary contributions consisted of prose, blank verse, and rhyme. Mitchell's thirty-seven literary publications began with prose and ended with poetry in both blank verse and rhyme. In 1859, he submitted to Oliver Wendell Holmes a poem, probably "The Hill of Stones," with the hope that it would be published in the *Atlantic Monthly*. It was not accepted but later appeared in an anthology of Mitchell's poems.

Mitchell and Holmes had a friendship that began in the 1850s and extended to the time of Holmes's death in 1894. Mitchell felt that he and Holmes were America's two most successful literary physicians. In 1892, Mitchell presented a portrait of Holmes to the College of Physicians of Philadelphia and wrote a poem for the occasion.

Mitchell's first literary publication, an anonymous short story titled "The Case of George Dedlow," appeared in the *Atlantic Monthly* in 1866. In the story, Dedlow, a Union Army officer, sustains sequential wounds in battle and eventually becomes a quadruple amputee. He is plagued by painful sensations from the amputated extremities. This was one of the earliest descriptions of phantom limb pain.

Medical issues are either integral or incorporated in many of Mitchell's literary works. "The Autobiography of a Quack," also published anonymously in the *Atlantic Monthly*, is the life story of a physician dying of Addison's disease (primary adrenal cortical insufficiency manifest by weakness and weight loss). The short story brings into focus the insecurities and temptations of the life of a doctor.

At the age of fifty, Mitchell increased his literary efforts. He had, by that time, become one of the country's most prominent and financially successful physicians, who also enjoyed an elevated social status. As a consequence of having developed preeminence as a physician, Mitchell felt free to identify himself as the author of literary works. Beginning in 1879, he spent half of the year away from Philadelphia and his practice in order to devote more time to his poetry and novels.

In 1884, Mitchell's first novel, *In War Time*, was published. The protagonist in that work is a physician, who, like Mitchell, was a contract physician at a military hospital on Filbert Street during the Civil War. The book describes the moral decline and eventual destruction of the mind and spirit of the central character. Mitchell's second novel, *Roland Blake*, was published two years later, and, by contrast, the main character is a patient who epitomizes bravery and gentlemanly behavior.

In the 1880s, Mitchell published three novels, two books of poetry, and more than fifty scientific articles. In his 1891 novel, *Characteristics*, the story is told in the first person by Dr. Owen North, whose description of himself is similar to that presented by Mitchell in his autobiography. North receives a bullet wound while performing an operation during the Civil War and becomes quadriparetic (weakness in all four extremities). He regains full sensation and returns to a consultative medical practice. *Dr. North and His Friends* was published as a sequel in 1900.

In 1897, Mitchell published two novels. *The Adventures of François* is about a foundling, thief, juggler, and fencing master during the French Revolution, and his most popular work, *Hugh Wynne, Free Quaker*, is the tale of a Quaker in the Revolutionary Army led by George Washington and includes Dr. Benjamin Rush as a minor character along with a description of senile dementia in the main character's father. *Hugh Wynne, Free Quaker* ranked second in readership on the *Bookman*'s best-seller list while *The Adventures of François* placed tenth. *Hugh Wynne, Free Quaker* sold more than five hundred thousand copies in the first decade after its publication and went through at least twenty-two editions.

Mitchell considered his work *Constance Trescot*, published in1905, to be his best novel. Constance is the wife of a lawyer who had served in the Union Army and practices in a Southern town, where he is shot dead by a legal opponent. The widowed Constance is dedicated to ruining the man who killed her husband and succeeds when her target shoots himself in her presence. *The Red City*, published in 1909, is a historical novel set in Philadelphia during the second term of George Washington's presidency when the city served as the temporary capital of the United States. Mitchell's last and nineteenth novel, *Westways* (1912), was published when he was eighty-four years old. It is replete with action-packed Civil War battle scenes and distinctive characters.

Mitchell's prose publications include four children's books. In 1864, he collaborated with Elizabeth Wister Stevenson on *The Children's Hour*. In 1866, he published *The Wonderful Stories of Fuz-Buz the Fly, and Mother Grahem the Spider.* In 1888, he published *Prince Little Boy and Other Tales*, and, in 1893, *Mr. Kris Kringle: A Christmas Tale.*

Mitchell's poems were not as well received as his prose. Walt Whitman, whom Mitchell offered medical consultation to after the famous poet had sustained a severe stroke and moved to Camden, New Jersey, stated, "Mitchell has written poems—a volume at least or two . . . they don't come to much—they are non-vital, are stiff at the knees, don't quite float along freely with the fundamental currents of life, passion." In 1889, Whitman commented, "Mitchell of late years has been bitten with the desire to compose, compose—that curse of curses: has written volumes: very bad, too-awful in their inadequacy: but personally he is a man to know."

Mitchell dedicated a volume of his poems to James Russell Lowell—poet, critic, Harvard professor, and editor of the *Atlantic Monthly*. In appreciation Lowell wrote Mitchell that his "The Swan-Women," "A Medal," and "The Miser: A Masque" were "particularly fine and even Masterly." Mitchell regarded "Ode to a Lycian Tomb," which was written as a memoriam for his daughter, to have been his best poem.

During his later years, Mitchell composed and presented a number of poems to highlight special moments. In addition to the previously mentioned poem honoring Oliver Wendell Holmes, he presented "Minerva Medica" for the commemoration of the fiftieth anniversary of the doctorate of D. Agnew

Hayes, professor of surgery at the University of Pennsylvania. His poems were also written in honor of his close friend, William Osler, and Abraham Jacobi, "the father of American pediatrics." In 1896, on the occasion of the fiftieth anniversary of the first public demonstration of surgical anesthesia, Mitchell wrote "The Birth and Death of Pain." In 1914, after his death, *The Complete Poems of S. Weir Mitchell* was published.

Mitchell is memorialized in a great many ways: a bronze portrait plaque of him was sculpted by Augustus Saint-Gaudens; a portrait was painted of him and hangs in the same hall as that of Oliver Wendell Holmes in the College of Physicians of Philadelphia; a neurological disease is named for him; a biological laboratory has been named the Weir Mitchell Station in honor of his exploration of the area on Mount Desert Island, Maine; the S. Weir Mitchell Award is given by the American Academy of Neurology; and the Weir Mitchell Oration is sponsored by the College of Physicians of Philadelphia.

SOURCES

Cervetti, Nancy. *S. Weir Mitchell, 1829–1914: Philadelphia's Literary Physician.* University Park, PA: Pennsylvania State University Press, 2012.

Walter, Richard D. *S. Weir Mitchell, M.D.: Neurologist.* Springfield, IL: Charles C. Thomas, 1970.

19

ROBERT SEYMOUR BRIDGES

The Lone Laureate

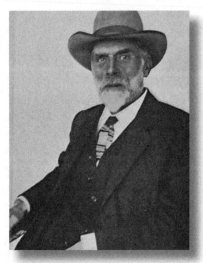

From 1913 until the time of his death on April 21, 1930, the calling card of the only medical graduate to be designated poet laureate of Great Britain read, "Robert Seymour Bridges, OM." The "OM" refers to the Order of Merit, which was established by King Edward VII in 1902 to recognize distinguished service in the armed forces, science, art, literature, or the promotion of culture. It is restricted to a maximum of twenty-four living recipients from the monarch's realm plus an occasional honorary member. The other physicians to be so honored were the Lord Lister, Sir Charles Scott Sherrington, Wilder Penfield, Sir Frank Mac-farlane Burnet, the Lord Florey, Sir Peter Medawar, Sir Magdi Yacoub, and Albert Schweitzer. Unlike the others, with the exception of Schweitzer, Bridges's recognition was not related to medical contributions but based solely on his reputation as a poet.

Bridges was born on October 23, 1844, in Upper Walmer, Kent, on the southeast coast of England. He was taught at home by a governess until he was ten years old, when he was sent to board at the exclusive Eton boarding school. He was in a subset of students referred to as "oppidans," whose parents paid full fees, allowing the students to live in residences outside the school. While he studied at Eton, his serious attitude toward religion intensified, while he also developed an interest in music, more particularly oratorio or setting poems to music. In 1863, he left Eton and entered Corpus Christi College at Oxford.

Early in his stay at Oxford, he developed a strong bond of friendship with Gerard Manley Hopkins, the Jesuit priest who was among the leading Victorian poets, and the friendship would persist throughout their lives. At Oxford, Bridges's adherence to the High Church of England intensified, and he was elected to the Brotherhood of the Most Holy Trinity (BHT). But as a result of his studies of philosophy, he drifted from his religious sympathies and resigned from the BHT.

In 1869, Bridges began his medical training at St. Bartholomew's hospital in London, and, in December 1874, he received his medical degree from Oxford. While he was still engaged in his medical training, Bridges's first published volume of poems appeared in *Poems* (1873). The table of contents was classified by content and verse form. The volume consisted of fifty-three poems, including elegies, descriptions of nature, philosophical statements, and four ballads.

In 1875, Bridges began an apprenticeship as a house physician to Dr. Patrick Black at St. Bartholomew's. That year, Bridges contributed an article on "A Severe Case of Rheumatic Fever Treated Successfully by Splints" to the *St. Bartholomew's Hospital Reports*. During his period of apprenticeship, he continued to write sonnets, some of which were included in *The Growth of Love: A Poem in Twenty-Four Sonnets*, published in 1874. *The Growth of Love* would be published as two subsequent editions, the last appearing in 1889 containing seventy-nine sonnets.

In 1876, Bridges passed the examination for membership of the Royal College of Physicians, resigned as house physician, and took a position in the relatively recently established St. Bartholomew's Casualty Ward. The role of the physician in the Casualty Ward was to treat minor ailments and determine which patients required admission to the hospital or outpatient management. In one year, Bridges saw almost thirty-one thousand patients in the Casualty Ward. In 1878, he worked three days a week at St. Bartholomew's and, in addition, served as an outpatient physician at the Children's Hospital and at the Great Northern (Royal Free) Hospital.

In time, he transferred his medical activities to the other hospitals and became an assistant physician at the Hospital for Sick Children, Great Ormond St., and a full physician at the Great Northern Hospital. He is credited with preventing an epidemic of smallpox in one area of London by isolating victims and creating a process of quarantine. In 1879, Bridges published another volume of poems that began with "A Hymn to Nature." The following year, another volume just titled *Poems* appeared. Gerard Manley Hopkins expressed his opinion of the work to Bridges: "If I were not your friend I shd. [should] wish to be the friend of the man who wrote your poems. They shew the eye for pure beauty." The volume contains some of Bridges's best lyrics.

The last three poems in the volume are in Bridges's version of "sprung rhythm" (attributed to Hopkins), in which the first syllable is stressed to be followed by a variable number of unstressed syllables, in order to imitate the rhythm of natural speech. "On a Dead Child" is the one poem in the volume that emanated solely from Bridges's medical experience.

> Perfect little body, without fault or stain on thee,
> With promise of strength and manhood full and fair!
> Though cold and stark and bare,
> The bloom and charm of life doth awhile remain on thee . . .

In June 1881, Bridges contracted a severe case of pneumonia, which extended over several months, forcing him to a warmer climate in Italy. In 1882, he published his first major work, *Prometheus the Foregiver*, subtitled *A Mask in the Greek Manner*. A reviewer wrote that Bridges accomplished "the first perfect imitation of Miltonic blank verse in two hundred years of experiment." The work depicts the change "in Christian belief from Old Testament attitudes and a basic questioning of religious faith, and includes an assertion that man's spiritual nature is an adequate guide to conduct."

That year, Bridges ended his medical ties and moved with his mother to Yattendon, a small village in Berkshire, where he would devote himself to his literary career. It was stated that Bridges became a doctor with the intention "to practice medicine until he was forty, when he would retire; the experience would give him knowledge of men for his work as a poet." In 1900, Bridges had been awarded fellowship in the Royal College of Physicians. On the occasion of receiving an honorary degree from the University of Michigan in 1924, he told the students, "First of all, the uncertainty of medical science and the possible complications in any difficult case gave me an intolerable anxiety—Then again since medicine was not nor could not ever be my sole or chief interest in life, I could not face the perpetual industry which was needful in order to keep up with continuing and rapidly expanding knowledge."

He initiated his literary activity in his new location with the writing of plays. The first of his plays, *Nero, Part I*, was not intended for the stage. The work was a historical tragedy, in which the complex characters were well defined, but the plot was weak and most of the action was reported rather than shown. The second of his completed plays, *The Return of Ulysses*, was a dramatization of the main scenes of Homer's *Odyssey*. It eventually appeared in 1890, preceded by another drama, *The Feast of Bacchus*, which had been started earlier. Unfortunately, none of Bridges's dramatic works gained critical acclaim.

In 1884, Bridges married, which prompted the production of several love sonnets that would be incorporated in later collections. His second major poem, *Eros and Psyche*, was first published in 1885. The review in the *Spectator* stated, "Yet, excellent as the whole poem is, it is the sort of thing that one may read with extreme pleasure and never desire to re-read." The theme is that the human being should be guided by love, in which sexuality is tempered with compassion.

During the latter half of the 1880s, Bridges concentrated on writing dramas. In 1890, *Achilles in Scyros*, *Palicio*, *The Return of Ulysses*, and *The Christian Captives* were published. Also, that year his *Short Poems* appeared in print. The reviewers generally regarded the plays as "modern-antiques which do not interest us very much," while a reviewer of *Short Poems* wrote, "Though extremely scholarly, he is at his best (as most men are at their best) a very simple writer. . . . His verse is, indeed, as full of thought as it is accomplished in form and melodious in sound; but it abides by the principal things, and does not busy itself with things that are not principals."

In 1893, the Oxford University Press published Bridges's first prose, *Milton's Prosody: With a Chapter on Actual Verse and Notes*, which underwent a final revision in 1921. The work is a detailed analysis of the verse found in John Milton's *Paradise Lost* and defines the changes in Milton's later poems. According to Bridges, in contradistinction to other analyses, Milton wrote a form of syllabic verse.

The last decade of the nineteenth century was significant for Bridges. In 1893, noted Victorian anthologist A. H. Miles titled the final volume of his Poets and the Poetry of the Nineteenth Century series as *Robert Bridges and Contemporary Poets*, and used a photograph of Bridges as the frontispiece. Bridges spent much of his time on musical collaborations, the first of which was the oratorio *Eden*, composed by Charles Stanford. Bridges published an essay, "A Practical Discourse on Some Principles of Hymn-Singing" (1901), and several hymnal books, including *Songs of Syon* (1904). One of Bridges's dirges caught the attention of British composer Gustav Holst, who in 1930 wrote *A Choral Fantasia Op. 51* based on Bridges's poem "Ode to Music."

In 1899, Bridges's *Small Hymn Book* and *Shorter Poems* were published. In 1893, the *Academy*, reviewing his achievements, stated, "Of metre Mr. Bridges is a master, as befits one who has written learnedly with insight on the rhythms both of Milton and Keats. . . . He has left the English lyric a far more flexible thing than he found it, and one seems already to trace his influence in the versifications of . . . younger writers."

Bridges experimented with quantitative verse, based on the duration of syllables without regard for accents or stresses. In 1902, he wrote a long poem, "Wintry Delights," which surveys humans' achievements in science and their effect on people's view of the world. A year later his poem "To a Socialist" presented arguments against the doctrine of socialism.

In 1910, Bridges became acquainted with Francis Brett Young, another poet and physician (see chapter 34), who asked Bridges to set some of his poems to music. Bridges declined but invited Young to visit him. In 1914, Young wrote the first critical book about Bridges's work.

In 1912, Bridges was awarded an honorary doctor of letters at Oxford. That year, Oxford University Press published their first edition of Bridges's *Poetical Works*, which included a selection from his previous works and a few additional poems.

In 1913, the *Journal of Education* polled its readership for the "three greatest poets in order of excellence." The result was first place for Rudyard Kipling, second place for William Watson, and third place for Robert Seymour Bridges. That year, after Britain's poet laureate Alfred Austin died, the two men considered to replace him were Kipling and Bridges. Bridges was selected because he was deemed more capable of writing for an occasion.

In 1916, an anthology of Bridges's works, *The Spirit of Man*, was published. It was extremely popular, requiring three reprints the following year. In 1918, Bridges arranged for the posthumous publication of the verse of his friend Gerard Manley Hopkins. The work established Hopkins as the superior poet. At the end of World War I, Bridges wrote a poem on the armistice for the *London Times*. In 1920, *October and Other Poems* was published, followed by *The Tapestry: Poems* in 1925, and *New Verse* in 1926.

Bridges began his long philosophical poem, *The Testament of Beauty: A Poem in Four Books*, on Christmas Day 1924, and it is generally regarded as his masterpiece. He put it aside for two years, and it was eventually published in October 1929, five months after he received the Order of Merit, one day after his eighty-fifth birthday, and six months before his death. In that work, he sought to place humanity within the natural world so that we could be compared with other species. Religion is reconciled with modern knowledge and concepts. Two basic instincts, "selfhood" and "breed," preservation of the self and the species, are identified and form the basis of compassion and passionate love.

In the introduction to *The Oxford Book of Modern Verse* 1892–1935, W. B. Yeats praised Bridges with these words: "His influence—practice not theory, was never deadening; he gave to lyric poetry a new cadence, a distinction as deliberate as that of Whistler's painting. . . . Every metaphor, every thought a commonplace, emptiness everywhere, the whole magnificent." Critic Albert Guérard in his literary study of Bridges's work wrote, "Bridges believed that man's instincts are the basis for his intellectual and spiritual achievements, that these instincts are intrinsically good, though the material for vice as well as virtue, that happiness depends upon a harmony of impulses effected through the agency of reason, and that man's ideal aspirations, without which his life is meaningless, find their finest support in physical beauty."

The publication of *The Testament of Beauty* was very successful. The first printing of two thousand copies sold out immediately, and, by 1946, it was estimated that about sixty-eight thousand copies had been printed. But despite the success of his final work and his lifelong multifaceted productivity, which included poetry, hymns, dramas, and prose, Bridges, currently, receives little attention and remains best known for his editing of *Poems of Gerard Manley Hopkins*.

SOURCES

Philips, Catherine. *Robert Bridges: A Biography*. Oxford: Oxford University Press, 1992.
Dictionary of National Biography (1967), s.v. "Bridges, Robert Seymour."

20

SIR WILLIAM OSLER

A Precedent from a Peerless Physician

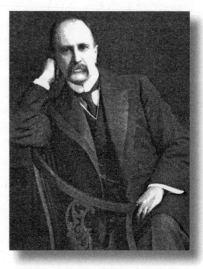

Physician and writer Sir Arthur Conan Doyle (see chapter 24), in the voice of Sherlock Holmes, wrote in *A Study in Scarlet*, "There is nothing new under the sun. It has all been done before." In fiction, throughout time, themes have recurred. The same applies to nonfiction, where previous reports of similar or identical subject matter are readily discoverable. In the case of writers with a medical background, a recent work titled *Doctors of another Calling*, a multiauthored series of essays about physicians who devoted their time to other pursuits, includes nine men who are featured in this current work. But the precedent for those twentieth-century physicians who have contributed significant nonmedical nonfiction literary works must be assigned to William Osler. In 1908, *Alabama Student and Other Essays*, based on Osler's presentations to the Johns Hopkins Historical Club and other invited lectures, brought attention to the medical backgrounds of four literary luminaries: Sir Thomas Browne, John Locke, John Keats, and Oliver Wendell Holmes.

Given that the word "clinician" derives from the Greek *klinikos*, meaning "belonging to a bed," and that, in Latin, *clinicus* was applied to a physician who visited patients at a bedside, Osler was certainly the premier clinician of the latter half of the nineteenth century and the early twentieth century. He was not only the consummate practicing clinician, but he also led the transformation of medical education by moving the emphasis of instruction from the lecture room to the patients' bedsides. His peerless medical stature was augmented by his humanistic literary contributions, articulated in addresses that found their way into print and have persisted as beacons of inspiration.

William Osler was born on July 12, 1849, in the backwoods of Canada, about forty miles north of Toronto. Eight years later, his family moved to the town of Dundas (at the head of Lake Ontario), where his father was designated canon of the parish. In 1866, Osler entered Trinity College School, which was advertised as the equivalent of Rugby in England, at Weston, a few miles west of Toronto. A year later, Osler matriculated at the University of Toronto College, intending to prepare for the ministry, but he shifted his attention to the study of medicine. In 1868, he enrolled in the Toronto School of Medicine, a private, for-profit institution. In 1870, Osler transferred to the McGill Medical School in Montreal and received a medical degree from that institution in 1872.

Shortly thereafter, Osler left for England and Europe, where he spent two years, mainly in London. There he focused on studying physiology and histology. His main graduate study consisted of the investigation of circulating particles in the blood that would later be identified as platelets. Although his research was neither innovative nor definitive, his work was noticed and he was considered for a faculty appointment at McGill. Within a year of his arrival at McGill, he was promoted to professor of the Institutes of Medicine to fill the vacancy of a recently appointed professor, who vacated the position because of heart trouble.

Osler supplemented his meager salary with the stipend he received as a physician to the smallpox ward at Montreal General Hospital. At the Institutes of Medicine, Osler was innovative from the onset, introducing a course on microscopy and histology, a first for Canadian medical education. He also added a new course on practical pathological demonstrations, which was conducted in the autopsy room of Montreal General Hospital. Osler rapidly became the most popular member of the faculty for the students and a leader to be followed by his colleagues. If these medical commitments weren't enough to keep him quite busy, he also served as a professor at Montreal Veterinary College. In spite of his relatively junior status, in 1878, he was appointed to fill the one vacancy as attending physician at Montreal General Hospital.

Osler was a prolific contributor to the medical literature, and, in 1881, the first year of his eligibility, he was elected a fellow of the Royal College of Physicians of London. That year, at an international medical congress held in London, Osler presented a well-received paper, in which he suggested that the vegetations within the heart in endocarditis were caused by bacteria. He returned to Europe in 1884, and, while in London, he was interviewed by Silas Weir Mitchell, the renowned Philadelphia physician (see chapter 19), for the position of professor of clinical medicine at the University of Pennsylvania. A few months later, Osler was formally appointed to that distinguished professorship. Despite Osler's translocation from Montreal to Philadelphia, he was elected to the presidency of the Canadian Medical Association for 1885. In Philadelphia, although Osler continued to emphasize the important correlation between clinical practice and research, his own professional direction became more focused on clinical medicine.

In September 1888, Osler accepted the position of physician in chief of the newly created Johns Hopkins Hospital and moved to Baltimore, Maryland, in May 1889, for the official opening of that facility. The board of Johns Hopkins University appointed him professor of the theory and practice of medicine. His final duty at the University of Pennsylvania was to deliver a farewell address to the students. That address, titled "Aequanimitas" ("Equanimity"), which invoked the classical era of medicine and offered advice to young physicians, was published and remains one of the most oft-quoted works of medical literature. In it Osler stresses the importance of imperturbability as a characteristic of a physician. Equanimity and infinite patience in the face of adversity are considered to be prime requisites for a physician.

In Baltimore, Osler was the driving force behind the immediate formation of a journal club, a medical society, and a historical club, as well as the publications known as the *Johns Hopkins Hospital Bulletin* and the *Johns Hopkins Reports*. Toward the end of 1890, while awaiting the opening of the medical school, Osler began writing a textbook titled *The Principles and Practice of Medicine*. This work of 1,050 pages, written by Osler alone, was published in 1892. He gave the first copy to Grace Linzee Revere Gross, a widow, whom he married that year.

It was the first great textbook of modern medicine and the last to be written by a single author. It had a long life span. In 1908, Osler produced the seventh edition, and, in 1912, the eighth edition credits Thomas MacCrae as coeditor. The textbook did not go out of print until after the sixteenth edition in 1947, and it was resurrected in 1968 as a multiauthored textbook of internal medicine.

While awaiting the opening of the newly created Johns Hopkins School of Medicine, Osler maintained an active schedule of lectures. The year after the publication of the first edition of *The Principles and Practice of Medicine*, he delivered a graduation address titled "Student and Teacher" at the University of Minnesota. In offering advice to the students, he invoked the classics and the writings of humanists. Weeks later, Osler spoke against medical specialization to the American Pediatrics Association, which would elect him to its presidency in 1892.

The Johns Hopkins School of Medicine opened in 1893, and the students did not come under the influence of Osler until they entered their third year. He initiated the clinical clerkship, which integrated students into the care of the patients at the hospital during their fourth year, and he soon became the students' favorite professor. At the same time, Osler developed a large and lucrative private practice that did not discriminate among socioeconomic groups. At the beginning of the twentieth century, he began to devote more of his time to medical history and philosophical issues, particularly those that pertained to education and his bibliophilia. Osler eventually accumulated all of the editions of Sir Thomas Browne's *Religio Medici*.

In 1905, one year after receiving an honorary doctor of science degree from Oxford University, which was sponsored by the British Medical Association, Osler was named Regius Professor of Medicine at Oxford. Soon thereafter, he began work on the multivolume, multiauthored *System of Medicine*, the first volume of which appeared in 1907. During his first year at Oxford, Osler spent time in London with his colleagues Drs. William Welch, William Steward Halsted, and Howard A. Kelly, all of whom sat for famed artist John Singer Sargent's *The Four Doctors*, which had been commissioned to immortalize the founding fathers of the Johns Hopkins Hospital. Osler is the central figure with pen in hand to denote his prolific writing.

In 1911, at the same time as the coronation of King George V, a baronetcy was conferred on Osler, who became Sir William Osler, Bart. The honor was indicative of the recognition and adulation that Osler enjoyed throughout the English-speaking world. Spanning the last two decades of the nineteenth century and the first two decades of the twentieth, Osler's reputation was unequaled in Canada, the United States, and the United Kingdom.

His reputation as a physician during his life, which ended on December 29, 1919, as a consequence of empyema (purulent plural fluid) and bronchopneumonia due to *Hemophilus Influenzae*, was based mainly on his role as a teacher of medicine. He made no major scientific discoveries, though his name is attached to two uncommon diseases: polycythemia vera (Vaquez-Osler disease) and hereditary hemorrhagic telangiectasia (Osler-Weber-Rendu

133

disease), as well as a condition known as "Osler's nodes" (painful spots on the hands and feet of individuals with subacute bacterial endocarditis). But word spread of his teaching, thanks to grateful students, those who benefited by his presence, and the thousands who read his textbook, which engrained his name in the history of medicine.

In the realm of literary legacy, Osler produced a significant body of essays related to medicine, many of which are the most often read and often quoted in that field. Osler was influenced by and contributed to the classical revival that took place in the second half of the nineteenth century. He listed in *Aequanimitas* "ten books which you may make good friends," and which would provide a "Liberal education." They are *Plutarch's Lives*, *Religio Medici* (Osler's favorite), *Don Quixote*, the Old and New Testaments, and works by William Shakespeare, Michel de Montaigne, Marcus Aurelius, Epictetus, Oliver Wendell Holmes, and Ralph Waldo Emerson. Robert Burns and John Keats were among Osler's favorite poets, while the tales of Boccaccio, Rabelais, Charles Dickens, George Eliot, Robert Louis Stevenson, and Arthur Conan Doyle provided Osler with pleasure.

Osler's library also included works by Maimonides, Erasmus, Pascal, Voltaire, Benjamin Franklin, and Robert Burton, the author of *The Anatomy of Melancholy*, which Osler regarded as "the greatest medical treatise written by a layman." Osler was definitely interested in dramatists' representations of physicians and included works by Molière, Henrik Ibsen, and George Bernard Shaw in his collection of books, currently held at McGill University under the name Bibliotheca Osleriana.

Osler's essays appear in print in two books: *Aequanimitas with Other Addresses to Medical Students, Nurses, and Practitioners of Medicine* and *An Alabama Student and Other Biographical Essays*. The first work was originally published in 1904; later, Osler added to a second edition (1906) three valedictory addresses delivered before leaving America.

In "Teacher and Student," a paper presented at the University of Minnesota in 1892, Osler stressed the importance of the art of detachment, the virtue of method, and the quality of thoroughness, alluding to the need for concentration on medicine and avoidance of distraction, the advantage of systematizing work, and the need to maintain a full acquaintance with the science upon which the practice of medicine is based. In that essay, one of Osler's aphorisms, "The practice of medicine is an art, based on science," appears.

"Physic and Physicians as Depicted in Plato" was a paper presented to the Johns Hopkins Historical Club in 1893, and it speaks to Osler's philhellenism. "Teaching and Thinking," delivered at McGill Medical School in 1894, details approaches to the "teaching" of students, while the "thinking" relates to enlarging "the boundaries of knowledge" by research. Osler stressed that teachers who impart current knowledge may not be investigators. Conversely, those who are consumed with scientific investigation should not be de-energized by teaching commitments. He opined that the two subsets are required in the table of organization of a university.

In "Books and Men," delivered at the Boston Medical Library in 1901, Osler stated, "The study of the phenomena of disease without books is to sail an uncharted sea, while to study books without patients is not to go to sea at all." His panoramic grasp of various subject areas can be seen in his presentations on "British Medicine in Greater Britain" and "Medicine in the Nineteenth Century." "Chauvinism in Medicine" was a presentation to the Canadian Medical Association in 1902. Osler defined "chauvinism" as "a narrow, illiberal spirit," and decried nationalism in medicine, referring to it as "the great curse of humanity." In that essay, he wrote that "the philosophies of one age have become the absurdities of the next, and the foolishness of yesterday has become the wisdom of to-morrow" and "the greater the ignorance the greater the dogmatism."

Osler referred to "The Hospital as a College" in addressing the New York Academy of Medicine in 1903, and he delivered "The Master-Word in Medicine" as a celebratory address at the University of Toronto in that same year. In the latter presentation, he implores his audience to remember that "the master word is Work, a little one, as I have said, but fraught with momentous sequences if you can but write it on the tablets of your hearts and bind it on your foreheads."

Just prior to Osler's departure from America to take up his post at Oxford, he addressed students at McGill and in Pennsylvania. That oration was published in *Aequanimitas* as "The Student Life." In this speech, Osler alludes to the requirement for lifetime learning in medicine. He concedes, "No human being is constituted to know the truth, the whole truth, and nothing but the truth. . . . In this unsatisfied quest, the desire, thirst . . . [and] the fervent longing are the be-all and the end-all. What is the student but a lover courting a fickle mistress who ever eludes his grasp?" Osler regarded education to be most animated when the teacher is "a senior student anxious to help his juniors," and when "there is no appreciable interval between the teacher and the taught."

The second publication of Osler's literary work is also a collection of lectures, but in this case all of them focused on individual physicians. *An Alabama Student and Other Biographical Essays* was published in 1908, and it is indicative of Osler's "lifelong interest in biography as a recreation" and of his "strong conviction of its value in education." The title stems from the first essay, which was read at the Johns Hopkins Hospital Historical Club in 1895. The author brings to the attention of his audience a physician of little distinction who left a small town in Alabama and his family to augment his medical education in Paris in 1836.

Also in January 1895, Osler read a paper, "Thomas Dover, Physician and Buccaneer," at the club. Dover received a bachelor of medicine degree from Cambridge in 1683 and began to practice in the southern English city of Bristol. In 1708, Dover was a promoter and third in command of a privateering expedition in the South Seas. The expedition became memorable because of the discovery of Alexander Selkirk, who had been stranded on an island for four years and four months, and came to be known as "Robinson Crusoe." Dover's around-the-world voyage lasted about three years and made him a rich man. In 1721, he was admitted to the Royal College of Physicians, and, in 1732, he published *The Ancient Physician's Legacy to His Country, Being What He Has Collected Himself in Forty-Nine Years of Practice.* The book went through eight editions, the last occurring in 1771.

In 1899, Osler's address to the Rhode Island Medical Society on Elisha Bartlett also appears in *An Alabama Student.* Bartlett was a native of Rhode Island and had received his medical degree from Brown University in 1826. He was a peripatetic teacher of medicine, having taught in several schools: the Berkshire Medical Institute, Dartmouth College, Transylvania University, the University of Maryland, Vermont Medical College, the University of Louisville, and the College of Physicians and Surgeons of New York (Columbia University). Bartlett was also a prolific contributor to the medical literature. His work on *Fevers* was one of the most notable contributions of American physicians to the subject.

Osler included among the essays in *An Alabama Student* a profile of William Beaumont, whose 1833 book titled *Experiments and Observations on the Gastric Juice and the Physiology of Digestion* detailed the experiments and observations on gastric juice and the process of digestion. It was the only medical work included in the Grolier Club's list of the one hundred most significant books published in the United States during the nineteenth century.

Osler also included an essay on the influence of the Parisian physician Pierre Charles Alexandre Louis on American medicine. Louis had a direct and personal influence on Oliver Wendell Holmes and a distinct but indirect influence on two Philadelphia physicians, who were profiled by Osler. William Pepper, professor of medicine and provost at the University of Pennsylvania, was the son of a professor of medicine at that school. The elder Pepper had considered himself to be the intellectual son of the great Louis. The other Philadelphia professor of medicine, who was included in the work by Osler, was Alfred Stille.

Osler's interest in Renaissance medical history is evidenced by the inclusion of an address he had given about the fifteenth-century Veronese physician Hieronymus Fracastorius. Fracastorius's reputation was established by his work *De Contagione*, in which the author proposed three classes of infection: diseases acquired by direct contact; infections transmitted by an intermediate agent, such as fomites; and infection that travels a distance through the air. Fracastorius's more momentous contribution was perhaps the most celebrated poem in medical history. *Syphilis Sive Morbus Gallicus*, published as a seventy-page quarto in 1530, gave the name to the disease, offered an alternative ("the French disease or pox"), and ascribed its spread to the return of Spaniards from the source in America. The remainder of *An Alabama Student* consists of essays about physician/literary figures we have already covered, such as Keats, Holmes, Locke, and Osler's exemplar Sir Thomas Browne. The book concludes with Osler's Harverian lecture on William Harvey and his discoveries.

After Osler died in 1919, his brain was displayed in the Wistar Institute in Philadelphia until it was moved to the Mútter Museum in that city. As Michael Bliss, Osler's most recent biographer, wrote, "Try as I might, I could not find a cause to justify the death of Osler's reputation. He lived a magnificent, epic, important, and more than saintly life." The appellation "Oslerian" identifies groups interested in the history of medicine throughout the English-speaking world. The name has been assigned to a building at the Johns Hopkins Hospital, several public schools in Canada, a library at McGill University, a student dining room at Oxford University, and the main hall of the Maryland State Medical Society building.

FROM MEDICINE TO MANUSCRIPT

SOURCES

Bliss, Michael. *William Osler: A Life in Medicine*. Oxford: Oxford University Press, 1999.
Cushing, Harvey. *The Life of Sir William Osler*. Oxford: Oxford University Press, 1940.

21

SIR FREDERICK TREVES

Extraordinary Edwardian with an Elephantine Association

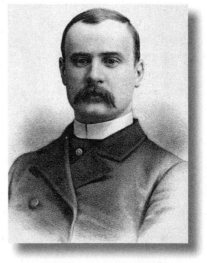

S ir Frederick Treves led a life that was divided into two distinct parts. In the first portion, he gained recognition as the leading anatomist and surgeon in England. He then abruptly moved away from surgery and gained celebrity as a literary figure. His literary works were well received by contemporary readers in the late-nineteenth century and early-twentieth century. One of his literary contributions has recently been reintroduced to the New York Broadway stage, and it is enjoying great appeal.

Treves was born in Dorchester, England, in 1853 and moved to south London in 1867, after his father died. He decided on a career in medicine, but since his societal class precluded gaining entrance into Oxford or Cambridge, which were the gateways to membership in the Royal College of Physicians, he set surgery as his goal. In 1871, he studied at University College London and did his clinical apprenticeship at the London Hospital, located in one of London's poorest areas. It was noted for having the largest surgical ward and several distinguished teachers.

In 1874, he qualified as a licentiate of the Society of Apothecaries (the lowest tier of England's tree of medical practitioners), and the following year he passed his membership examinations for the Royal College of Surgeons. After serving four months as a house officer at the London Hospital, Treves joined his brother at the Royal National Hospital for Scrofula (a form of tuber-culosis manifest by enlarged lymph nodes) at Margate. That experience led to the publication of Frederick's first book, *Scrofula and Its Glands Diseases*, in 1882.

Treves spent several months as a partner in a general medical practice in a small town in Derbyshire before returning to London, where, in 1878, he passed the fellowship examination (as a second step) of the Royal College of Surgeons. He accepted the lowly post of a surgical registrar at the London Hospital and supplemented his income as a demonstrator in physiology and as an assistant at the Royal Orthopaedic Hospital. In less than one year, he was promoted to assistant surgeon and became a demonstrator in anatomy and a lecturer in practical anatomy.

In 1881, he published ten articles in medical journals and was designated Erasmus Wilson Professor of Pathology. His professional rise continued to be meteoric. In 1883, he published *Surgical Applied Anatomy*, the last edition of which appeared in 1962. In 1883, Treves was appointed head of the anatomy school, and, a year later, he became a full surgeon at the London Hospital. He remained prolific in his medical publishing; *The Anatomy of the Intestinal Canal and Peritoneum* came out in 1885, and a three-volume *Manual of Surgery* appeared the next year. By 1887, he had become one of the leading surgeons in London.

Between 1890 and 1895, Treves published four more books. *A German-English Dictionary of Medical Terms* was poorly received. By contrast, his two-volume *A Manual of Operative Surgery* and its abridgement, *The Student's Handbook of Surgical Operations*, were very successful. The latter went through ten editions and twenty-seven printings between 1892 and 1957. His last medical text, *A System of Surgery*, was published in 1895.

At the age of forty-five, he retired from the London Hospital and focused on his extensive and highly remunerative private practice. Shortly after the onset of the Boer War in October 1899, Treves established a privately financed surgical team to participate in the medical care of the British forces in South Africa. He was designated as consulting surgeon, and, for several months, he cared for the wounded and diseased at several military engagements, which were disastrous for the British army. After about three months of active par-ticipation, Treves became ill and returned to London. His experiences during the Boer War constituted the basis for his first nonscientific book, *The Tale of a Field Hospital*, published in 1900.

Shortly after his return to England and a hero's welcome, the *Times* news-paper began a journalistic campaign that was severely critical of the medical care provided by the Royal Army Medical Corp (RAMC). In a letter, which appeared in the *British Medical Journal*, he countered the criticism and indicated that the RAMC provided excellent care for the troops. Subsequently, at a royal commission inquiry, Treves was rewarded for his service when King Edward VII made him a knight commander of the Royal Victoria Order in May 1902. He also received the South Africa Medal and was made a Companion of the Order of Bath. In 1903, a royal commission on the war in South Africa was held. On that occasion, Treves completely contradicted his previous testimony and presented damning evidence against the RAMC.

Treves's stature is evidenced by the high regard in which he was held by British royalty. In 1897, he was made surgeon in ordinary to the Duke of York, who would later become King George V. In 1900, he received the same appointment to Queen Victoria. After King Edward VII assumed the throne, Treves was appointed sergeant surgeon. In June 1902, during the period of preparation for the coronation, Treves, who was the accepted British authority on appendicitis or, as he usually referred to it, "perityphlitis," drained the monarch's appendiceal abscess at Buckingham Palace. In 1903, Treves was made a baronet.

Treves had a multifaceted and, at times, ironic association with appendicitis, which became appropriately recognized as a serious medical condition during the time that he was engaged in surgery. In 1886, Reginald Fitz, professor of pathology at Harvard Medical School, provided evidence that the inflammatory process, previously ascribed to the cecum (first portion of the large intestine), actually was located in the appendix. He suggested that the term "appendicitis" replace "typhlitis" and "perityphlitis," and advised early removal of the appendix when the symptoms and signs indicated the diagnosis.

In 1892, in response to an article that appeared in an American periodical assigning priority to Thomas G. Morton for the first removal of the appendix on April 23, 1887, Treves reported his experience. On February 16, 1887, he operated on a patient with "relapsing typhlitis" and corrected a distortion of the appendix without removing it. He indicated that he reported the case to the Royal Medical and Chirurgical Society in September 1887, at which time he advised removal of the appendix during a quiescent period rather than in an emergency situation.

In1900, Treves's eighteen-year-old daughter developed abdominal pain, which proved to be due to appendicitis. He did not suspect the diagnosis, and she developed peritonitis due to perforation of the appendix. Treves operated on his daughter, but she died shortly after the procedure.

When Treves was fifty years old, he abruptly retired from private practice. In 1903, he was made rector of the University of Aberdeen for five years. Two years later, he was designated a knight grand cross of the Victorian Order. In 1910, Treves signed the death certificate of King Edward VII and was appointed sergeant surgeon by King George V. Treves's close association with royalty coupled with the durability of his medical publications made him the most famous surgeon in Great Britain and throughout the world after the death of Lord Lister in 1912. Treves was given the honor of representing the king at Lister's funeral.

Treves's interest in literature and his becoming a presence in the literary world have been ascribed to his early association with William Barnes and Thomas Hardy in Dorset. As a youth, Treves was a student of Barnes, who was a poet, naturalist, archeologist, and a stimulating educator. Thomas Hardy, the famous English naturalist, novelist, and poet, was thirteen years older than Treves, but the two shared a youthful development in Dorset and a mentoring by Barnes. Coincidentally, Hardy bought his first writing desk from Treves's father's shop and used the desk throughout his life.

With a single significant exception, Treves's literary contributions were confined to travel books. He was directed, specifically, to that genre by his good friend Newman Flower of the London publishing house of Cassel & Co. The first of his travel books, *The Other Side of the Lantern: An Account of a Commonplace Tour Round the World* (1905), was a consequence of a trip he made with his wife and surviving daughter. It is generally regarded as his best in that category. The first printing rapidly sold out and was reprinted five times in four months. It remained in print for twenty-eight years. Portraits in prose, which were narratives of Treves's travel, were stylistically modern, while descriptions of India, China, Japan, and Malay were presented with a perspective of time.

Treves's second travel book, *Highways and Byways in Dorset* (1906), was commissioned by Macmillan Publishers for their Highways and Byways series. The book, illustrated by the American-born Joseph Pennell, was an account of the towns and villages where the author had spent his youth. *The Cradle of the Deep* (1908) is a fanciful approach to the West Indies. Treves considers the West Indies, measuring them by English standards, and consequently is often critical. He sympathizes with the slaves but has a low opinion of the natives. *Uganda for a Holiday* (1910) brings into focus the native tribe, which Treves deems praiseworthy, and the sociological effects of building and completion of the Uganda railway.

The Land That Is Desolate: An Account of a Tour of Palestine (1912), although highly regarded as one of Treves's better literary contributions, was somewhat somber, and it confronted organized religion and "priestcraft." He considers much of the pageantry of the Holy City to be fraudulent and expresses admiration for the Jews praying at the Western Wall. Treves, admittedly, indulged himself by writing *The Country of "The Ring and the Book"* (1913), in which he uncovered all the sites where the action of Robert Browning's poem "The Ring and the Book" took place.

The Riviera of the Corniche Road (1921) includes observations on the indolence of the leisured class in Monte Carlo and the south of France. *The Lake of Geneva*, which was written from the vantage point of a tourist, was published in 1922, the year before Treves died as a consequence of peritonitis in Lausanne, Switzerland.

The name of Frederick Treves lives on, not as the eponymous attachment to an internal hernia between the ileum and appendix, or a bloodless fold from the antimesenteric border of the terminal ileum to the appendix, or a sheet of peritoneum passing from the ventral surface of the mesentery of the terminal ileum to the anterior surface of the ascending colon near the cecum. Rather, his name enjoys broader recognition for his last book, *The Elephant Man and Other Remembrances* (1923).

Treves first encountered Joseph Merrick, who was presented as "the Elephant Man," at a freak show in London in 1884. Treves arranged for Merrick to visit the London Hospital and undergo an examination at his direction. Treves anticipated making a presentation of his findings to the Pathological Society. The description was briefly mentioned in the abstract section of the *British Medical Journal*. Merrick moved on to exhibitions in Leicester and Brussels before returning to London in 1886 when Treves arranged for Merrick to be housed in two rooms on the ground floor of the hospital.

In his hospital residence, Merrick was visited by society ladies, including the Princess of Wales, who would become Queen Alexandra. In 1890, Merrick died in his sleep in his hospital room at the age of twenty-seven. Treves's book, in which Merrick was the central subject, was published twenty-three years later and received critical acclaim.

In 1977, the play *The Elephant Man* by Bernard Pomerance premiered in London. Two years later, it opened in New York City, where it received numerous awards, including the Tony Award for Best Play. The following year, a movie was released. In 2014, the play was revived and had a limited engagement in New York City.

SOURCES

Dictionary of National Biography (1967), s.v. "Treves, Sir Frederick."
Trombley, Steven. *Sir Frederick Treves: The Extra-Ordinary Edwardian*. London:
    Routledge, 1989.

22

ARABELLA MADONNA KENEALY

Female Physician Fosters Medical Feminism in Fiction

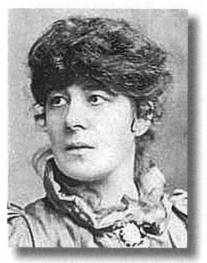

The fact that there are only two women physicians included among the deceased medical individuals who are deemed to have had a significant literary career is to have been anticipated. The licensing of female physicians in Europe and the United States is a relatively recent development. Perhaps Dorothea Erdeben, who, having received dispensation to study medicine from Frederick the Great of Germany and who graduated with an MD from the University of Halle in 1754, merits recognition as the first European licensed female physician. The first woman in the English-speaking world to be awarded a medical degree was Margaret Ann Bulkley. An early example of transgenderism, she lived her entire adult life as a man under the name James Barry and graduated from the University of Edinburgh Medical School in 1812. Dr. Barry was commissioned in the British army and rose to the rank of inspector general.

The acceptance of women in modern medicine is, more appropriately, considered to have occurred in the middle of the nineteenth century. Elizabeth Blackwell, who graduated from Geneva College in Geneva, New York, with an MD degree in 1849, is generally regarded to be the first female English-speaking licensed physician. In 1865, Elizabeth Garrett Anderson became the first English woman to be permitted to practice medicine, subsequent to becoming a licentiate of the Society of Apothecaries in London. In 1874, she cofounded the London School of Medicine for Women, which was the only British school to offer courses in medicine for women when Arabella Kenealy, the senior of the two women to be considered, pursued her studies. At the time, medicine represented the pinnacle of feminine scientific achievement.

Arabella Madonna Kenealy was born on April 11, 1859, in Portslade, Sussex, England, the second of eleven children of an Irish barrister. She was initially educated at home but later proceeded to study at the London School of Medicine for Women. She practiced as a physician among the poor in London and a few miles northwest of the city in Watford between 1888 and 1894. During the Victorian Age, female physicians were obliged to limit their practice to the care of women and children. After suffering a severe attack of diphtheria and having experienced the successful publication of her first novel in 1893, Kenealy retired from medicine and devoted herself to writing and the cause of women's rights.

Kenealy's first and most successful novel, *Dr. Janet of Harley Street*, was published in 1894. A reviewer for the *Dial* magazine wrote, "Everything about it is, of course, in the highest degree absurd, while a hysterical method and . . . much dismally irrelevant matter deprive the book of its last hope of arousing interest." Like several of Kenealy's fourteen subsequent novels, *Dr. Janet of Harley Street* concerns dysfunctional marriage and the abuse of women. Kenealy used fiction to complement her scientific writing to communicate her theories.

In the novel, Dr. Janet, who works at a hospital for women, is described as a mature, large, unfeminine senior physician. "The forehead was large and massive, the chin broad and resolute. He would be a bold man who opposed the firm and fiery will of this big woman." Dr. Janet presents herself to her guests as a "neuter" and opines that, when a woman develops masculine mental traits and an athletic body, it detracts from the role as mother of the race.

Dr. Janet rescues a young and attractive Phyllis Eve from an older degenerate husband before the marriage is consummated. Phyllis is taken in by Dr. Janet and supported while Phyllis trains to become a doctor. There are lesbian undertones on the part of Dr. Janet, who develops "a violent affection" for Phyllis. As Dr. Janet helps shape Phyllis into becoming a doctor, she stresses to her mentee the importance of maintaining her natural femininity. Janet advises Phyllis to study only moderately in order to sustain her womanly emotions. The attitude expressed by Janet is in concert with Kenealy's concept of feminism, as expressed in her essays.

Kenealy avoids the issue of Janet's homosexuality by calling her a "neuter" and presenting her protagonist as asexual and without deviant behavior. Phyllis, on the other hand, experiences love for a man and for motherhood, which is deemed by Kenealy to be woman's highest function.

Kenealy's other works of fiction include *Molly and her Man of War* (1894), *Some Men Are Such Gentlemen* (1894), *The Hon. Mrs. Spoor* (1895), *Woman and the Shadow* (1898), *A Semi-Detached Marriage* (1899), *Charming Renée: A Novel* (1900), *The Two Loves of Richard Herrick* (1902), *His Eligible Grace, the Duke* (1903), *An American Duchess* (1906), and *Dr. Smith of Queen Anne Street* (1907).

Some Men Are Such Gentlemen is the tale of a young, innocent girl and her struggle with life, and how she learns by experience to judge men. *Charming Renée: A Novel* pivots on a beautiful girl's marriage with a lord, who is under an obligation to have no heirs. *The Love of Dr. Herrick* tells of a young, attractive painter who spurns Herrick's love because she wants to remain independent. Herrick marries a simple girl who goes mad; he has an affair with a widow; and after his wife dies, he finally marries his repentant first love. A reviewer of that novel wrote, "One is always amused by Miss Kenealy, but on this occasion it is impossible to help wishing that she had not used her characters so often as phonographs to air her views on that tedious subject, the position of women." *An American Duchess* is a novel about the decadence of high society. *Dr. Smith of Queen Street* is a collection of stories that deals with the motifs of the woman who doesn't know what she wants and the woman who marries to free herself of debt.

The most notable of Kenealy's short stories is "A Beautiful Vampire," which was published in *Ludgate Magazine* in 1896. The story focuses on an aristocratic lady who maintains youth and beauty by sucking vitality and energy rather than blood from young servants and her personal nurses. She is the widow of two rich husbands, whom she entrapped and from whose incomes she continues to live lavishly. Eventually, the menopausal vampire is foiled by a nurse, and the older woman shrivels and withers to her "natural" state.

Kenealy's nonfiction was about medical and sexual issues. Her anti-vivisectionist conviction was published in a book titled *The Failure of Vivisection*, which was published in 1909. Her major concern, however, was eugenics. In 1891, her article "A New View of the Surplus of Women" appeared in *Westminster Review*. In that essay, Kenealy advocated for the entry of women into all professions. The opportunity of economic independence outside of marriage would sift a significant percentage of women from the marriage market and, thereby, give those who chose to marry a greater choice. Kenealy proposed that this would result in genetically superior babies.

Over the years, her views regarding feminism and eugenics were modified and were eventually published in 1920, in her most famous book, *Feminism and Sex-Extinction*. She articulated a contrarian view in the contemporary corpus of literature on feminism. Kenealy believed that only through women could the race be salvaged and improved. She wrote, "Nature made women ministrants of Love and Life, for the creation of an ever more healthful and efficient, a nobler and more joyous Humanity. Feminism degrades them to the status of industrial mechanisms." She wrote that masculine women bred weakling sons, and that education and work outside the home had a detrimental effect on the health and beauty of women and on their role in sustaining and improving the human race. The book has been referred to as "the classic case against the disruptive effects of women claiming equality with men."

In her later years, she became more interested in occultism and the effect of the gyroscopic rotation of the earth on human evolution. This consideration was the subject of her last book, *Gyroscope*, which was published two years before she died on November 18, 1938. Although her contributions have become obscure, Bram Dijkstra, emeritus professor at the University of California, San Diego, who wrote about sexuality, stated that Kenealy is "still a bedrock of our own sense of sexual identity."

SOURCES

Richardson, Angelique. "Kenealy, Arabella Madonna (1859–1938)." In *Oxford Dictionary of National Biography*. Oxford University Press, 2018–. http://www.oxforddnb.com/view/10.1093/ref:odnb/9780198614128.001.0001/odnb-9780198614128-e-50057?rskey=HLYym6&result=1.

Swenson, Kristine. "The Menopausal Vampire: Arabella Kenealy and the Boundaries of True Womanhood." *Medical Women and Victorian Fiction* 10, no. 1 (2003): 27–46.

23

MARGARET GEORGINA TODD

Contemporary Champion
of Common Cause

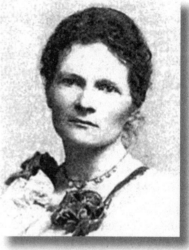

Margaret Georgina Todd is paired with Arabella Kenealy as a female physician who championed the movement of women into the medical profession. Todd, like Kenealy, is notable for having produced period medical fiction that attempted to redefine social attitudes concerning female doctors in Victorian culture. These two female physicians are discussed in a chapter titled "The New Woman Doctor Novel" in Christine Swenson's *Medical Women and Victorian Fiction*.

Although the exact date and place of Todd's birth is not known, it is thought that she was born around 1859, the same year as Kenealy, in or near Glasgow, Scot-

Photo courtesy of National Book League (Great Britain).

land. Todd had literary ambitions before she entered the Edinburgh School of Medicine for Women in 1886. The school was established that year by Dr. Sophia Jex-Blake, with whom Todd had a long-term romantic relationship.

Todd took eight years to complete a designated four-year course of medical studies because she divided her time between studying and the writing of her first novel. Her medical course work was focused on the restricted care of women and children. After graduating from the Edinburgh school in 1894, she obtained an MD in Brussels and accepted an appointment as an assistant medical officer at the Edinburgh Hospital and Dispensary for Women and

Children. Five years later, Todd resigned her medical position and concentrated on writing.

Todd's first and most popular novel, *Mona Maclean, Medical Student*, was published in 1894, under the pseudonym "Graham Travers." The novel imparts an optimism regarding the recently evolved situation of women in medicine. The protagonist achieves happiness and professional fulfillment without compromising herself. The novel deals with the education and holistic development, including that of empathy, of a woman physician. Men in the book support medical women as social and professional partners. While the novel celebrates female independence and provides fulfilling alternatives to marriage, the heroine achieves a happy marriage with a doctor who treats her as a professional equal and, in one symbolic instance, considers her more qualified than himself.

The book was well received and was reprinted several times. It shared with Kenealy's *Dr. Janet of Harley Street* the characterization of representing "a hysterical method [see last chapter]." Unlike Kenealy, however, Todd was praised for her skill and charm. One reviewer wrote, "It stands forth by itself as one of the freshest and brightest novels of the time."

Todd produced five more novels and several short stories that appeared in magazines. *Fellow Travellers* and *Kirsty o' the Mill Toun* were published in 1896. *Windyhaugh*, in which the heroine succumbs to morphine addiction during a trying period but ultimately triumphs over the addiction and succeeds, was published in 1899. *The Way of Escape*, published in 1902, concerns an unfortunate heroine who was betrayed by men. She regards herself as a "moral leper," and her "escape" comes when she loses her life while saving children in a school fire. The last of Todd's novels, *Growth*, was published in 1907. All of the novels bore the name of Graham Travers as the author. Todd's final publication, *The Life of Dr. Sophia Jex-Blake*, was published under her own name in 1918, five years after her companion died.

Three months after the publication of that biography, Todd herself died. It is believed that she committed suicide. Although her name has faded into obscurity, she retains some permanence due to a scholarship that bears her name at the London School of Medicine for Women, along with the credit she is given for suggesting the name "isotope" for a radioactive element that has more than one atomic mass.

SOURCES

"Obituary: Dr. Margaret Todd." *Times* (London, England). September 5, 1918. p. 9.

Swenson, Kristine. "The Menopausal Vampire: Arabella Kenealy and the Boundaries of True Womanhood." *Medical Women and Victorian Fiction* 10, no 1 (2003): 27–46.

24

SIR ARTHUR IGNATIUS CONAN DOYLE

A Modicum of Medicine— a Mass of Manuscripts

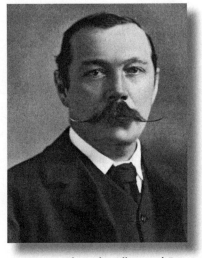

Photo by Elliot and Fry.

The honors list, which accompanied the coronation of England's Edward VII, included the names of two doctors, both of whom served in the Boer War but were knighted for distinctly different contributions. The previously considered Sir Frederick Treves (see chapter 21), the senior by six years, was the most distinguished surgeon in Great Britain, and had recently increased the esteem in which he was held by draining the king's appendiceal abscess just prior to the coronation. At the time of the ceremony, Treves had not delved into the literary field, but would subsequently establish his reputation as a writer. By contrast, Sir Arthur Conan Doyle had, over a decade earlier, left behind a brief and undistinguished career as a practicing physician and a failed eye specialist to rapidly become the most popular, most financially successful, and easily recognizable English author of that era.

Doyle was born in Edinburgh, Scotland, on May 22, 1859, to parents with an Irish Catholic heritage. He received his early education at Stonyhurst, a highly regarded Jesuit school in Lancashire. The finishing touches of classical studies and adding the German language to his capabilities took place while he spent a year in Feldkirch, Austria. During that period, he was exposed to the mysteries of Edgar Allan Poe, and there was early evidence of his literary skill in the *Feldkirch Newspaper*, a student's periodical, which he edited and which was largely filled with his prose. At the age of seventeen, Doyle entered Edinburgh University to study medicine, a determination that had been made by his mother, who would remain a dominant factor throughout his life.

While Doyle studied at Edinburgh, his major focus was completing the requirements for a medical degree and assimilating the broad scope of scientific knowledge, for which he would be tested in order to be licensed to practice. But the years at Edinburgh were also critical to Doyle's literary career. Among the lecturers to whom he was exposed were those of Joseph Bell, a surgeon, whose deductive skills served as an inspiration for Doyle's most famous literary character, Sherlock Holmes. Another literary experience that Doyle enjoyed while he expanded his medical knowledge was the first publication of one of his short stories, "The Mystery of Sasassa Valley," which appeared anonymously in *Chambers' Journal* in October 1879.

In early 1880, Doyle left on a seven-month sealing and whaling trip in the role of the nominal ship's surgeon. On his return, he successfully passed the examinations required for his bachelor of medicine and master of surgery degrees. After another sea voyage as ship's surgeon along the west coast of Africa, Doyle began a general medical practice in September 1882, at Southsea, a suburb of Portsmouth.

His eight years at Southsea constituted a period during which Doyle proceeded along dual and disparate paths, one being medicine, the other writing. His medical practice was modest, assisted in part by acquaintances he made while excelling at cricket, football (soccer), and a lawn game called bowls in addition to his participation in the local Literary and Scientific Society. His impressive physical presentation of six feet two inches in height and about 210 pounds in weight was doubtless another attraction. He continued medical studies at home, and, in 1885, he returned briefly to Edinburgh, where he successfully passed the examinations for the doctor of medicine degree. That year, Doyle married the sister of one of his patients.

The income generated from Doyle's medical practice barely sustained his modest lifestyle; from the onset of his stay at Southsea, his income was augmented by monies earned from his published works. He had received small stipends for short stories that appeared in cheap London magazines, but his literary stature rose when his "J. Habakuk Jephson's Statement," a tale of a derelict mystery ship, appeared in the highly regarded *Cornhill Magazine* in 1884.

It was published as an anonymous contribution, which one critic attributed to Robert Louis Stevenson and compared with works by Edgar Allan Poe.

This success increased Doyle's pace of writing. He sent several stories to the *Cornhill Magazine*, but the early ones were rejected. In 1885, "The Great Keinplatz Experiment," in which Herr Baumgarten of Stonyhurst became Professor von Baumgarten of Keinplatz, was published in the magazine *Belgravia*. The same year, he completed a novel, *The Firm of Girdlestone*, which was twice rejected, and he began the first of his Sherlock Holmes stories. That work, "A Study in Scarlet," was started in March and finished in April 1886. It was rejected initially by the *Cornhill Magazine*, but accepted to appear in *Beeton's Christmas Annual* for 1887. Doyle contracted for the measly sum of twenty-five pounds for the complete copyright for the British publication of that work.

The first of Doyle's published novels was *The Mystery of Cloomber*, which appeared in December 1888, but was dated 1889. The first of his historical novels, *Micah Clarke*, was published in February 1889 and received an enthusiastic reception. It is a coming-of-age work about Micah, a young man during the Monmouth Rebellion in England toward the end of the seventeenth century. The protagonist is sent into battle by his forceful Protestant father in an attempt to replace Catholic King James. In the end, Micah preaches religious toleration.

The second of the Sherlock Holmes tales, "The Sign of the Four," appeared in both the English and American editions of *Lippincott's Monthly Magazine* for February 1890 and was published in book form several months later. Toward the end of that year, Doyle's second historical novel, *The White Company*, his personal favorite, was accepted as a serial for the *Cornhill Magazine*. The story takes place during the One Hundred Years War, in 1366 and 1367, when Edward, the Black Prince, attempted to restore Peter of Castile to the throne of that kingdom. Also in 1890, *The Firm of Girdlestone*, which followed the chicanery of a father and son as they struggled to maintain their previously distinguished firm, appeared in print. In addition, a volume of Doyle's short stories, *The Captain of Polestar, and Other Tales*, was published.

With the success of the publication of four novels, two collections of short stories, and two episodes of Sherlock Holmes to his credit, Doyle planned a radical change in his medical practice. After spending two months in Paris and Vienna to become an eye specialist, he established his office and residence in Russell Square, London, but was unable to attract any clientele. This resulted in Doyle's decision to end his medical career and support himself and his family solely with the proceeds of his literary publications. Between April and August 1891, Doyle sent six Sherlock Holmes short stories to the *Strand Magazine*; "A Scandal in Bohemia," "The Adventure of the Red-Headed League," "A Case of Identity," "The Bascombe Valley Mystery," "The Five Orange Pips," and "The Man with the Twisted Lip" appeared sequentially beginning in July. Doyle's popularity and fame were rapidly propelled to the highest level of the English literary world.

At that point, he had little interest in continuing production of Sherlock Holmes tales. Rather, he planned to concentrate on a new historical novel but was enticed by a lucrative contract to provide the *Strand Magazine* with six additional short stories, which maintained Sherlock Holmes and Dr. John H. Watson in the public eye. The six episodes, which, combined with the initial dozen, would constitute the 1892 publication *The Adventures of Sherlock Holmes*, were "The Adventure of the Blue Carbuncle," "The Adventure of the Speckled Band," "The Adventure of the Engineer's Thumb," "The Adventure of the Noble Bachelor," "The Adventure of the Beryl Coronet," and "The Adventure of the Copper Beeches." In *Arrowsmith's Christmas Annual* for 1892, "The Great Shadow," Doyle's first Napoleonic story, appeared.

Between December 1892 and December 1893, twelve more Sherlock Holmes stories were published in the *Strand Magazine* and compiled as *The Memoirs of Sherlock Holmes* in 1894. They included "The Adventure of Silver Blaze," "The Adventure of the Cardboard Box," "The Adventure of the Yellow Face," "The Adventure of the Stockbroker's Clerk," "The Adventure of Gloria Scott," "The Adventure of the Musgrave Ritual," "The Adventure of the Reigate Squire," "The Adventure of the Crooked Man," "The Adventure of the Resident Patient," "The Adventure of the Greek Interpreter," "The Adventure of the Naval Treaty," and "The Final Problem," in which Watson reports the death of Sherlock Holmes.

Doyle's literary productivity during 1892 provides evidence of his diversity and the rapidity with which he could complete a project. In addition to the output of Sherlock Holmes short stories, he completed a play and the second of his historical novels. The one-act play "Waterloo" was an adaptation of his short story "A Straggler of '15" and was first performed by the theatrical idol Henry Irving in London in 1894. Doyle had previously completed a three-act play, "Angels of Darkness," in which Dr. Watson appears without Sherlock Holmes. That drama, which takes place in San Francisco, remained unpublished for over a century until 2000. The novel *The Refugees: A Tale of Two Continents*, written in 1892, is a story that takes place in Europe and America during the reign of Louis XIV. In 1893, the light opera "Jane Annie or the Good-Conduct Prize," produced by D'Oyly Carte, with lyrics by J. M. Barrie (of Peter Pan fame) and Arthur Conan Doyle, opened in London at the Savoy Theatre.

The year 1894 was particularly hectic. That year also witnessed the publication of *Round the Red Lamp*, a collection of short stories, including several with a medical theme, and a novelette, *The Parasite*, in which a young physiology student is confronted with the occult.

That year, Doyle went on an invited speaking tour of the United States, which included New York, several Midwestern cities, and a visit with Rudyard Kipling, who was living in Brattleboro, Vermont, with his American wife. During the tour, Doyle read to the large audiences "The Medal of Brigadier Gerard," the first of a series of comic stories about an overly vain, and at the same time brave, French officer during the Napoleonic Wars. After Sherlock Holmes and Dr. Watson, Brigadier Gerard is considered to be Doyle's most successful literary creation, and he has been credited as the novelist who, in the corpus of his works, provides the most "vivid and intimate" depiction of Napoleon Bonaparte. In 1895, Doyle's epistolary novel *The Stark Munro Letters*, based on his own experiences in setting up a medical practice with an unorthodox physician, was published.

In 1896, *The Exploits of Brigadier Gerard*, a book including all the stories that appeared in the *Strand Magazine* the two previous years, was released. The same year, the gothic mystery and boxing novel *Rodney Stone* appeared. A year later, another Napoleonic novel, *Uncle Bernac: A Memoir of the Empire*, was published. This was followed by *The Tragedy of the Korosko*, a novel that takes place in 1895 in Egypt. In that work, a group of Europeans sailing up the Nile are abducted by marauding dervishes. The narrative includes a defense of British imperialism in North Africa and expresses concern for a spreading Islam.

In 1898, a new series of Doyle stories, called "Round the Fire Stories," appeared in the *Strand Magazine* and included "The Story of the Lost Special," in which the voice of Sherlock Holmes is heard offstage. The next year, *A Duet with an Occasional Chorus*, a novel about an ordinary suburban English couple, was published. The book, which focuses on the couple's reciprocal love, was attacked by critics on the grounds of immorality.

From April to July 1900, Doyle served as a physician in the volunteer Langman Hospital during the Boer War. His patients worshipped him for his total involvement in their care. That year, *The Green Flag*, a collection of thirteen of his short stories, some of which had previously appeared in serial form, was published as a bound volume. Toward the end of the year, Doyle's standard history of the war appeared. It went through sixteen editions before the war ended in 1902. On his return to Great Britain, Doyle ran for a seat in Parliament to represent the Central Division of Edinburgh, but lost, in part because of his Catholic birth and Jesuit schooling, despite the fact that he had indicated he did not accept Catholicism.

From August 1901 through May 1902, Sherlock Holmes reappeared as a serial in *The Hound of the Baskervilles* in the *Strand Magazine*. In 1902, Doyle published a pamphlet, which has been regarded as one of his most important contributions. *The War in South Africa: Its Cause and Conduct*, a detailed factual narrative, was written to counter the German press's criticism of British conduct during the Boer War, labeling it as barbaric. The book, priced at sixpence, sold 600,000 copies in six weeks. On August 9 of that year, a "Sir" was permanently appended to Doyle's name.

The next year, *Adventures of Gerard*, including eight previously serialized tales of the brigadier, appeared in book form. Beginning in October and extending to December 1904, tales of Sherlock Holmes were serialized. They constituted a 1905 book, *The Return of Sherlock Holmes*, which includes "The Adventure of the Empty House," "The Adventure of the Norwood Builder," "The Adventure of the Dancing Men," "The Adventure of the Solitary Cyclist," "The Adventure of the Priory School," "The Adventure of Black Peter," "The Adventure of Charles Augustus Milverton," "The Adventure of the Six Napoleons," "The Adventure of the Three Students," "The Adventure of the Golden Pince-Nez," "The Adventure of the Missing Three-Quarter," "The Adventure of the Abbey Grange," and "The Adventure of the Second Stain."

In 1906, Doyle once again unsuccessfully stood for Parliament, this time for the Border Burghs of Hawick, Selkirk, and Galashiels in Scotland. At the end of that year, *Sir Nigel* was published. This constituted a work to which Doyle ascribed great significance in establishing his reputation as an important novelist, rather than merely the author of tales about Sherlock Holmes. *Sir Nigel* is an inverted sequel of Doyle's favorite novel, *The White Company*, in that it followed the life of Nigel Loring as a youth during the chivalrous Middle Ages, the period about which Doyle most enjoyed writing.

The year 1906 was also a period in which Doyle applied the deductive skills that characterized Sherlock Holmes to come to the aid of an innocent convicted person. In what has been referred to as "The Great Wyrley Outrages," George Edaji, in 1903, had been found guilty of slashing horses, cows, and sheep in Staffordshire in the West Midlands. The convicted party was a solicitor and the son of the local vicar, who emigrated from Bombay and had converted from Parsi to Christianity. Doyle proved that George Edaji was the framed victim of racial prejudice. The solicitor was allowed to resume his legal practice, and Doyle chronicled the event in a small volume, *The Story of Mr. George*, published in 1907.

Through the Magic Door was published in 1907, a work in which Doyle takes the reader to meet writers of the past. The next year, his collection of sixteen stories titled *Round the Fire Stories*, which mainly focused on the "grotesque and terrible," reached the public. In 1909, he once again made use of his literary skill to address a cause. In this case, he was championing the oppressed natives in the Congo Free State who had been mercilessly abused by King Leopold II of Belgium. To gain public awareness of the situation, Doyle published a sixty-thousand-word booklet titled *The Crime of the Congo*, for which he accepted no compensation.

At the same time, he began to concentrate on writing plays. Doyle's morality play dramatization of his novel *The Tragedy of the Korosko* was performed in 1909 as *The Fires of Fate*, and it was well received at the Lyric Theater. At the end of that year, the Adelphi Theater was the venue for Doyle's *The House of Temperley*, a production that thrilled the audience with a formal bare-knuckle fight in a ring. A month after that play closed, the same theater became the site of the opening of *The Speckled Band*, which enjoyed a long run and had several touring companies. The appearance of several new short stories kept Doyle and his audience of voracious readers busy in 1910. The *Strand Magazine* published "The Terror of Blue John Gap," "The Marriage of the Brigadier," and "The Adventure of the Devil's Foot," while "The Last Galley" and "The Last of the Legions" appeared in the *London Magazine*. *The Last Galley* is the title of a 1911 collection that includes eighteen of Doyle's short stories, and, the same year, thirty-one examples of Doyle's verses were brought together to form *Songs of the Road*.

Doyle adopted a prehistoric era as the backdrop of a story that appeared serially between April and November of 1912 in the *Strand Magazine*. In *The Lost World*, a quartet of intriguing and quite distinctive men, with Professor Challenger as their leader, takes part in adventures with dinosaurs, ape-men, and pigmy elephants.

Between 1908 and 1913, five short stories specifically about Sherlock

Holmes, that particular one among all of his literary characters who Doyle continuously regarded as anathema, appeared in various periodicals. These tales included "The Adventure of Wisteria Lodge," "The Adventure of the Red Circle," "The Adventure of the Bruce-Partington Plans," "The Adventure of the Dying Detective," and "The Disappearance of Lady Frances Carfax," to which "The Adventure of the Devil's Foot" and "His Last Bow" would be added to comprise Doyle's 1917 publication of the book *His Last Bow*.

In 1913, Professor Challenger and his friends reappear in the sci-fi novella *The Poison Belt*, referring to a belt of poisonous ether through which the earth moves. Not long thereafter, Doyle wrote his last and what is generally regarded to be his best detective novel, *The Valley of Fear*. And in the same year, he published his short story "Danger! Being the Log of Captain John Sirius," in which he prophetically describes a flotilla of enemy submarines that brings England to terms.

When World War I was declared, Doyle attempted, unsuccessfully, to enlist as a private. However, he did continue to chronicle military events throughout the war. This began in 1914 with *The German War*, a volume of essays on various phases of the Great War. In 1916, he published *A Visit to Three Fronts* and the six-volume *The British Campaigns in France and Flanders*. His eight-volume sequel, *The British Campaigns in Europe 1914–18*, was published in 1928.

Doyle publicly asserted, in 1916, that he believed in spiritualism, a subject that he had studied for almost thirty years. The contention of spiritualism is that, when a person dies, both the body and soul journey to a world beyond and that communication with those who have passed might be established. Doyle's announcement appeared in the October 21 edition of the psychic magazine *Light*. Two books by Doyle on the subject of psychic phenomena, *The New Revelation* and *The Vital Message*, were published in the next two years. Throughout the remainder of his life, Doyle traveled over fifty thousand miles, including tours of the United States and Australia, and addressed over a quarter million people on the subject. In 1926, his previously serialized novel *The Land of Mist* presented the psychic adventures of Professor Challenger and his friends. That same year, he published the two-volume *History of Spiritualism*, and in 1930, the year of his death, he brought out *The Edge of the Unknown*.

Tales of Sherlock Holmes had begun to reappear in the *Strand Magazine* in 1921, and continued through 1927, when they were brought together to constitute *The Case-Book of Sherlock Holmes*. Included were "The Adventure of the Illustrious Client," "The Adventure of the Blanched Soldier," "The Adventure of the Mazarin Stone," "The Adventure of Three Gables," "The Adventure of the Sussex Vampire," "The Adventure of the Three Garridebs," "The Problem of Thor Bridge," "The Adventure of the Creeping Man," "The Adventure of the Lion's Mane," "The Adventure of the Veiled Lodger," "The Adventure of Shoscombe Old Place" (the last of the fifty-six Sherlock Holmes stories), and "The Adventure of the Retired Colourman."

The incredible enormity of Doyle's literary corpus is unmatched by any other physician I know of who made literary contributions. His reputation is generally based on the fifty-six short stories featuring the most recognizable detective in all of literature. Arguably, Sherlock Holmes remains the most famous character in English literature. Recent authors have attempted to replicate Holmes. He continues to be presented on the cinema screen and in television series. Devotees periodically join one another as "Baker Street Irregulars."

But the adventures of Sherlock Holmes and Dr. Watson, while the most financially rewarding of Doyle's works, were the least emotionally satisfying for him. Also, when considering word count and the number of pages devoted to Holmes, these are a small part of Doyle's literary corpus. They must be weighed against a total of 239 works of fiction, including more than a dozen novels unrelated to Sherlock Holmes, definitive chronicles of the Boer War and World War I, four collections of poems, seven plays, four books on spiritualism, and innumerable published essays. The "incredible" becomes the truth because, as Doyle himself wrote, "When you have eliminated the impossible, what remains, however improbable, must be the truth."

SOURCES

Carr, John Dickson. *The Life of Sir Arthur Conan Doyle*. Garden City, NJ: Doubleday, 1949.
Dictionary of National Biography (1967), s.v. "Doyle, Sir Arthur Ignatius Conan."
Locke, Harold. *A Bibliographical Catalogue of the Writings of Sir Arthur Conan Doyle, 1879–1928, M.D., LL. D.* Kentish Mansions, London Road: D. Webster, 1928.

25

ANTON CHEKHOV
Fusion of Fiction and Medicine

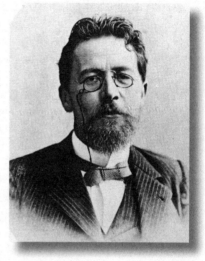

No writer incorporated his or her experiences and personal inter-relationships with the medical profession within his or her literary contributions to a greater extent than Anton Chekhov. This selfless physician, who persisted in his devotion particularly to the care of patients and improving public health, never shed his medical mantle. Although his income could be attributed more to his literary publications than to his clinical work, he managed to include medicine, patients, and physicians as essential elements in many of his short stories, novellas, and plays. For years he viewed himself as a doctor first who considered his literary contributions to be inconsequential.

Chekhov was born on January 17, 1860, in Taganrog, a town on the Azov Sea in southern Russia, and spent the first nineteen years of his life in that area. At age seven, he was enrolled in a preparatory school run by Greek expatriates. Because of the school's inadequacies, a year later, he was transferred to the Taganrog Gymnasium, where he received a classical education. The school now bears his name.

Chekhov's father, Pavel Egorovich, was born a serf, whose grandfather had bought freedom for the family from his landed master. Pavel eventually established himself as a grocer in Taganrog, Russia's leading port at the time. Anton was obliged to spend many hours working in the store and was exposed to his father's insistence on extraordinarily pious behavior. Pavel was a despotic father who abused his children with frequent beatings.

FROM MEDICINE TO MANUSCRIPT

In 1876, Pavel declared bankruptcy and fled to Moscow to avoid being confined to a debtor's prison. Anton and his brother Ivan were left behind to complete their education. As a teenager, using the monies he acquired by tutoring while he remained in Taganrog, Anton assumed financial responsibility for his destitute family. In 1879, he moved in with his family while he matriculated at the medical school of the University of Moscow.

At the time, several comic journals were growing in popularity among the rapidly expanding literate Russian population. Shortly after moving to Moscow, Chekhov submitted his first story, "The Alarm Clock," to one of the periodicals. It was rejected, but his next story, "The Dragonfly," was accepted by another magazine. Because only a pittance was paid per line for such stories, the quantity of acceptances an author received was critical. Six of his stories were published in 1880. While still a medical student, Chekhov continued to churn out stories, which, when appearing in print, were written under pseudonyms, in order to avoid tainting his reputation as a future physician. He most frequently used the name "Antosha Chekhonte," which had been given to him while he was a student in Taganrog.

There is evidence that Chekhov's first play, *Platonov*, was submitted and rejected in 1881. It was found among his papers and later published by the Soviet government in 1923. The long melodrama, containing references to notable writers of the past, a failing estate, and a physician's failure to abort a suicide, foretold the future of many of Chekhov's dramatic productions.

Between 1881 and 1882, during the short life of the periodical known as the *Spectator*, Chekhov had eleven stories published in that journal. By 1882, his writings brought in three times the amount of his father's salary. In 1883, while preparing for several examinations in clinical sciences, including surgery and gynecology, he wrote a weekly article for the *Spectator* as well as one for the more prestigious St. Petersburg periodical *Fragments*. Later in his life, Chekhov disowned all of his early stories (two hundred of which had been written when he was a student), and did not include them in his collected works.

In 1884, Chekhov graduated from the university with a class of about two hundred students, and he was qualified as a general practitioner. At the time, there were about sixteen thousand physicians in all of Russia, which was still medically backward. Chekov began his practice in Moscow as an enthusiastic doctor tending mainly to the needs of friends and the poor and, consequently, receiving little compensation. Early in his medical career, he wrote in a letter, "Medicine is my lawful wife and literature my mistress." Toward the end of

1887, he considered completely abandoning literature for his medical career. This was obviated by his early literary success and the need to support his family.

Medicine would persist as a topic in his prose throughout his life. In an autobiographical entry compiled for the Moscow University almanac in 1900, he wrote,

> I do not doubt that my medical activities have had a powerful influence on my work as a writer; they have significantly expanded my field of observation, enriched my knowledge, and only people who are doctors themselves will be able to appreciate the true value of all this. . . . My acquaintance with the natural sciences and the scientific approach has always kept me on my toes, and I have tried, whenever possible, to deal with scientific facts.

In 1884, Chekhov published, at his own expense, his first book titled *Tales of Melpomene* (muse of tragedy), which contained six stories by "A. Chekhonte," and he also began publishing stories in the *Petersburg Newspaper* and, subsequently, in *New Times*, Russia's most popular newspaper. Also in 1884, he started coughing up blood, the first manifestation of his tuberculosis.

In autumn of the year that Chekhov embarked on his medical practice in Moscow, his first and only novel, *A Shooting Party*, began to appear as a serialization, which would extend over thirty-two issues. This, the longest of Chekhov's works, is generally not held in the same esteem as his short stories and plays. It is a parody of contemporary detective novels and tells of a murder at a shooting party that takes place in provincial Russia.

In 1885, Chekhov visited St. Petersburg, the cultural center of Russia and the location of the more highly regarded publications, in which many of his writings had appeared. On that occasion, he met Alexsey Suvorin, a wealthy publisher and owner of the nation's major newspaper. Suvorin would become a father figure for Chekhov, who, in turn, would become the protégé of the influential businessman. Their strong friendship and business relationship persisted until the end of 1897, when Chekhov joined French novelist Émile Zola in defense of Alfred Dreyfus while Suvorin's publications were anti-Dreyfus and strongly anti-Semitic.

From the time that Suvorin became Chekhov's "manager," Chekhov's stories would no longer be published with a variety of pseudonyms but under his own name. "The Requiem," the first short story written under the spon-sorship of Suvorin and with the name of Anton Chekhov as the author, appeared in February 1886. Fifty-five stories, published under pseudonyms, had appeared in 1885. Seventy-six were published in 1886, and fifty-seven in 1887, the year in which *Motley Tales*, the first collection of his stories, was reviewed. One reviewer wrote, "[Mr. Chekhov] will like a squeezed-out lemon, inevitably die, completely forgotten, in a ditch. . . . Mr. Chekhov's book is a very sad and tragic spectacle of a young talent's suicide."

Shortly thereafter, a second collection of stories titled *In the Twilight* was published, which became the basis for awarding Chekhov the Russian Acad-emy's prestigious Pushkin prize in 1888, "for the best literary production distinguished by high artistic worth." The book was reprinted twelve times and reissued in 1891, followed by eleven reprintings. In 1887, Chekhov also launched his career as a dramatist with the first performance of his play *Ivanov*. Unfortunately, it proved to be an embarrassment for the author, but after being revised, the play premiered in St. Petersburg in January 1889, at which time it was viewed as a great success. In 1888, two of Chekhov's one-act farces, *Swan Song* and *The Bear*, were produced. *The Bear* was a resounding success and con-tinued to be performed over the years.

In 1889, a landmark year occurred in Chekhov's life when his masterpiece novella *The Steppe* appeared in print. It was the first of his works to be included in an important literary review, which gained for him immediate fame. That year, he announced he would no longer seek compensation for the medical care he rendered, but he would continue to attend patients gratis and would continue to participate in public health issues.

In January 1890, Chekhov left home for one year, spending several of the summer months on the island of Sakhalin in Siberia, where he conducted a study of the infamous penal colony there, which consisted of ten thousand prisoners and ten thousand men and their families who guarded them. He gathered data and anecdotal information that would form the basis of his monograph *The Island of Sakhalin*, which would first appear as a serial publica-tion in 1893 and as a book in 1895. A century later, the work was the subject of a poem, "Chekhov on Sakhalin," by the poet laureate Seamus Heaney. In March 1892, Chekhov moved his immediate family, including his father, mother, and sister, to a small country estate at Melikhovo. They would live there for about seven and a half years. Located forty miles south of Moscow, eighteen miles from a post office, and six miles from the train station, Melikhovo is currently the site of the Chekhov museum, recognizing that many of the author's famous stories and plays, including *The Seagull* and *Uncle Vanya*, were written there.

Five months after the move to Melikhovo, Chekhov wrote to his manager, Suvorin, "I have been busy being sole doctor of the Serpehovskovo district, and trying to catch cholera by the tail and organize health services. I have in my district 25 villages, 4 factories, and 1 monastery. In the morning I see patients and in the afternoon I go on house calls." Added evidence of his continued interest in medicine appeared in 1895, when he helped save the Moscow medical journal *Surgical Chronicle*, which was in financial distress.

But he spent most of his time at Melikhovo writing. In an 1894 letter to a lady friend, Chekhov stated that "not for a minute am I free from the thought that I must, am obliged to write, write, write." By 1897, the recent publications of his novella *My Life* and multiple short stories, particularly "Peasants," established Chekhov as the Russian writer second only in importance to Tolstoy, with whom he was friendly.

But Chekhov was disheartened when his play *The Seagull* opened at a jubilee benefit in October 1896, at the Alexandrinsky Theatre in Petersburg. The audience's hoots and hisses expressed displeasure, and the critics were equally negative. This was offset by the enthusiastically favorable reception of the very same play in Moscow and other cities in Russia, as well as the triumphant opening of *Uncle Vanya* in Moscow a few years later in October 1899.

Between the Petersburg and Moscow openings of *The Seagull*, Chekhov changed his residence. Because of the progression of his tuberculosis and the difficult winter weather, he sold the Melikhovo property and moved with his mother and sister, after his father had died, to Yalta in the latter half of 1899. In January 1901, the Moscow opening of his play *Three Sisters* firmly established Chekhov as Russia's leading playwright. Later that year, Chekhov married Olga Knipper, a Russian stage actress who had appeared in several of his shows. *The Cherry Orchard* opened in Moscow on January 17, 1904. On July 15, 1904, Chekhov died in the spa town of Badenweiler in the German Empire, and *The Cherry Orchard* appeared in print posthumously that year.

Chekhov has been referred to as the father of the modern short story and, along with Norwegian playwright Henrik Ibsen and Swedish playwright August Strindberg, as a parent of the modern drama. The first English translation of his short stories, under the title *The Black Monk and Other Stories*, appeared in 1903. The story "The Black Monk" includes a medical description of the manifestations of tuberculosis and a form of psychosis. In Chekhov's works, the use of the stream-of-consciousness technique, the concentration on mood and psychic projection rather than plot, influenced James Joyce, Franz Kafka, Ernest Hemingway, and others.

As indicated by Jack Coulehan, who edited a collection of Chekhov's medical tales, the inclusion of all of Chekhov's doctors in the collection would have resulted in an unwieldy and heavy book. Doctors play significant roles in almost three dozen Chekhov stories. Consideration of medical settings, diseases, and psychological disorders would add additional weight. Among the titles of short stories in a contemporary collection of Chekhov's works are "The Doctor," "Sleepy," "A Nervous Breakdown," "Ward. No. 6," and "A Doctor's Visit."

The inclusion of medical issues and personalities in his writing was unequaled by any other physician who published fiction. While in medical school, Chekhov wrote "Intrigues," in which a pompous attending physician is profiled. In "Malingerers," extreme compassion that extends beyond medical treatment characterizes the protagonist, a female homeopathic physician. In "Excellent People," a young doctor appears who, after her husband's death, attempts suicide and eventually gives up medicine. After living with her brother for a period of time, during which she feels an absence of purpose, she takes off to do vaccination work in the provinces. In "Enemies," Dr. Kirilov's dedication to duty takes him on a needless house call, requiring him to leave his wife and recently deceased son's body. Dr. Tsvyetkov in "The Doctor" attends the dying child of an unmarried mother while he tries to learn if he fathered the child. "A Nervous Breakdown" focuses on reconciliation between the necessity for a physician to maintain objectivity and emotional detachment while, at the same time, recognizing others' feelings.

In "The Grasshopper," the saintly Dr. Dymov, who is deceived by his wife, contracts erysipelas (an acute skin infection) and later dies of diphtheria as a consequence of his work. "The Head-Gardner's Story" is a tale of another selfless doctor. An elderly and beloved physician is murdered, and the murderer is found guilty but is later freed by the judge because he couldn't believe that any man would sink so low as to murder the doctor. The judge regards his acquittal as an expression of faith in humanity.

Dr. Ragin, in "Ward No. 6," cares for emotionless psychiatric patients and finds himself transformed into the state of his patients. Eventually he becomes one of them. In "A Doctor's Visit," a young doctor aids a patient with no organic illness by guiding the patient through the existential elements that have caused her to suffer. By contrast, the change that can occur in a young physician who becomes callous and focused on affluence is described in "Ionitch."

The only physician to appear in one of the five novellas that Chekhov wrote attempts to mediate the conflicts of the antagonists in *The Duel*. Physicians are also characters in several of Chekhov's plays. The first lines spoken in *Platonov*, Chekhov's first play, come from a doctor. In *Ivanoff*, a physician constantly reminds others that he is an "honest man," and he informs Ivanoff that his wife is dying of tuberculosis. The title character of *The Wood Demon* is a landowner who holds the degree of doctor of medicine. In *The Seagull*, which is a play within a play, all are ridiculed in the drama, with the exception of the physician.

Constantin Stanislavski, the Russian actor and director whose "system" was used throughout the world of stage performers, played one of the central roles, that of Dr. Astrov, in the original production of *Uncle Vanya*. In *The Three Sisters*, Chebutykin is a burned-out, alcoholic physician. The most famous of Chekhov's plays, *The Cherry Orchard*, is devoid of a medical character, but contains an aphorism that physicians still invoke: "If there is any illness for which people offer many remedies, you may be sure that particular illness is incurable."

Chekhov's legacy in drama lives on. George Bernard Shaw, who was generally critical of other playwrights, praised Chekhov's dramatic contributions. In 1960, a Socialist statue of Chekhov was erected in Alexandrovsky Square in Taganrog (the town where he had been born) to mark the centenary of his birth. In 1981, Tennessee Williams adapted *The Seagull* for his play *The Notebook of Trigorin*. As recently as 2013, the Yale School of Drama paid tribute to Chekhov with a production of *Platonov*.

Two American physicians have expressed admiration for Chekhov's short stories, particularly as they refer to medical issues. William Carlos Williams (see chapter 33) said, "Read Chekhov, read story after story of his. . . . I turn to [Chekhov] all the time." Walker Percy (see chapter 41) writes, "I think of Chekhov as the deservedly revered father of all of us who have turned to the typewriter to let others know what goes on when you are dueling with death, hoping to win for the sake of your patients, and for the sake of yourself as well: Chekhov is the master of letting us all know that!"

SOURCES

Coulehan, Jack, ed. *Chekhov's Doctors*. Kent, OH: Kent State University Press, 2003.

Rayfield, Donald. *Anton Chekhov: A Life*. New York: Henry Holt, 1997.

26

ARTHUR SCHNITZLER
Perceived to Be Pornography

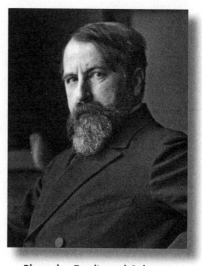

Photo by Ferdinand Schmutzer.

I n a time during which Sigmund Freud transformed psychiatry, a Viennese medical colleague wrote plays and works of fiction that focused on psychological reactions. The writer's contributions had introspective themes, and he introduced stream-of-consciousness narration. The eroticism and frank description of sexuality that were pervasive throughout his works labeled the author a pornographer.

Arthur Schnitzler, the son of a distinguished Austrian laryngologist, was born in Vienna on May 15, 1862. As a youth, he demonstrated artistic tendencies. He was a competent pianist and wrote poetry that was published in a leading newspaper. Following in the footsteps of his father, he studied medicine at the University of Vienna and received his doctorate of medicine in 1885. Sigmund Freud preceded him as a student by four years. Like Freud, Schnitzler began his postgraduate training at the Allgemeines Krankenhaus der Statdt Wien (Vienna General Hospital), where he focused on psychiatry.

Schnitzler attended patients at the city hospital and cared for a few private patients among Vienna's Jewish bourgeoisie. Early in his career, he authored a paper on the use of hypnosis and suggestion as treatments for aphonia (loss of voice), a disorder for which his father was considered an expert. But, as a young physician, Schnitzler spent most of his time writing plays and stories.

His earliest published works were short stories. After his father died in 1893, he gave up his hospital post but kept a few private patients.

Schnitzler's first published play, *Anatol*, appeared in 1893, but it did not premiere until 1910. The seven-act play, set in nineteenth-century Vienna, depicts a series of shallow relationships between a young playboy and a variety of women. The nature of the relationships changes during the course of the play and leads to the conclusion that the protagonist fears intimacy and is unable to establish a permanent relationship. The play resulted in Freud's designation of Schnitzler as a "psychological depth researcher." In 1921, Cecil B. DeMille directed the film *The Affairs of Anatol*, starring Gloria Swanson.

The first play of Schnitzler to be produced premiered on October 5, 1895, in Vienna. *Liebelei* (*Flirtation*), which deals with extramarital love and class differences, brought immediate recognition to its author. There have been four cinematic and three television renditions of the work between 1913 and 1969. Schnitzler continued to write short stories, which, over time, have been considered to be more important than his plays. "Sterben" ("Dying"), published in 1895, is an early example of the stream-of-consciousness technique that gained him fame. The literary technique that James Joyce perfected in *Ulysses* (1922) characterized several other Schnitzler stories, including the 1900 work *Leutnant Gustl* (*Lieutenant Gustl*).

That novella consists of an inner monologue that is critical of the Austrian Hungarian military code of honor and of the main character, a military officer. As a reflection of the rising tide of anti-Semitism at that time, Schnitzler was stripped of his commission as a reserve officer in the medical corps.

In the first decade of the twentieth century, he wrote sixteen plays. The most notable of these is *Das Reigen* (*La Ronde* or *The Cycle*), which was printed for private circulation in 1900, published in Vienna in 1903, and premiered in 1920. The play consists of a cycle of ten dialogues that take place before and after coitus, which is marked by asterisks in the text. The theme focuses on sexual morals and how they transcend the boundaries of class. Beginning with an encounter between a prostitute and a soldier and ending with the same prostitute's contact with a count, the cycle involves ten individuals, each of whom appear in two consecutive scenes.

The book form of the play was banned by censors a year after publication. It was translated into French in 1917 and into English in 1920. The production of the play in Berlin in 1920 and in Vienna the next year created one of the biggest scandals in the history of the German theatre and provoked large anti-Semitic riots in Berlin. Schnitzler bore the label of "a Jewish pornographer." A Berlin court trial, which considered the charge of obscenity, ended in acquittal for the author.

During this period of turmoil, Freud wrote to Schnitzler in a complimentary tone: "You have learned through intuition—though actually as a result of sensitive introspection—everything that I have had to unearth by laborious work on other persons." More than a dozen films based on the play have appeared over the years, including during the present century.

Schnitzler's *Der Weg ins Freie* (*The Road into the Open*), which was published in 1908, has been dubbed "the great novel of Freud's Vienna" and is, in part, autobiographical. The plot consisting of a composer who impregnates a singing teacher but avoids commitment to his lover, who calmly accepts his decision, parallels a segment of Schnitzler's life. The narrative speaks to the issue of the Jewish longing for social and intellectual freedom.

Between 1910 and 1919, Schnitzler published eight plays and several short stories and novellas. His 1912 play, *Professor Bernhardi*, is supposedly modeled on his father and is distinctive among Schnitzler's plays in that it is devoid of sex. The plot revolves around a Jewish physician caring for a woman who is dying of sepsis following an abortion. The physician refuses admission of a priest because he, as a physician, believes it would indicate to the patient that she is dying and undermine her state of euphoria. The play was suppressed until 1918 by an anti-Semitic populace, which was outraged by the main character being unwilling to compromise his convictions.

Schnitzler maintained a devoted readership that was attracted by sexual intrigues. In his 1918 work *Casanovas Heimfahrt* (*Casanova's Homecoming*), an elderly lover evinces disgust for his sexual partners, his friends, the church, and himself. The book was the focus of a court case, in which the plaintiff was the New York Society for the Suppression of Vice. The charges were dismissed.

Several of Schnitzler's stories are psychoanalytical assessments of erotic crises or aberrations. His play *Paracelsus*, set in the time of the famous sixteenth-century physician and alchemist, focuses on psychoanalysis and psychological insight into one's self. Schnitzler's use of dreams and stream of consciousness in several of his works suggests a relationship with Freud, but there was little actual or written contact between the two men, though Freud certainly seemed to take note of Schnitzler's perceptiveness about human psychology.

A notable exception was a letter that Freud wrote to Schnitzler on the latter's sixtieth birthday. In it Freud stated, "Your determinism as well as your skepticism—what people call pessimism—your preoccupation with the truth of the unconscious and of the instinctual drives in man, your dissection of the cultural conventions of our society, the dwelling of your thoughts on the polarity of love and death; all moves me with an uncanny feeling of familiarity."

While in his sixties, Schnitzler wrote three of his most popular works: *Fräulein Else* (1924), *Traumnovelle* (1926), and *Therese* (1928).

Fräulein Else is a novella written as the stream-of-consciousness mono-logue of a nineteen-year-old girl who is forced to show herself in the nude to offset her father's debt. She articulates her sentiments and ends by committing suicide. Several cinematic adaptations of the work have appeared.

Traumnovelle (Rhapsody: A Dream Novel) was the basis of the 1999 film *Eyes Wide Shut*, directed by Stanley Kubrick. The original work, which was set in early-twentieth-century Vienna, deals with sexual desires during marital life and the consequences of those desires. *Therese. Chronik eines Frauenlebens (Therese: The Chronicle of a Woman's Life)* is the tale of a woman who gives birth to an ille-gitimate son and is confined to a life of poverty. A succession of lovers affords no relief, and the potential for marriage to a wealthy man ends with his unex-pected sudden death. Her life ends when she is killed by her ungrateful son.

Schnitzler was representative of the last gay years of the "Donaumon-archie" (Danube monarchy) of Vienna. His works embody the traditional past but are also modern and forward-looking. As an accurate analyst of the human mind, he presented dialectics of intimacy versus detachment, cerebra-tion versus sentimentality, and societal corruption versus the individual's basic moral concern.

Schnitzler died in Vienna on October 21, 1931. Two years later, his stories and plays were banned in Austria and in Germany by the Nazis. That year, his works joined those of Freud, Albert Einstein, Franz Kafka, and other Jews at Joseph Goebbels's infamous, anti-Semitic book burning in Berlin. Disagreement persists regarding Schnitzler's status as a literary figure. His reputation fluctuates between being viewed as a major author, based on his insight, modernity, and artistic control, whose greatness was not recognized, and that of a skillful, second-rate peripheral writer who produced few meaningful works in a great literary age. In a eulogy, Thomas Mann paid homage to Schnitzler's "extraordinary literary sensibility sharpened by the experience of a doctor." In a 1992 article in the *New York Times*, Schnitzler is referred to as "the doctor who left to literature his diagnoses of a society in crisis, the doctor in attendance at the birth of the 20th century."

SOURCES

Swales, Martin. *Arthur Schnitzler: A Critical Study*. Oxford: Oxford Clarendon Press, 1971.

Wolff, Larry. "The 20th Century: Dr. Schnitzler's Diagnosis." *New York Times*. November 8, 1992. https://www.nytimes.com/1992/11/08/books/the -20th-century-dr-schnitzler-s-diagnosis.html (accessed April 27, 2018).

27

R. AUSTIN FREEMAN

Scientifically Superior to Sherlock

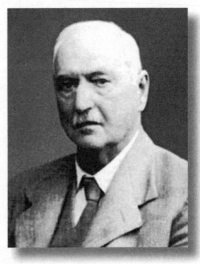

R. Austin Freeman's central literary character, Dr. John Evelyn Thorndyke, was first revealed to his readership in 1907. Over the course of thirty-six years, Dr. Thorndyke acquired the designation of "the greatest scientific detective." He followed in the footsteps of Edgar Allan Poe's C. Auguste Dupin and Arthur Conan Doyle's Sherlock Holmes, and surpassed them scientifically. As was the case for Holmes's creator, the author of the Dr. Thorndyke stories preceded his literary presence with a brief medical career.

R. Austin Freeman was born on April 11, 1862, in the Soho district of London, about two miles from Hampstead, the location of many of his stories. At age eighteen, he began his medical studies at the Middlesex Hospital in London. His name first appeared in print as the author of a two-hundred-word communication published in *Naturalist's World* in 1886, while he was a student, on the small mammals known as moles. He qualified as a physician and surgeon in 1887 and entered the Colonial Service to attain financial security. In June of that year, he sailed to Accra on the Gold Coast to take up the position of assistant colonial surgeon.

In 1888, he joined an expedition to Bontúku (Bondoukou, Cote d'Ivoire). During the trek, he conducted a survey and created a map of that area that was published in 1893. He remained in the squalor of Bontúku for about two months before journeying back to Accra, where he resumed his medical duties, spending much of his time treating malaria. Freeman suffered several attacks of the disease. In 1891, he traveled to the disputed boundary between the British territory and German Togoland. Shortly thereafter, he contracted a complication of malaria known as blackwater fever and became so disabled that he had to return to England.

The next phase of his life as a physician is vague. During the ten years between his return to England and his settling in Gravesend in northwest Kent in 1902, most of his time was spent as a temporary replacement (*locum tenens*) covering other physicians' practices. In 1895, he set up practice in Wimbledon, but he attracted few patients. His main source of income came from tutoring several youths and from his writings, which, prior to 1900, consisted of magazine articles and a book, *Travels and Life in Ashanti and Jaman*, that chronicled his African experiences. That beautifully bound volume, which contains maps, photographs, and drawings by the author, received praise from the critics. Between 1900 and 1902, Freeman served under Dr. John James Pitcairn as an assistant medical officer at Holloway Prison in London.

One of the rarest volumes of twentieth-century detective stories is ascribed to Freeman, who coauthored the book with Dr. Pitcairn in 1902. *The Adventures of Romney Pringle* first appeared as a series in *Cassell's Magazine* and, subsequently, as a bound book, only eight copies of which have been found. It was written under the pseudonym "Clifford Ashdown." The following year, *The Further Adventures of Romney Pringle* was published under the same pseudonym, but with a copyright shared by R. Austin Freeman. Between December 1904 and May 1905, "Clifford Ashdown" also appeared in *Cassell's Magazine* as the author of a series of short stories containing medical sleuthing, titled "From a Surgeon's Diary."

In 1905, Freeman's name appeared for the first time as the author of a book of fiction when *The Golden Pool* was published. This lengthy, slow-moving adventure story takes place in the part of Africa with which the author was well acquainted. The book received little enthusiasm, thus prompting Freeman's decision to embark on writing detective stories. He began by deliberately inventing a protagonist, probably based on Dr. Alfred Swaine Taylor, the author of multiple editions of *Principles and Practice of Medical Jurisprudence*, the authoritative work on the subject.

The characters of Dr. John Evelyn Thorndyke, along with his persistent associates—Nathaniel Polton and Dr. Christopher Jervis—appear for the first time in the 1907 novel *The Red Thumb Mark*. This book was published by Collingwood and was the only novel published by the company, which was known for producing commercial directories. Therefore, it is likely that the author paid to have the book published. The story is based on the erroneous premise that fingerprints can be forged. Nevertheless, in *Fingerprints: Fifty Years of Scientific Crime Detection*, which points out the fallacy of fingerprint forgery, the authors refer to Thorndyke as "the first truly scientific detective in fiction, a medico-legal expert who in technical attainments, extreme thoroughness, lucidity of mind and speech, and even physical appearance, foreshadowed the late Sir Bernard Spilsbury [a great forensic pathologist]."

The two characters, who would accompany Dr. Thorndyke on his adventures over the next thirty-five years, enjoy a harmonious relationship with the protagonist. Polton was a jack-of-all-trades who primarily managed Thorndyke's bachelor quarters, but also evidenced ingenuity in the laboratory, where he invented eyeglasses that allowed the wearer to see behind him, a periscope walking stick, and a device to photograph through a keyhole. He was devoted to "the Doctor," who had saved his life. Dr. Jervis is the analog of Sherlock Holmes's Dr. Watson. He is the recorder and narrator of many of the stories. He himself fails to perceive the significance of the observations but loyally accompanies the one individual who is capable of resolving the case.

Although *The Red Thumb Mark* was not a best seller, the sales justified releasing a paperback edition in 1908. It was the basis upon which *Pearson's Magazine* accepted a set of eight Dr. Thorndyke stories. The first to appear was "The Blue Sequin" in the Christmas issue of 1908. Almost all of the stories in the set were published in book form in 1909. Between the publication of the first group of stories and the next group, Freeman created his literary invention, the inverted type of detective story, in which the secret of the crime is told at the beginning of the narrative, and the reader's attention is maintained until the final page by the ingenuity of the detective and the excitement engendered by the deductive process. In all of the inverted stories, the first part is narrated in the third person by one of the participants, often the murderer. The second part is related by Jervis, who describes Thorndyke's involvement and the solution of the case. The first of Freeman's efforts in this genre was the story known as "The Case of Oscar Brodaki," which is generally regarded to be the best. Other examples of inverted mysteries are "A Wastrel's Romance," "The Echo of a Mutiny," "A Case of Premeditation," "The Dead Hand," and "The Scarred Finger."

In 1911, during the interval between the appearances of the first two books of Dr. Thorndyke short stories, *The Eye of Osiris* was published. It's regarded to be one of the major detective stories of the twentieth century, with much of its action taking place in the Egyptology section of the British Museum. In

1913, *The Unwilling Adventurer* was published. Rather than another detective tale, this novel is a historical nautical romance. The next year, *The Uttermost Farthing: A Savant's Vendetta* was first published in America. It represents one of the least satisfying of Freeman's novels. By contrast, *A Silent Witness*, the last of the Dr. Thorndyke tales to appear before World War I, was one of the best. The assessment of critics was that a steady improvement was evident when the Dr. Thorndyke stories were considered chronologically.

Freeman entered the Royal Army Medical Corps in 1915 as a lieutenant at the age of fifty-two and was assigned to the Home County Field Ambulances. A year later, he was promoted to captain and placed in charge of one of the regional units. In 1916, *The Adventures of Danby Crocker*, a series of adventures unrelated to Dr. Thorndyke, was published. It was deemed to be of little literary value. Before the war ended, two more of Freeman's inverted stories were published, bringing the total to six. In "The Missing Mortgagee," there is undeniable evidence of Freeman's dislike of Jews. In that tale, the Jewish moneylender and his clerk are presented with distinctly unpleasant physical and moral characteristics. The 1918 publication of *The Great Portrait Mystery* contains the novella of that name and three short stories, none of which were of the detective genre.

Freeman's efforts were next directed to social issues and eugenics. He contributed to the periodical *Eugenics Review*, and, in 1921, his theses were published as a book titled *Social Decay and Regeneration*. The introduction was provided by Havelock Ellis, the renowned British physician who was a social reformer and is known for his studies of human sexuality. Freeman's conclusions were that machines impacted negatively on human culture and society, and that eugenic reform was required to sustain the human race and provide for evolutionary improvement. He referred to the fact that the immigration of inferior people from Eastern Europe had lowered the standard of English life.

Beginning in 1922, the decade in which Freeman entered his sixties, was his most prolific. It began with the publication of *Helen Vardon's Confession*, the longest of the Dr. Thorndyke stories. During the 1920s, three collections of short stories appeared: *Dr. Thorndyke's Case Book*, *The Puzzle Lock*, and *The Magic Casket*. In the first collection, "The Funeral Pyre" concentrates on medical jurisprudence. In addition to the three collections, an average of one novel per year was published during the decade. The first to appear was *The Cat's Eye*, followed by *The Mystery of Angelina Frood*, which is based on themes in Charles Dickens's unfinished novel, *The Mystery of Edwin Drood*. In 1925, a novel titled

The Shadow of the Wolf was published, followed the next year by *The D'Arblay Mystery*.

In 1927, two novels appeared: *The Surprising Experiences of Mr. Shuttlebury Cobb*, which the author referred to as a "resuscitated pot-boiler," and *A Certain Dr. Thorndyke*. Two more novels were published during the following year: *Flighty Phyllis*, which centered on a young lady who became a man-about-town, and *As a Thief in the Night*, regarded by critics to be one of the best Dr. Thorndyke tales. In 1928, Freeman's name appeared in *Who's Who* for the first time. In 1929, *The Dr. Thorndyke Omnibus*, consisting of thirty-seven of the character's criminal investigations, was published in London. This marked the end of Freeman as a writer of short stories, but he would continue to produce some of his finest Dr. Thorndyke novels.

Mr. Pottermack's Oversight remains a favorite of fans of the Dr. Thorndyke character and is relatively unique in that it is a full-length inverted story. *Pontifex and Son* and *Thorndyke* replicate the situation found in *Helen Vardon's Confession* in that the murderers are East London Jews. In 1932, *The Dr. Thorndyke Omnibus* was published in New York and a new Dr. Thorndyke novel titled *When Rogues Fall Out* appeared in England. In Freeman's next book, *Dr. Thorndyke Intervenes*, a real case was used as the basis of the novel. It was followed by *For the Defence: Dr. Thorndyke* and *The Penrose Mystery*. Freeman's next novel, *Felo de Se (Suicide)*, was published in America with the title *Death at the Inn*. *The Stoneware Monkey* was the last of Freeman's books published before Great Britain entered World War II. *Mr. Polton Explains* was published in 1940, while *Dr. Thorndyke's Crime File*, an omnibus that included some novels and several essays, was published in 1941. The last of the Dr. Thorndyke novels, *The Jacob Street Mystery*, appeared in 1942, a year before Freeman died. A series of television productions titled *Thorndyke* aired in 1964. In 2011, the BBC presented several radio adaptations of Dr. Thorndyke short stories.

When Vincent Starrett, who wrote a weekly book column for the *Chicago Tribune*, learned of Freeman's death, he wrote, "The best of the Thorndyke stories will live on—minor classics on the shelf that holds the good books of the world." E. F. Bleiler, in his introduction to *The Best Dr. Thorndyke Detective Stories*, published in 1973, wrote, "For the first twenty-five years of his career, at least he dominated the world of British detective fiction." Raymond Chandler, a highly regarded American writer of detective stories, wrote, "This man Austin Freeman . . . has no equal in his genre." Christopher Morley, American journalist, novelist, and poet, stated, "When in doubt, stick to Dr. Thorndyke."

SOURCES

Binyon, T. J. *Murder Will Out: The Detective in Fiction*. Oxford: Oxford University Press, 1989.

Browne, Douglas Gordon, and Alan St. Hill Brock. *Fingerprints: Fifty Years of Scientific Crime Detection*. London: G. G. Harrap, 1953.

Donaldson, Norman. *In Search of Dr. Thorndyke: The Story of R. Austin Freeman's Great Scientific Investigator and His Creator*. Bowling Green, OH: Bowling Green University Popular Press, 1971.

Freeman, R. Austin. *The Best Dr. Thorndyke Detective Stories* (Dover Edition). Mineola, NY: Dover Publications, 1973.

28

HARVEY WILLIAMS CUSHING

Honors Galore—a Pulitzer Prize and More

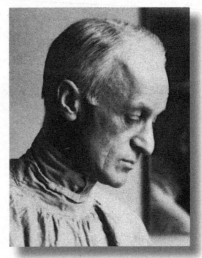

Apropos Harvey Cushing's pres-ence in medicine and his concur-rent contributions as a literary figure is a letter he received from a former student and then dean of the Johns Hopkins Medical School, stating, "I read one of your papers and addresses. I think you should do nothing else but write; when I see you operate I think you should do nothing else but operate; and when I see you experiment I think you should do nothing else but experiment."

Harvey Williams Cushing, referred to as a painstaking perfectionist, was born on April 8, 1869, in Cleveland, Ohio, bearing the paternal genes of three generations of physicians. The progenitor of the family in America arrived in the Massachusetts Bay

Photo courtesy of Yale University, Harvey Cushing / John Hay Whitney Medical Library.

Colony in 1638. The first physician in the family, David Cushing Jr. (1768–1814), practiced at Stafford Hill, a town in the Berkshire Mountains of Massachusetts. His son Erastus (1802–1893) received a diploma from the Berkshire Medical School at Pittsfield, the Medical Department of Williams College. He practiced in Lanesboro, Massachusetts, and in 1835, he traveled to the Western Reserve, where he established a practice in Cleveland. Erastus's son Henry Kirke (1827–1910), who would become Harvey Cushing's father, was educated at Union College and the Cleveland Medical College, where he would serve as professor of midwifery, diseases of women, and medical jurisprudence.

Harvey, the tenth and youngest child in the family, after graduating Central High School in Cleveland as class president, entered Yale University in 1887. His academic performance was creditable but was outshined by his athleticism. His standing as a student and membership on the highly regarded Yale baseball team was strikingly similar to that of his future surgical mentor, William Stewart Halsted.

In 1891, Cushing entered Harvard Medical School, where his first significant contribution occurred. As a consequence of having a patient, whom he had etherized, die under his management, he, and a classmate who had a similar experience, developed the "ether chart." The measurement and charting of a patient's pulse, respirations, and temperature during an operation under inhalation anesthesia was first applied in 1895. Cushing refined the "ether chart" fifteen years later by adding measurements of blood pressure using a modification of the Riva-Rocci inflatable cuff, to which Cushing was exposed during his European tour of 1900–1901.

Cushing graduated from Harvard Medical School cum laude in June 1895. During his internship at the Massachusetts General Hospital, he began working with X-rays, within months of Wilhelm Conrad Roentgen's announcement of his discovery. In 1896, Cushing moved to Johns Hopkins to become an assistant resident under William Stewart Halsted, America's most highly acclaimed surgeon. Cushing's maiden clinical study employed the use of X-rays to study a woman with a gunshot wound to her neck and presenting neurologic manifestations. This led to an exhaustive review of the literature on spinal cord injury and Cushing's first publication in a national journal.

In 1898, Cushing reintroduced block anesthesia produced by cocaine infiltration, a technique that had been pioneered by Halsted prior to his arrival at Johns Hopkins, but abandoned. This type of local anesthetic was used by Cushing for amputation of extremities and, more liberally, for hernia repair, in order to obviate operative death due to inhalation of anesthesia. In 1899, he modified the approach to include removal of the Gasserian ganglion to erase the excruciating pain of trigeminal neuralgia. The report of the case in a medical journal was accompanied by illustrations that Cushing himself created. The operation was hailed in the press as "probably the most daring operative procedure ever attempted by a surgeon."

This introduction into the realm of neurosurgery provided a point of focus as he embarked on a fourteen-month period of travel abroad. He visited the most notable surgeons in England and Europe who had expressed interest in the neurologic system, and spent time in their laboratories and conducted research. There, Cushing demonstrated that an increase in intracranial pressure results in a concomitant rise in systemic pressure. While in Berne, Switzerland, he developed an admiration for Albrecht von Haller (see chapter 8) and later presented a paper on Haller's contributions to the Johns Hopkins faculty. In the physiology laboratory at Berne, Cushing conducted perfusion experiments on the blood supply to frog muscle and demonstrated that both calcium and potassium must be added to sodium chloride to maintain a state of normal responsiveness. During his visit to the laboratory of future Nobel laureate neurophysiologist Charles S. Sherrington, he trephined (bored holes in) the skulls of an orangutan and a gorilla.

On his return to Baltimore, Cushing was given the title of "assistant" in surgery and initiated a course on animals in which third-year medical students performed operations on animals that replicated procedures actually performed on patients. This was formalized as the Hunterian Laboratory for Experimental Surgery, and the idea spread throughout medical schools in the United States.

Modern neurosurgery was fathered by Cushing during the first decade of the twentieth century. In 1901, he was given his desired assignment to neurosurgery by Halsted, and, initially, he was allotted one day per week for neurosurgical operations. By 1908, Cushing had performed over three hundred neurosurgical procedures, mainly for decompression, and he detailed his techniques, accompanied by his own illustrations, in a chapter called "Surgery of the Head," which appeared in W. W. Keen's *Surgery*.

The same year, he began his lifelong focus on the pituitary gland, and, in 1909, he removed a pituitary tumor from a patient with acromegaly (abnormal growth of the hands, feet, and face), the first successful case performed in the United States. In the course of presenting his work on the subject, he introduced the terms "hyperpituitarism" and "hypopituitarism." Cushing's 1912 book, *The Pituitary Body and Disorders*, detailed the histories of forty-eight patients he had managed. In that book, he introduced the concept that the pituitary secretions controlled growth.

His acclaim was enhanced in 1910 when he successfully removed a vascular tumor (a meningioma) from within the cranium of Major General Leonard Wood, chief of staff of the US Army. The following year saw the appearance of his seminal paper on the use of silver clips to control cerebral bleeding during an operation. Cushing's reputation was firmly established throughout the sixteen years that he spent at Johns Hopkins. He had been offered several professorships of surgery at distinguished universities, but consistently declined before accepting the appointment as the Mosely Professor of Surgery at Harvard and surgeon in chief at Boston's Peter Bent Brigham Hospital, which was under construction. Cushing moved to Boston in 1912.

After World War I began, Cushing left Boston in March 1915 for a two-month period as the head of a Harvard unit, consisting of thirteen surgeons and four nurses, attached to a French hospital in Paris. He would return to the war in May 1917 as a member of a base hospital, which was initially associated with the British Expeditionary Force and, subsequently, with the American Expeditionary Force until the end of hostilities in 1918. During its first tour of duty, the Harvard unit performed many serious and diverse surgical procedures at Neuilly, on the outskirts of Paris.

In 1917, Cushing's second book, a monograph on tumors of the acoustic (or auditory) nerve, was published. It was a report on twenty-nine cases, the largest number ever studied. After he returned to France and the war, his life was hectic and, at times, exhausting. He cared for the wounded at the front during the battle at Passchendaele (the third battle of Ypres) and at several field hospitals, and he rose to the rank of lieutenant colonel. Throughout his military experiences, he kept meticulous notes, often accompanied by his sketches. A distilled version taken from the almost one quarter of a million words he had written was published in 1936 under the title *From a Surgeon's Journal: 1915–1918*. This significant literary contribution, considered to be "one of medical history's Great War journals," received high acclaim.

Cushing's next major literary contribution came after the death of Sir William Osler (see chapter 20), who had been a colleague, a mentor, an intellectual father figure, and a stimulus and guide for Cushing's bibliophilia and its accompanying scholarship. Osler's widow called upon Cushing to produce a biography of Osler's life. When Cushing arrived at Johns Hopkins in 1896, he was twenty-seven years of age and Osler was forty-seven. Their relationship over the ensuing two decades remained very close. *The Life of Sir William Osler* was published in 1925, containing 1,371 pages and bound as two volumes, and provides evidence of the extent of the undertaking. Reviews were positive, and Cushing was awarded the Pulitzer Prize in biography in 1926, the only surgeon ever to be so honored.

During the years that Cushing worked on the biography, he continued his extensive clinical activities and served as the president of the Society of

Neurological Surgeons (1920, 1921); the president of the Association for the Study of Internal Secretions, later to become the Endocrine Society (1921); the Society of Clinical Surgery (1921); the American College of Surgeons (1922); and the American Neurological Association (1923). In 1927, he would serve as president of the American Surgical Association.

The year in which Cushing was awarded the Pulitzer Prize also found him publishing two new books: one coauthored by Percival Bailey, on gliomas, and the other a compilation of three lectures that Cushing presented in Edinburgh when he received the Cameron Prize (Pasteur was a previous recipient). In 1928, a volume collecting fourteen of Cushing's essays was published as *Consecratio medici* [*Commitment of Medicine*] *and Other Papers*. The review in the *Boston Globe* stated, "Once again he wields the pen that commemorated Osler—in *Consecratio medici and Other Papers* he takes lay readers on an enchanting stroll through the humanism of a noble profession—essays and addresses which are a mosaic of medical history, reminiscence, humor and philosophy. . . . The hand, which can wield both the scalpel and pen, can make the reader forget the doctor in the man of letters."

In 1931, Cushing removed the two thousandth brain tumor of his career. That year, a group of young neurologists and neurosurgeons formed the Harvey Cushing Society, which, in 1965, changed its name to the American Association of Neurological Surgeons, and has become the leading professional organization of neurological surgeons in the United States. In 1932, Cushing permanently etched his name in the lexicon of medical disorders when he described the manifestation of hypersecretion of pituitary hormones (Cushing's disease).

In 1932, Cushing's appointment at the Peter Bent Brigham Hospital came to an end, and, a year later, he moved to New Haven, Connecticut, where he assumed the title of Sterling Professor of Neurology at Yale University. He initially devoted his time to completing a monograph on meningiomas that is considered to be "a masterpiece, a classic, an epic of neurosurgery. . . . [I]t contained a whole philosophy of surgery and of the doctor-patient relationship."

Cushing's final addition to the literary field was a by-product of his bibliophilia, *A Bio-Bibliography of Andreas Vesalius*, the father of modern anatomy. The book was published posthumously in 1943, on the four hundredth anniversary of the publication of Vesalius's monumental work, *De humani corporis fabrica*.

Cushing died on October 7, 1939, and to commemorate his seventieth birthday, which had occurred earlier in the year, the publisher Charles C.

Thomas Co. brought out a 108-page octavo that listed Cushing's publications. In 1941, the redesigned Yale Medical History Library opened as the Harvey Cushing / John Hay Whitney Library. It houses Harvey Cushing's collection of rare books, his desk, and other memorabilia. In 1988, the US Postal Service issued a commemorative stamp bearing his portrait. Four pages of small font sizes that constitute an appendix in John F. Fulton's *Harvey Cushing: A Biography* enforce the assertion that Cushing was the most honored surgeon of the twentieth century and, perhaps, in all of history.

SOURCES

Bliss, Michael. *Harvey Cushing: A Life in Surgery*. Oxford: Oxford University Press, 2005.

Fulton, John F. *Harvey Cushing: A Biography*. Springfield, IL: Charles C. Thomas Press, 1946.

29

WILLIAM SOMERSET MAUGHAM

Maintaining Medical Status while Producing Profitable Prose

A biography of the long, complex, unorthodox, and highly productive life of William Somerset Maugham reads like a novel. If it had been a novel, it would have been criticized as improbable and overly convoluted. The fact that he was a licensed doctor is rarely appreciated, in part because it is obscured by his enormous literary stature. Although he never practiced medicine, Maugham completed his medical education and contended that the lessons learned from science and the exposure to human strife, while he was in training, contributed to his literary output.

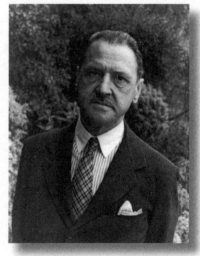

Photo by Carl Van Vechten.

William Somerset Maugham was born on January 21, 1874, within the walls of the British embassy in Paris to protect him from potential conscription in the French army had he been born on French soil. His father was a British lawyer, who had established a successful practice among expatriates in Paris, and served as a legal advisor at the British embassy. William disliked his own name and would later be published as W. Somerset Maugham. He did, however, like his close friends to call him "Willie." He had three brothers, who were significantly older, which left him to be the focus of his mother's adoring attention.

For Somerset, tragedy struck early. When he was eight years old, his mother died of tuberculosis. Two years later, his father died of cancer of the stomach. The combined losses had a significant psychological impact on the young boy. As a ten-year-old orphan, he was placed in the care of his paternal uncle, the Reverend Henry MacDonald Maugham, the Anglican vicar of Whitstable in Kent. This only intensified the boy's psychological trauma. Somerset's surrogate parent was cold, cruel, bigoted, and created miserable memories that persisted throughout Somerset's life.

After a year at a local school, Maugham entered the King's School in Canterbury, the same school where Thomas Linacre (see chapter 2) had received his early education three centuries earlier. Maugham won prizes at that school, despite being compromised by having French as his primary language. His performance at school and his relationship with his fellow students were also adversely affected by his small stature and his stuttering, both of which persisted throughout his life. As he stated, "the accident of a physical infirmity . . . separated me to a greater extent than would be thought likely from the common life of others."

As a sixteen-year-old, Maugham began a two-year stay at Heidelberg University in Germany, where he wrote his first book, a biography of composer Giacomo Meyerbeer, in celebration of the one hundredth anniversary of the composer's birth. That work has been lost. After he returned from Germany, Maugham was confronted with the need to select a profession and continue his education accordingly. He was not interested in following his father and three older brothers into the legal profession, and instead opted to study medicine. His early experience with the death of his parents, particularly his mother, coupled with a sense that his stammering would be less limiting, are thought to have influenced his selection.

On September 27, 1892, he entered St. Thomas's Hospital, a medical school of King's College London. At that venue, he experienced the atmosphere of the anatomy dissecting rooms, which he vividly described in *Of Human Bondage*. He was particularly affected by his obstetrical clerkship, during which he cared for women and babies in the most appalling slums of London. This would provide the background for Maugham's first novel.

In 1897, Maugham passed a series of final examinations and was awarded two diplomas: Licentiate of the Royal College of Physicians and Member of the Royal College of Surgeons. He never initiated a medical practice but maintained a lifelong subscription to the British medical journal *Lancet* and completed an annual questionnaire in order to maintain a listing in the *Medical Directory*. In 1961, at the age of eighty-seven, he was still qualified as a physician, listed in the directory, and in that year he prescribed medication for his friend Lord Beaverbrook. In his autobiographical work *The Summing Up*, Maugham wrote, "I do not know a better training for a writer than to spend some years in the medical profession."

In addition to his medical experience, another factor that influenced Maugham's writings was his dominant homosexuality, which became manifest during his early school days and was temporarily modified by a period of bisexuality that included a marriage and his fathering a child. As a consequence of the British law declaring homosexuality a crime, which was in effect during almost all of his life, Maugham was in constant fear of exposure. As a literary disguise, he often used women, rather than homosexual characters, to express his ideas.

The year Maugham became a licensed physician, before he completed his qualifying exams, he witnessed the publication of his first major work, a novel titled *Liza of Lambeth*. For that work, he drew from his medical experience with midwifery in the slums of London to tell the lurid tale of a young factory worker living in a London slum who becomes attracted to a married man, gets pregnant, and is assaulted by the man's wife, all of which leads to miscarriage, sepsis, and death. Nobel laureate V. S. Naipaul, who indicated that he was positively influenced by Maugham's writings, stated, "Maugham describes the slum people with a detachment that is not without humor. . . . The women, especially, are interesting. . . . For them life is a messy monotony of motherhood and maulings . . . a normal part of their existence." The book was an immediate success. The first print sold out in weeks, and his next ten works failed to achieve equivalent sales.

After the success of his first novel, Maugham began his pattern of frequent travel with long stays by residing in Seville, Spain, for over a year, during which he wrote the first of his five travel books. Over the years, travel books constituted a minor category of Maugham's prose, which included essays, screenplays, novels, plays, stories, and an autobiography.

The first of his novels written after he returned to London was *The Hero*, in which the main character develops enteric fever and is cared for by his fiancée. Doctors appear frequently in Maugham's early novels. In his 1904 work, *The Merry-Go-Round*, Dr. Frank Hurrell confronts the view that humans are ennobled by pain, and he blames inhumane doctors for allowing patients to needlessly suffer. In *The Magician*, published in 1908, one of the central characters is a renowned English surgeon.

That year, *Lady Frederick*, Maugham's first success on the London stage and the first to be performed in New York, appeared. In 1909, his theatrical contributions played a major role in establishing his reputation, particularly early in his career. At one time, four of his plays were running in theaters simultaneously. Maugham wrote a total of twenty-nine plays, eighteen of which were included in *Collected Plays* (1931–34).

When Great Britain entered World War I in 1914, Maugham joined the British Red Cross, which became notable for the "Literary Ambulance Drivers" John Dos Passos, E. E. Cummings, and Ernest Hemingway. While involved in that activity, which took him into the center of battles in France where he witnessed mass carnage, he worked on the novel for which he is best known, *Of Human Bondage*. Published in 1915, the work is autobiographical in many respects. The mother of the protagonist, Philip Carey, dies after giving birth to a stillborn baby. Maugham's mother gave birth to a stillborn baby and died a few years later of tuberculosis. Carey moves to the house of his uncle, the vicar of Blackstable, another similarity. At school, Carey is humiliated, in part related to a clubfoot, which is thought to be a symbolic replacement for Maugham's impairment of stammering. When Carey, an aspiring artist, realizes that he does not have sufficient talent, he elects to follow in his late father's footsteps and enters medical school, where he struggles. He drops out, returns after a long interval, and becomes licensed as a physician. He is offered an attractive partnership with another physician, but refuses.

Early in the war, in 1915, Maugham was recruited by British intelligence and was stationed in neutral Switzerland. A year later, he was sent to the South Seas to acquire information about Samoa, where Britain had a strategic interest. He spent time in Tahiti, where the seed was sown for *The Moon and Sixpence*, based in part on the life of primitivist artist Paul Gauguin. That book, which was published in 1919, was Maugham's first commercial success. In 1917, he went to Russia as the chief agent for British and American intelligence. He participated in an attempt to maintain the existing provisional government so that Russia would remain an ally in the war against Germany. Two months after his arrival, the Bolsheviks gained control. His book of stories titled *Ashenden*, which was popular and well received by critics, drew from his experiences as a spy.

As Maugham's popularity grew rapidly after the war, he continued sporadically to incorporate medical personalities and issues into his writings. In his most famous story, "Rain" (also presented on the stage and in film as *Miss Sadie Thompson*), a physician, Dr. Macphail, is a witness to the evolving drama. In Maugham's play *The Constant Wife*, the main character is married to a famous surgeon who has sexual relations with patients in his office, manipulates patients into accepting operations, and extends surgical procedures for his own satisfaction. A seemingly homosexual physician, who lost his license due to unethical behavior, is the main character in the short story *The Narrow Corner*, a novel published in 1932.

In addition to the doctors, disease—particularly cholera—plays a role in several of Maugham's works. Such is the case in *The Painted Veil*, which also presents a physician/bacteriologist as a central character. The setting of that work provides evidence that Maugham was the first modern English author to write about China, which he visited in 1920 and 1921. In another story, "Mirage," which takes place in China, an older Maugham, as the narrator, is approached by a fellow St. Thomas's Hospital medical student whom Maugham eventually recalls was dismissed for fraud.

By the mid-1920s, Maugham had become the most prosperous English writer, outselling many of his contemporaries, such as George Bernard Shaw, Rudyard Kipling, H. G. Wells, John Galsworthy, and P. G. Wodehouse. He had previously been a participant in the hedonism of Capri and, in 1926, established his base in Cap Ferrat on the French Riviera by purchasing the lavish Villa Mauresque. The villa was Maugham's home until his death, with the exception of five years at the time of World War II. At the villa, he continued his prolific production of prose. Between 1923 and 1929, he published twenty-nine stories in *Cosmopolitan* and *International Magazine*. During that period, he entertained his diverse and distinguished guests in sybaritic style that was marked by overt homosexuality. The visual appeal of the villa was enhanced by an important art collection, which included works by Gauguin, Lautrec, Renoir, Utrillo, Matisse, Monet, Pissarro, Sisley, Vuillard, Bonnard, and Picasso.

The most recent of Maugham's biographers, Jeffrey Meyers, considers *Cakes and Ale, or the Skeleton in the Cupboard*, published in 1930, to be Maugham's masterpiece. Maugham also felt that it was his best novel. It draws from the life of novelist Thomas Hardy, who had died in 1928, and the work addresses the quest for a literary reputation, an issue that Maugham shared.

Elements of Maugham's life are readily identifiable in his works. In

"The Buried Talent," which appeared in the *International Magazine* in 1934, Maugham, as narrator, describes his time at Heidelberg as a medical student and his experiences in Paris, Russia, and at Cap Ferrat, with references to his own art collection. In 1938, his autobiographical *The Summing Up* included his medical training at St. Thomas's Hospital. That year, after returning from India, Maugham initiated therapy to prevent and reverse aging. He was treated by Dr. Paul Niehans, a Swiss doctor. The regimen consisted of the injection of freshly harvested fetal lamb cells. Maugham repeated the treatment in 1958 and 1962.

In the fall of 1940, Maugham moved to the United States, where he spent the remainder of World War II. During that time, he had close ties with Hollywood. Over the course of his life, his association with motion pictures was probably unmatched by any other author. Either as the author whose story was adapted for film, as the author of a story and script written specifically for film, or as a writer called in to modify a script, Maugham was involved in almost fifty motion pictures. Seven of his novels were adapted for the screen: *The Razor's Edge* and *The Painted Veil* twice, and *Of Human Bondage* three times. Many of his plays and short stories also reached the screen; "Rain" (*Miss Sadie Thompson*) was the subject of three iterations.

After the war, Maugham returned to his villa at Cap Ferrat, where, a month before his ninety-second birthday, he suffered a stroke and died in a hospital in Nice on December 15, 1965. During his life, he was well aware of his literary status. He considered himself to be on the top of the second rung of the literary ladder. He wrote, "I have never pretended to be anything but a story teller. . . . It is unfortunate for me that telling a story just for the sake of a story is not an activity that is in favour with the intelligentsia."

As a storyteller, Maugham has few peers. His books have sold almost forty million copies, and he had earned almost forty million dollars in royalties. At one point in his career, he was paid five dollars per word, more than any other contemporary author. Within twelve years of its publication, his best-selling novel *The Razor's Edge* had sold almost 1,400,000 copies. He wrote seventy-eight books and twenty-nine plays. Penguin Books has published over 100,000 copies of ten of his books. In his own opinion, Maugham gained more fame from the film versions of his work, which were also more highly remunerative than the original publications. His plays continue to be performed, and about eighty of his stories have been shown on television.

His ashes were buried on the grounds of the King's School that he had attended and disliked during his attendance. His legacy is a large corpus of engrossing plots and a large number of memorable characters and scenes. In the realm of medicine, a number of his quotations have been incorporated in the standard *Familiar Medical Quotations*:

> "The normal's the one thing you practically never get. That's why it's called the normal."
> "You will have learned many tedious things . . . which you will forget the moment you have passed over your final examination, but in anatomy it is better to have learned and lost than to never have learned at all."
> "What makes old age hard to bear is not the failing of one's faculties, mental and physical, but the burden of one's memories."
> "Dying is the most hellishly boresome experience in the world! Particularly when it entails dying of 'natural causes.'"

SOURCES

Hastings, Selina. *The Secret Lives of Somerset Maugham: A Biography*. London: John Murray, 2009.

Meyers, Jeffrey. *Somerset Maugham: A Life*. New York: Alfred A. Knopf, 2004.

Strauss, M. B. *Familiar Medical Quotations*. Boston: Little, Brown, 1968.

Swinton, W. E. "Physicians in Literature: Part IV: Somerset Maugham, Talented But Troubled." *CMA Journal* 114 (January 10, 1976): 61–67.

30

JAMES JOHNSTON ABRAHAM

Surgeon, Soldier, Author, and Publisher

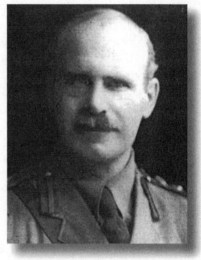

The "In Memoriam," which appeared in the *Annals of the Royal College of Surgeons of England* on the occasion of the passing of James Johnston Abraham, referred to the "very full life as surgeon, soldier, author and publisher" of a loyal member, who died seven days before his eighty-seventh birthday. Although his name and accomplishments currently are recognized by but a few, his presence as a surgeon was of great significance and his contributions to literature had enjoyed an appreciable readership.

Abraham was born on August 16, 1876, in Coleraine, County Derry, Northern Ireland, the descendant of an officer in Cromwell's army. He received his early schooling at the Coleraine Academical Institution and proceeded to Trinity College, Dublin, in 1894 to prepare himself for a career in medicine. While at Trinity College, he received the New Shakespeare Society Prize and the Gold Medal in Natural Science. He graduated in 1898 with a bachelor of arts in English. The chair of English counseled Abraham to pursue a career in medicine rather than literature, invoking Charles Lamb's advice, "Literature is a bad crutch but a good walking stick."

Abraham qualified MB BCh and BAO after an internship at Dr. Steevens' Hospital in Dublin. For a brief period, he was a medical officer at the private asylum Farnham House in Dublin, and later practiced venereology in County Clare, but, in 1901, he moved to become senior house surgeon to Mr. C. B. Keetley at the West London Hospital. After contracting a nonspecific illness in his lungs, Abraham spent six months as a ship's surgeon traveling to Japan and Java.

While preparing for the final examination for a fellowship at the Royal College of Surgeons of England, Abraham worked as a resident medical officer (RMO) at the London Lock Hospital for Women on Harrow Road. During his time as RMO, the bacterial cause of syphilis was discovered and the Wasserman blood test was introduced. These advances led to Abraham's selection of the subject for his thesis "Recent Advances in the Diagnosis and Treatment of Syphilis," which, when accepted, qualified him for an MD degree.

He next became house surgeon to Mr. Ernest Miles of eponymous fame at the Gordon Hospital, and, subsequently, he was appointed registrar at the London Lock Hospital, an institution with which he had a forty-five-year association. That hospital became part of Paddington Hospital until it closed in 1952. Abraham completed the requirements and became a fellow of the Royal College of Surgeons of England.

His first book, *The Surgeon's Log: Being Impressions of the Far East*, which stemmed from his travels as the ship's surgeon aboard the *Clytemnestra*, was published in 1911 and received favorable reviews. Over the ensuing fifty years, it appeared in thirty editions and sold over a half million copies. Also in 1911, Abraham was appointed assistant surgeon at Princess Beatrice Hospital, Earls Court.

Two years later, Abraham's one novel, *The Night Nurse*, appeared. His name does not appear as the author, rather "by the author of *The Surgeon's Log*." The work is a romance about a physician in training and a nurse. It was set in Dr. Steevens' Hospital and drew from the author's personal experiences. Stephen Brown referred to the novel in *Ireland in Fiction*, which was first published in 1919. He wrote that *The Night Nurse* "deals with the problem of 'the greater and lesser love' against the background of undesirable Catholics and disreputable Irishry (four plagues of Ireland being priests, politicians, pawnbrokers and publicans)." The novel, which was banned by the matrons of all the London hospitals, except Guy's Hospital, underwent four editions, the latest appearing in 1932. Two years later, a motion picture adaptation, *Norah O'Neale*, was produced in 1934.

In 1914, when World War I began, Abraham had an established London surgical practice with an office on Wimpole Street. At the age of thirty-six, he was deemed too old for the Royal Army Medical Corps (RAMC). But with the assistance of Sir Frederick Treves (see chapter 21), he was placed in charge of the largest No. 1 Hospital of the First British Red Cross Serbian Mission. That service earned Abraham the honorary rank of senior captain, and he was awarded the Order of St. Sava and the Croix Rouge de Serbie.

In 1915, again with Treves's help, he joined the RAMC as temporary lieutenant. He was second-in-command of the 24th Stationary Hospital at Kantara, where he handled the many casualties from the battles of Gaza. He rose to the rank of lieutenant colonel and was awarded CBE (Commander of the Most Excellent Order of the British Empire) and DSO (Distinguished Service Order), and elected a Knight of St. John. After the war, he became a consulting surgeon, as a general surgeon, urologist, and venereologist, at Princess Beatrice Hospital, and had a private practice on Caledonian Road.

Throughout his career as a practitioner, he lectured to students and postgraduates at several London hospitals. Abraham's contributions to medical literature include a paper on the treatment of syphilis with Compound 606 ND (salvarssan) and a fascicle containing lectures describing gonorrhea in women and children. Abraham thought that his best work was *Lettsom: His Life, Times, Friends, and Descendants* (1933), a biography of the eighteenth-century Quaker physician and philanthropist John Coakley Lettsom, who founded the Medical Society of London. The review of the biography in the *Times Literary Supplement* occupied the two front pages.

My Balkan Log, published in 1921, details Abraham's experiences during his service in Serbia. The work chronicles the medical care he provided in the face of inadequate and primitive supplies. He dealt with outbreaks of typhoid, scarlet fever, malaria, smallpox, and a typhus epidemic that killed "tens of thousands of Serbian and Austrian soldiers and civilians." He was the first one on the scene to make the diagnosis.

In 1937, a book of Abraham's essays, *Ninety-Nine Wimpole Street*, which had originally appeared as a series in *Nash's Magazine*, was published. Among the subjects considered were what doctors think of novelists; Harley Street, where physicians' offices dominated; the evolution of the doctor; pioneers of medicine; the romance of medicine; and the fear of death.

Several of Abraham's works written after 1937 were directed at counteracting the disturbing effect on the confidence of the public in the medical profession that was provoked by A. J. Cronin's *The Citadel*. To counter Cronin's criticism of the medical profession, Abraham used the pseudonym "James Harpole," derived from the first and last syllables of two notable sites of medical practice (Harley Street and Wimpole Street), for his next four publications.

Leaves from a Surgeon's Case-Book, which was published in 1937, draws from

Abraham's reminiscences to offer encouragement and to allay the fear of the average patient about to undergo an operation. Seven editions were printed within a year. It was then published in the United States and translated into nine languages. A second volume, mainly of short medical stories, came out the following year. It was titled *The White Coated Army*, referring to the surgeons, pathologists, physicians, nurses, and others working in the hospitals. It was published in the United States as *The Body Members*.

In 1941, with the onset of World War II, Abraham began writing and broadcasting for the BBC. A year later, he became the chairman and managing director of the medical company of Heinemann's publishing house, which published the works of W. Somerset Maugham (see chapter 29). In 1944, Abraham gave the Vicary Lecture, founded in honor of Thomas Vicary, sergeant surgeon to Henry VIII and the first master of the barber surgeons of London. The lecture was titled "The Early History of Syphilis."

Abraham was the chairman of the library committee of the Atheneum and a trustee of the Hunterian Collection. He was the recipient of a DLitt, honoris causa, from the University of Dublin and the Arnott Memorial Gold Medal of the Irish Medical Schools and Graduates Association. The last of his reminiscences, *Surgeon's Journey: The Autobiography of J. J. Abraham*, was published in 1957.

Abraham died on August 9, 1963. His eulogist wrote, "Seldom has a surgeon contributed more to the scientific side of his profession, and more rarely still to advancing the esteem of his profession in the eyes of the public." J. B. Lyons (see chapter 43) specifically credited Abraham as his model, indicating that *The Surgeon's Log* stimulated his sabbatical year as a ship's surgeon and his interest in doctors and medical students who were also distinguished writers.

SOURCES

Abraham, J. Johnston. *Surgeons Journey: The Autobiography of J. Johnston Abraham*. London: Heinemann, 1957.

Brown, Stephen J. *Ireland in Fiction: A Guide to Irish Novels, Tales, Romances and Folklor.* Dublin and London: Maunsel and Company, Limited, 1919.

"J[ames] Johnston Abraham (1876–1963)." Ricorso.net. http://www.ricorso .net/rx/az-data/authors/a/Abraham_JJ/life.htm (accessed April 5, 2018).

"In Memorium." *Annals of Royal College of Surgeons England* 33, no. 6 (December 1963): 392–95.

31

OLIVER ST. JOHN GOGARTY

A Diverse and Demonstrative Dubliner

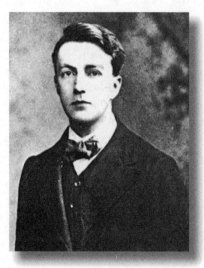

At Trinity College and among Irish physicians who contributed to literature, he was compared to Charles Lever (see chapter 16). In genealogic consideration, he followed the pattern of Harvey Cushing (see chapter 28) as the fourth generation of physicians in his family. Like another Dublin native, Arthur Conan Doyle (see chapter 24), he had some of his early education at Stonyhurst in London, but unlike Doyle, he became a successful specialist in a surgical field and a visible member of the government. As a writer, he held Rabelais (see chapter 3) in esteem, and his own verse is similarly frolicsome and, at times, Rabelaisian. But, despite comparisons to others, Oliver St. John Gogarty remains uniquely legendary at Trinity and stands out for his diversity of accomplishments as an otolaryngologist, senator, poet, playwright, novelist, and a highly regarded associate of the great Irish contributors to twentieth-century literature.

Gogarty was born on August 17, 1878, the first child of an affluent Irish Catholic family, which was among Dublin's elite. That status was unusual for the time when the Protestants possessed the wealth and dominated the professional class in the community. It was rare that his father, a successful doctor and a fellow of the Royal College of Surgeons in Ireland, could claim two previous generations of physicians, and that his mother's father was a prosperous Galway miller. This would account for the absence of any insecurity, beginning in the early years and continuing throughout Gogarty's life.

FROM MEDICINE TO MANUSCRIPT

Gogarty's father died of a ruptured appendix when the boy was nine years old, but the family's finances and his mother's strong influence compensated for the loss. After spending five years boarding at Stonyhurst, which Gogarty disliked and regarded as religious imprisonment, he was educated for a year at Clongowes Wood, a Jesuit school located near Clane in County Kildare. During his early schooling, he gained recognition as an outstanding athlete in football (soccer) and cricket. Next he enrolled to study medicine at the Royal University because the church considered that university preferable to Trinity College, a Protestant institution. In 1898, his lack of progress led him to transfer to Trinity.

At Trinity, over the extended eight years required to complete his studies (the so-called "Long Course"), Gogarty established a reputation as an athlete, a literary figure, a raconteur, and a prankster that persisted long after he left the school. The legend that he left behind him at Trinity was said to be equaled only by one other student, Charles Lever, who had preceded him by seven decades. Gogarty excelled at everything with the exception of his medical studies, as evidenced by the three years he required to pass an anatomy examination and the cumulative length of his time at Trinity.

During his medical studies, he turned his athletic attention to cycling and won almost all the cycling events at the college races. He was victorious in the Irish national championship, and, in London, he beat the English champion. His cycling career ended abruptly in 1901 when he was suspended for inappropriate language. That year, he won a university prize for verse, an achievement he would repeat during the subsequent two years.

Outside the walls of Trinity, a literary renaissance was taking place in Dublin. Gogarty would become a friend or acquaintance with almost all of the participants. He met poet William Butler "W. B." Yeats in 1901, and the two maintained a lifelong friendship. In 1904, at Yeats's request, Gogarty provided him with a translation of the verse *Oedipus Rex*, which Yeats would use for his dramatic work with the same title. When Yeats died in 1939, Gogarty wrote his obituary in the *Evening Standard*, in which he indicated that Yeats was the greatest conversationalist he had ever met and "Ireland's greatest most powerful voice."

Gogarty's circle of friends included George Moore, the leading English novelist of his time, and "Æ" (George William Russell), the mystic writer, painter, and nationalist. Among his fellow medical students, Gogarty was the leader of their pursuits of the city's bars and brothels. He embellished the escapades with limericks and ballads. The complex relationship between Gogarty and James Joyce, who was three years his junior, began in 1901. Initially, although they had totally dissimilar backgrounds and Joyce was a student at University College Dublin, the two were the closest of friends. Gogarty lent Joyce money, gave him clothes, and, in 1904, invited Joyce to live with him in the Martello Tower in Sandycove, on the shore of Dublin Bay. After living together for several days, they quarreled and Joyce left.

Although they corresponded in1907, and met briefly and without satisfaction at Gogarty's home, in 1909, their friendship terminated. When Joyce's *Ulysses* appeared in 1922, it was apparent that "Buck" Mulligan was patterned after Gogarty. Although the character was handsome, witty, and brilliant, Gogarty took umbrage. At the time of the publication, Gogarty, who had become a leading surgeon and a senator, did not wish to be associated with the wild Rabelaisian character of Mulligan.

In January 1904, Gogarty left Trinity for two semesters at Worcester College, Oxford, in order to work on his poetry. At Oxford, he was an entertaining Irishman in constant demand. When Gogarty returned to Trinity, he became involved in the new Sinn Fein Irish separatist movement and spoke at the first annual convention in 1905. Arthur Griffith, who defined the principles that led to Sinn Fein's election thirteen years later and, ultimately, self-government for Southern Ireland, was impressed with the young Gogarty, and the two remained friends until Griffith died in 1922. Just before Griffith died, he asked Gogarty to be governor general of the new Irish state, but it would not come to pass because Griffith died before the appointment could be made.

In June 1907, ten years after beginning his medical studies, Gogarty qualified as a doctor. In the final six months, as a student living in the Richmond Hospital, he came under the influence of Sir Robert Woods, an eminent ear, nose, and throat surgeon. Shortly after Gogarty qualified, he went to Vienna to enhance his knowledge so that he could specialize in ear, nose, and throat surgery. He and his wife leased rooms that had belonged to Richard von Krafft-Ebing, the psychiatrist and author of *Psychopathia Sexualis (Sexual Psychopathy)*. Gogarty could not resist writing a parody of Keats's *On First Looking into Chapman's Homer*, titled *On First Looking into Krafft-Ebing's Psychopathia Sexualis*.

After spending about six months in Vienna, in March 1908, Gogarty established his practice as a surgical specialist in Dublin. In a 1960 lecture to the Royal Academy, in which he was highly complementary of Gogarty's poetry, Professor A. Norman Jeffares referred to Gogarty as the "ear, nose, and throat specialist with an ear for melody, a nose for the ridiculous, and a throat unashamed of emotional speech and song." In fact, Gogarty was highly regarded among members of his profession and specialty.

He brought a bronchoscope back from Vienna and was the first to use one in Great Britain. In 1914, his paper "Latent Empyema of the Nasal Accessory Sinuses" was published in the *British Medical Journal*, and he became the first to report on the medical occurrence. He developed a large and highly remunerative practice that he conducted mainly as a member of the staff of Dublin's Meath Hospital. His colleagues referred to him as "a brilliant surgeon," "lightning with his hands," and "top-notch surgeon—good judgment and good hands." He was kind and generous, never charging poor people, and reduced his fees for clergy of all denominations. He occasionally introduced a dramatic flair by tossing excised tonsils across the operating room. When, as a thirty-three-year-old, he performed the second laryngectomy in Ireland, he flipped the specimen to the gallery.

In 1922, his medical skills were also called into play when he performed the autopsy on Arthur Griffith and, shortly thereafter, on Michael Collins, an Irish revolutionary leader, who was ambushed and killed during the Irish Civil War. That year, Gogarty, was elected an original Free State senator. It was a hazardous position, in that the rebels had ordered the death of senators. In January 1923, Gogarty was kidnapped at gunpoint by the political opposition. He escaped his captors by diving into the Liffey River, swimming across, and seeking shelter at the local police station. The occasion generated a contemporary popular ballad.

> Cried Oliver St. John Gogarty, "A Senator am I!
> The rebels I've tricked, the river I've swum and sorra
>   the word's a lie."
> As they clad and fed the hero bold, said the sergeant
>   with a wink:
> "Faith, thin, Oliver St. John Gogarty, ye've too much
>   bounce to sink."

Shortly after the kidnapping, the Gogartys' country estate, Renvyle House, in County Galway, was burned down by the rebels. It was rebuilt as a hotel, which opened in 1933 and used by Gogarty to entertain guests. In 1923, he found it dangerous and difficult to conduct his medical practice. He temporarily moved his practice to London and returned to Dublin, weekly, to attend the Senate meetings. In 1924, in keeping with a pledge he made related to the role the Liffey River played in his escape, he released two swans into the body of water. He was accompanied by William Thomas "W. T." Cosgrove, president of the Executive Council of the Irish Free State, and W. B. Yeats, and the event gained national attention. Gogarty served as a senator until 1936 when the upper house of the legislature was abolished. As a senator, he endorsed expansion and improvements of roads, reforestation, sanitation, and education. He strongly opposed reinstating the Irish language.

A critical medical colleague said that Gogarty was "a first-class writer, a second-class senator, and a third-class surgeon." The last assessment was false, the second has elements of truth, and the first was true throughout his lifetime, but has faded over the years. Gogarty's versatility in life is paralleled by his literary versatility. Although he is best known for his verse, he produced prose and contributions to the theatre.

While a student at Trinity, Gogarty produced humorous limericks, parodies on verse by famous poets, and romantic verse. In 1900, on the occasion of the return of Irish troops from the Boer War, his "Ode of Welcome," written under a pseudonym, was published in the leading social magazine, *Irish Society*. Popular appreciation of the poem was enhanced by the fact that, when it was read vertically down, the first letters of the lines create the sentence "The whores will be busy." Association with the dons at Trinity exposed him to Greek and Roman literature and molded him into a classical poet who used classical meters.

Gogarty gained the reputation of the prime poet of medical students as they caroused outside the walls of Trinity in Dublin. At a time when he indicated that "he was really sick of his medical studies," Gogarty would amuse himself by writing related verse, such as "To John Kidney Who Died of Nephritis" and "To His Friends When His Prostate Shall Have Become Enlarged." His first published work, a collection of verse, *Hyperthuleana (Beyond the Beyonds)*, had only five copies printed in 1916. Within the next two years, Gogarty published two more small collections of poetry, *Secret Springs of Dublin Song* and *The Ship and Other Poems*. During the same period, his first play, *Blight*, was performed at the Abbey Theatre. The authorship was ascribed to "Alpha and Omega" on the program. The drama dealt with the slums of Dublin and caused a sensation. It contained the poetic aspects of the language of the Dublin poor and included an endorsement for the prevention of venereal disease.

FROM MEDICINE TO MANUSCRIPT

In 1919, Gogarty's second play, *A Serious Thing*, was also produced at the Abbey Theatre. It was written under the pseudonym of Gideon Ouseley and used the Roman occupation of the Holy Land in the Augustan Age to satirize the contemporary British rule in Ireland. Also, that year, under the same pseudonym, his comedy *The Enchanted Trousers* was presented at the Abbey. In 1924, during a time when Gogarty was at his peak as a surgical specialist, his first major book of poetry, *An Offering of Swans*, containing eighty-one poems, was published. The collection of Gogarty's lyrical, classical, and metaphysical works, for which Yeats wrote the preface, was awarded the Gold Medal for poetry at the Tailteann Games for 1924.

Two more publications of Gogarty's poetry, *Wild Apples* (awarded the 1928 Tailteann Gold Medal for poetry) and *Selected Poems*, appeared before the 1936 publication of Yeats's *Oxford Book of Modern Verse*. Seventeen of Gogarty's poems were included in that compendium, and, in the introduction, Yeats referred to Gogarty as "one of the greatest living poets of our Age." Two years later, another collection of Gogarty's poems, *Others to Adorn*, appeared. The work was distinctive in that it used the mock-myth form in which myth is expressed, using the rhythmic theme of a nursery rhyme. The following year, another group of poems appeared in *Elbow Room*. A collected edition of Gogarty's verse was published in 1952.

When Gogarty was in his fifties, he became less interested in medicine and emerged as a writer of prose. His first novel, *As I Was Going down Sackville Street*, presents, in reverse chronologic order, interconnected semifictional anecdotes that occur in Dublin. The city itself assumes the role of the novel's hero. Gogarty's second novel, *I Follow St. Patrick*, in which the reader is guided by the patron saint through his historical travels, was published in 1938 and provides a geographic and romantic profile of the country. The two books found on the desk of James Joyce, after he died in 1940, were Gogarty's work about St. Patrick and *Greek Lexicon*, ostensibly to be used to translate the Greek quotations in Gogarty's work. In 1939, *Tumbling in the Hay*, a hilarious comedy, which draws from Gogarty's life, relates activities of medical students in early-twentieth-century Dublin.

In 1939, when World War II broke out, Gogarty volunteered for the Royal Army Medical Corps, and, when rejected, he volunteered for the Royal Air Force and, again, was turned down because of his age. In 1939, he left on a lecture tour in America; he remained without returning for five years and adopted the United States as his main residence. After moving to America that year, he intended to practice medicine, but decided against taking the necessary examination.

He was a frequent contributor to *Vogue, Harper's Magazine, Esquire,* and *Atlantic Monthly.* He published two novels: *Mr. Petunia,* a tale of an eighteenth-century schizophrenic New England watchmaker, and *Mad Grandeur,* which takes place in eighteenth-century Ireland. He also published two poetry books: *Perennial* and *Unselected Poems,* a collection of Rabelaisian verse. In 1954, his autobiographical *It Isn't This Time of the Year at All* appeared.

Gogarty died at the Beth David Hospital in New York City on September 22, 1957. His body was returned to Ireland, where it was buried in Connemara near Renvyle in Galway. His multifaceted accomplishments remain manifest in his diverse legacy: an expensive pub in Dublin, an annual literary festival in Connemara, and a surgical ward in the Adelaide and Meath Hospital, often referred to as Tallaght Hospital in Dublin.

SOURCES

Lyons, J. B. *Oliver St. John Gogarty.* Lewisburg, PA: Bucknell University Press, 1976.
O'Connor, Ulick. *The Times I've Seen.* New York: Ivan Obolensky, 1966.

32

SIR GEOFFREY LANGDON KEYNES

Keynesian Contributions to Surgery and Literature

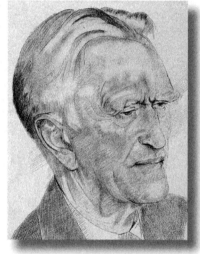

The aftermath of intense brilliance is generally deep darkness. The fraternal sequence of an extraordinary older brother is characteristically completed by an inconsequential and, at times, troublesome younger sibling. Eponymous fame of the senior is generally augmented by obscurity of the junior. In the case of the two Keynes brothers, a striking exception is manifest. Geoffrey Langdon Keynes contributed significantly to surgery and literature at the same time that his older brother, John Maynard Keynes, was the most recognizable name in modern economics.

Geoffrey's second name, Langdon, came from a great uncle, Dr. Langdon Down, who was the first to describe the

Photo from Wikimedia Creative Commons, author: G. Shaw; licensed under CC BY 4.0.

congenital mental deficiency known as "Down syndrome." Both brothers, doubtless, gained genetically from their father, John Neville Keynes, who majored in moral science at Pembroke College, Cambridge, and University College, London. He became secretary to the Council of the University of Cambridge and administered the affairs of that university for thirty-three years.

John Maynard was born on June 5, 1883; Geoffrey Langdon was born on March 25, 1887. While the older brother demonstrated exceptional intelligence at the beginning and throughout his schooling, Geoffrey's performance was average, and, in 1901, he was enrolled at Rugby, where he bonded with Rupert Brooke, a classmate, who played a significant role in Keynes's development as a literary figure. Keynes entered Pembroke College, Cambridge, in October 1906. Early in his college days, Keynes developed an appreciation of John Donne and a fixation on developing a collection of the writings of Sir Thomas Browne (see chapter 5). In 1908, Keynes sent a letter to Sir William Osler (see chapter 20), who had possessed the largest private collection of Browne's work, and received an invitation to stay at Osler's home. Keynes would persist in assembling Browne's works for about sixty years. The collection was ultimately bequeathed to the Royal College of Physicians of London. During Keynes's second year at Pembroke, he discovered William Blake, the mystic poet and artist, who would become the major focus of his literary life. Another of Keynes's associates at Cambridge was George Leigh Mallory, who took Keynes rock climbing and who would later die on his third attempt to reach the top of Mt. Everest.

In 1910, Keynes began his medical studies at St. Bartholomew's Hospital, known as Bart's, just outside the walls of London. After he passed the qualifying examination for the Royal Colleges and had received prizes for surgery in his class, in 1913, he was accepted as house surgeon at Bart's. His first contribution to literature was to insert a rubber tube and wash out the stomach of Virginia Stephen, who resided in the same lodgings as Keynes and had just made her first attempt at suicide by ingesting a large amount of narcotics. He saved the life of the woman, who married Leonard Wolff and authored her writings as Virginia Wolff. During the year as house surgeon, Keynes continued to satisfy his passion for bibliography and completed *A Bibliography of Dr. John Donne*, which was published in 1914 while he was serving as a junior officer in the Royal Army Medical Corps in Versailles.

Keynes spent a year at the front in Flanders in World War I and then practiced surgery on a large scale in casualty clearing stations in France. During that experience, he became acquainted with and applied the newly developed technique of the transfusion of preserved blood. After the war ended, he was appointed second assistant in the new professorial surgical unit at Bart's, the first of its kind in England. Keynes failed the Primary Fellowship Examination at the Royal College of Surgeons on his first two attempts, but, on his third try, he scored the highest marks among all candidates. He went on to receive the degree of MD after submitting a thesis called "The Diagnosis of Gunshot Wounds of the Abdomen."

Keynes joined the senior staff of the surgical unit at Bart's, and his first significant contribution to the field of surgery was his championing of blood transfusion, which, at the time, was used infrequently in England. In 1922, he published *Blood Transfusion*, the first textbook on the subject printed in Great Britain. On October 22, 1927, Keynes's broadcast, the first public appeal for donation of blood, aired on the BBC radio network. In 1949, a second larger textbook was published, for which Keynes provided the first chapter, "History of Transfusion." The book contained, for the first time, the blood types of fifty individuals in four generations of Keynes family members and members of his wife's family, the famous Darwins.

Keynes's second and most significant contribution to surgery was related to the treatment of breast cancer. In 1922, he began treating breast cancer with implantation of small needles containing radium to destroy the tumor and reported preliminary results five years later. He then challenged the logic of the standard radical operation (removal of the breast, underlying muscles and axillary lymph nodes) and championed conservative surgery and early diagnosis. From 1929 on through the remainder of his medical career, he advocated conservative treatment for breast cancer, and his position was met with strong disapproval. He started to assemble data but was thwarted when, in 1939, he became a consulting surgeon to the Royal Air Force and had to abandon his hospital and private practice. Decades after Keynes's initial suggestion, George Crile Jr. of Cleveland, Ohio, published a book on the conservative management of breast cancer and dedicated the book to Keynes, whose concept is now universally accepted. The dedication states, "To Sir Geoffrey Keynes, whose wisdom and foresight made him the first to resist the trend towards ever more radical treatment of breast cancer."

In 1928, Keynes was appointed assistant surgeon on the staff at Bart's, and it had been hoped that he would follow an academic career. He wrote, "I decided not to attempt this, the main consideration being that the practice of surgery was the central passion of my life. I was a craftsman by instinct, not a teacher, an administrator, a committee man, a politician, as I had noticed a professor had to be." In addition, he pointed out that his outside interests and growing family required a larger income.

During World War II, in his capacity as a consulting surgeon to the Royal

Air Force, Keynes organized an orthopedic service to care for downed pilots. This significantly improved care, as did changes that Keynes brought about for the treatment of burns. At the end of the war, acting air vice marshal Keynes returned to London, where his third significant medical contribution took place. As a consequence of his having developed a large practice of thyroid surgery, at times requiring intrathoracic extension, Keynes was called upon to perform removal of the thymus for myasthenia gravis, an operation that had been introduced by Alfred Blalock at the Johns Hopkins Hospital and later abandoned. Keynes developed the largest surgical series and reported favorable results.

In 1945, Keynes was elected to the council of the Royal College of Surgeons of England and, in time, received the title of honorary librarian and curator of pictures. He retired from the staff of Bart's in 1951, and, over the ensuing six years, his private surgical practice disappeared. In summarizing his surgical life, Keynes reflected, "Though my friends had often thought that literature and bibliography were my first loves, with surgery as a background, in reality it had been the other way round." In 1958, he was elected as a fellow of the Royal College of Physicians. The knighthood, which was conferred upon him in 1955, specifically, was "for surgical distinction by recommendation of the Royal College of Surgeons of England." This was followed by another honor in 1956 when he was appointed to the office of Sims Commonwealth Professor, resulting in visits to medical schools in Africa and Canada.

Keynes's bibliophilia began while he was a college student, still in his teens. By his own confession, the bibliophilia evolved into "bibliomania," and he also merits the sobriquet of "bibliographiliac" because his output in that literary genre was extraordinary and, perhaps, unequaled. His first publication, *A Bibliography of Dr. John Donne*, appeared in 1914. Three subsequent editions have been published. In 1924, *A Bibliography of Sir Thomas Browne*, which the author had begun in 1908 while a student at Cambridge, was published by the Cambridge University Press. In 1929, *Jane Austen: A Bibliography* appeared, followed by *Selected Essays of William Hazlitt* in 1930. The following year, *The Works of Sir Thomas Browne; Certain Miscellany Tracts, Repertorium, Miscellaneous Writings* and *The Works of Thomas Browne: Letters* were published. In 1937, *John Evelyn: A Study in Bibliophily and a Bibliography of His Writings* was published jointly by the Grolier Club of New York and the Cambridge University Press.

In 1931, Keynes was named literary executor of the estate of Rupert Brooke. Brooke's legendary status as a poet was intensified by his death in 1915.

Before seeing any active service, Brooke died of cellulitis and sepsis aboard a French ship on the way to Gallipoli. After his death, Winston Churchill wrote a valediction, which included a famous quotation from Brooke: "If I should die, think only this of me; / That there's some corner of a foreign field / That is forever England." In 1946, Keynes edited *The Poetical Works of Rupert Brooke*. In 1954, he compiled the complete *Bibliography of Rupert Brooke*. In 1968, Keynes published *The Letters of Rupert Brooke*.

William Blake remained a lifelong focus for Keynes. His first publication about Blake, a massive and handsome volume with a print run of 250 copies, was produced by the Grolier Club of New York in 1921. In 1948, Keynes published *Poetry and Prose of William Blake*, the first complete edition of Blake's writings. Keynes would continue to bring forth publications about Blake: *The Tempera Paintings of William Blake* (1951); *A Study of the Illuminated Books of William Blake: Poet-Printer-Prophet* (1964); *On Editing Blake* (1964); *Blake: The Masters 6* (1965); *Blake: Complete Writings with Variant Readings*, edited by Keynes (1966); *William Blake: Songs of Innocence and of Experience, Ed. by Sir Geoffrey Keynes* (1967); *William Blake Engraver* (1969); *Drawings of William Blake: 92 Pencil Studies* (1970); *William Blake's Water-Colours Illustrating the Poems of Thomas Gray* (1972); and *The Marriage of Heaven and Hell* (1975). And, as a conjunction between Keynes's confessed "Balletomania" and focus on Blake, he produced a ballet, *Job: A Masque for Dancing*, with Ralph Vaughan Williams's score, which premiered in June 1931 and has appeared at the Opera House, Covent Gardens, over sixty-five times. In 1979, it was stated by Kathleen Raine Berkeley, in *Blake and the New Age*, "The editorial and bibliographical labours of Sir Geoffrey Keynes over the last half-century have made Blake accessible, but not comprehensible." In 1942, Keynes was appointed a trustee of the National Portrait Gallery in London. In 1928, he first published *A Bibliography of the Writings of William Harvey*, which was revised as a second edition in 1953. In 1948, while preparing for a lecture on William Harvey, the author of *De Motu Cordis*, in which the circulation of blood was first described, Keynes discovered the only contemporary portrait of Harvey. The following year, Keynes published *The Personality of William Harvey* and, in 1958, *Harvey through John Aubrey's Eyes*. In 1966, *The Life of William Harvey* was awarded the John Tait Black Memorial Prize for biography. A second edition appeared in 1978 in celebration of the four hundredth anniversary of Harvey's birth. Another physician about whom Keynes wrote was Thomas Bright, whose *Treatise of Melancholie* (1586) was the source of several passages in Shakespeare's *Hamlet*. Keynes's *Thomas Bright 1510–1615, A Survey of His Life with a Bibliography of his Writings* was published in 1962.

Extending his focus, in 1951, Keynes published *A Bibliography of John Ray*, the great seventeenth-century naturalist, and, in 1976, *A Bibliography of Bishop Berkeley*, the Anglo-Irish philosopher who proposed a theory of "immaterialism," which contends that objects of perceived substance are only ideas in the minds of the perceivers.

In June 1965, Keynes received the honorary degree of doctor of letters within a period of five days from both the Universities of Oxford and Cambridge, an honor matched previously by only one other physician who also contributed notably to literature, Oliver Wendell Holmes (see chapter 17). In 1980, Keynes was awarded honorary fellowship in the British Academy. In 1981, he borrowed from Blake for the title of his autobiography, *The Gates of Memory*, which was published when the author was ninety-four years old. He died a year later.

If we were to create a "paroperative panthcon" of surgeons with literary contributions in which "paroperative," a neologism, reflects equal productivity in the operating room and in a field totally disparate from surgery, Keynes would certainly merit at least equal stature with the great Theodor Billroth, who contributed significantly to musicology, and two surgeons, previously considered in this work, Sir Frederick Treves and Harvey Cushing, who contributed meaningfully to literature.

SOURCES

Keynes Kt., Geoffrey. *The Gates of Memory*. Oxford: Clarendon, 1981.

33

WILLIAM CARLOS WILLIAMS

Passionate about Poetry while Persistently Providing Medical Care

Among twentieth-century literary figures, none sustained a medical practice in an uncompromised manner as well as William Carlos Williams. As he wrote in *The Autobiography of William Carlos Williams*,

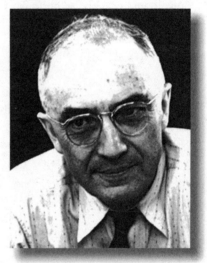

> [A]s a writer I have never felt that medicine interfered with me but rather it was my very food and drink, the very thing that made it possible for me to write. Was I not interested in Man?
>
> Five minutes, ten minutes, can always be found. I had a typewriter in my office desk. . . . If a patient came in

Photo courtesy of the Stonybrook School of Medicine.

> at the door while I was in the middle of a sentence, bang would go the machine—I was a physician. When the patient left, up would come the machine. . . . Finally, after eleven at night, when the last patient had been put to bed, I could always find time to bang out ten or twelve pages. In fact, I couldn't rest until I had freed my mind from the obsessions which had been tormenting me all day.
>
> And my "medicine" was the thing that gained me entrance to these secret gardens of the self. . . . I was permitted by my medical badge to follow the poor, defeated body into the gulfs and grottos. And the aston-

ishing thing is that at times in such places—foul as they may be with the stinking ischiorectal abscesses of our coming and goings—just there, the thing, in all its greatest beauty, may for a moment be freed to fly for a moment guiltily about the room.

His son, who was also a physician, wrote of his father: "He was a capable and respected physician. He was an active and honest reporter in his poetry. The trained observer physician complemented the vibrant imagist in the poet. Either occupation for most men would be a full-time job. Fortunately, he had at hand an inexhaustible well of energy that made it possible to do both jobs well. The doctor nurtures the poet through his privileged admission into the lives of his patients. The poet returned into the physician the distillate of his observations, making the doctor a more humane and altruistic ministrant to the sick."

William Carlos Williams was born in the small country town of Rutherford, New Jersey, on September 17, 1883. His father was born in England and grew up in St. Thomas, Virgin Islands. He never became a citizen of the United States. The same pertained to his mother, who was born in Puerto Rico and brought up in the Dominican Republic. Williams was educated in Rutherford until, as a fourteen-year-old, he was sent to study in Geneva and Paris for two years. On his return, he completed his high school education at Horace Mann in Manhattan, to which he commuted five days each week.

At the time, it was possible to enter medical school without a college degree, and, in 1902, Williams enrolled in the University of Pennsylvania School of Medicine, from which he graduated four years later. Before entering medical school, Williams had developed an interest in writing, particularly poetry. Williams had stated that "all writing starts and ends with poetry." While engaged in his medical studies, he developed what would become lifelong relationships with two students who would join Williams as leading American modernist poets, Ezra Pound and Hilda "H. D." Doolittle. At the same time, Williams and painter Charles Demuth became close friends, and for a while Williams flirted with painting.

One week after graduating from medical school, Williams became an intern at the French Hospital, located in Lower Manhattan. During his internship, he decided on general practice with an emphasis on pediatrics and obstetrics. He continued to write poems, but his early poetry was generally romantic, in sonnet form, and was not initially influenced by his medical experience. After almost two years of training at the French Hospital, Williams continued to enhance his medical development at the Nursery and Child's Hospital, in uptown Manhattan.

The female patients at that hospital were considered by many to be the dregs of the city. After several months, Williams became the chief resident and was called upon to sign off on the hospital demographics for an obligatory monthly report to the state. The hospital administrators refused to provide him with substantiating data, and, in protest, Williams resigned before he had completed a year at the hospital. He continued advanced studies in pediatrics for one year in Leipzig, Germany. Before returning home, Williams visited Ezra Pound in London and became exposed to several famous literary figures.

On September 10, 1910, Williams put out his medical shingle in Rutherford, New Jersey. Initially, he ran the office alone. In 1912, he married Florence Herman who would assist in the practice. Williams rapidly gained a reputation as one who truly cared for patients, and one who was more than reasonable regarding fees, often not charging those who could not afford it. He made frequent house calls, delivering patients' babies at their homes. During World War I, his father's illness gained Williams a deferment. His practice became hectic, particularly when the flu pandemic hit the United States in 1918, requiring Williams to make up to sixty house calls a day.

In June 1923, Williams took a one-year sabbatical from his practice, which was covered by a cousin. The first six months were spent with his wife in New York City, socializing with his literary colleagues and carrying out research in the New York Public Library for *In the American Grain*, a long poem extolling heroic figures in early American history. The second six months were spent abroad, during which he met James Joyce, Hungarian sculptor Constantin Brancusi, novelist and poet Ford Mattox Ford, visual artist Man Ray, British modernist writer Mina Loy, Hilda "H. D." Doolittle, Ezra Pound, and Ernest and Sally Hemingway.

Six months after Williams and his wife returned to America in June 1924, he expanded his practice by joining the staff of the Passaic General Hospital, in Passaic, New Jersey, and established a second office in that city. World War II impacted significantly on Williams's practice because several of the local physicians were drafted. Williams made patient rounds seven mornings a week as chief of pediatrics at the Passaic hospital. Afternoons were spent making house calls, and evenings were spent seeing patients at his Rutherford office. Over one two-week period in 1942, he recorded performing fourteen obstetrical deliveries.

Williams's tenure at the Passaic hospital extended over more than twenty years, during which he served not only as head of pediatrics but also as president of the Medical Board. He retired from his hospital duties in 1948 after he had suffered a heart attack. He retired from medical practice two years later.

Williams's poems and stories about his patients and medical issues reveal how intimately his two vocations were enmeshed. He wrote, "I would learn so much on my rounds, or making home visits. At times, I felt like a thief because I heard words, lines, saw people and places—and used it all in writing!" One of his most famous stories, "The Use of Force," in which the force emanates first from a child being examined by a doctor to determine whether she has diphtheria, and then by the physician to complete his examination. The poem "A Cold Front" focuses on a woman with eight children who decides to abort a pregnancy. The story "Old Doc Rivers" traces the complexities of a once skillful doctor, who deteriorates over time. Although "Doc Rivers" becomes the town's scandal, he continues to maintain a core of worshipers, who hold him in high regard because of his previous personal contributions to sustaining their health.

As a literary figure, Williams wrote short stories, plays, novels, essays, and translations, but he is best known for his poems. In 1908, he published his first book, a twenty-two-page pamphlet titled *Poems*, paying $32.45 for the printing himself. He criticized himself, commenting, "The poems were bad Keats, nothing else." In 1913, Ezra Pound arranged for Williams's second book of poems, *The Tempers*, to be published in London. The work presents evidence of a poet attempting to distance himself from the generally admired Romantic poets, such as Keats and Wordsworth.

Beginning in 1912, Williams commuted three days a week to New York City, which was only five miles from Rutherford, New Jersey, to further his training in pediatrics at Babies' Hospital and Post-Graduate Clinic. He lingered during the late afternoons and evenings with friends, who were regarded to be "rebels" in literature and art. The poets in the group erased the format of capitalizing the first letter of each line. Rhyme was removed, and the structure of the poem was changed to be more in line with the pattern of common speech. To achieve this goal, Williams invented a line-break pattern, termed the "variable foot." Also referred to as "triadic line poetry," it consists of three staggered lines that constitute a stanza.

Williams wrote, "But, we argued, the poem, like every other form of art, is an object that in itself presents its case and its meaning by the very form it assumes. . . . The poem being an object (like a symphony or cubist painting) it must be the purpose of the poet to make of his words a new form. To invent, that is, an object consonant with his day. This is what we wish to imply by Objectivism, an antidote." For Williams, "the syllable and the line, they make a poem."

The syllable "rules and holds together the line," and "the line comes from the breathing of the breathing of the man who writes, at the moment that he writes."

Williams's poems often were initially published in the recently launched avant-garde magazines, such as *Poetry*, the *Dial*, and *Others*, for which he edited one issue. In 1917, Williams's third collection of verse, *Al Que Quiere! (To Him Who Wants It!)*, was published. The book offered a description and interpretation of life in Rutherford and the personalities of the inhabitants. In 1920, *Kora in Hell: Improvisations*, combining poetry and prose, evoked severe criticism from his colleagues. In that work, he points out, "Imagination though it cannot wipe out the sting of remorse can instruct the mind in its proper use," and "There is nothing sacred about literature, it is damned from one end to the other. There is nothing in literature but change and change is mockery. I'll write as I damn and it'll be good if the authentic spirit of change is on it."

That year, Williams and Robert McAlmon, a modernist poet who was about twelve years younger, launched the literary magazine *Contact*, which Williams edited. The periodical gained significance by including contributions from Ford Mattox Ford, Ernest Hemingway, James Joyce, Ezra Pound, H. D., and Gertrude Stein. In 1923, Williams published a collection of his poetry, *Spring and All*, in which "The Red Wheelbarrow," his most anthologized poem, first appeared. In that work, he referred to his goal of being an innovator, creating new methods of writing. Also, in that year, *The Great American Novel*, which consists of only sixty-odd pages and could hardly be classified as a novel, was published. It included reminiscences of the author's medical and social experiences, in addition to episodes from American history. In 1924, Williams received the Governor's award from the magazine *Poetry*.

Williams's focus on America was expanded three years later with the publication of *In the American Grain*, a compilation of twenty essays focusing on the discovery and early history of the land of his birth, in an attempt to determine a cause for its distinctive fabric.

In 1926, Williams began writing his magnum opus, *Paterson*, which was published as an epic poem in five segments between 1946 and 1958, and in one volume with a fragment of a sixth segment in 1963. An embryonic form appeared as a poem with the same name in the 1926 edition of the *Dial*. Part 1 stands out as the premier segment and is generally regarded to be the best of Williams's work. Poet laureate Robert Lowell considered it to be the "best poetry by an American," and critic Randall Jarrell indicated that it "has an extraordinary range and reality, a clear rightness that sometimes approaches perfection."

Paterson is the personification of a New Jersey city that had been envisioned by its founder, Alexander Hamilton, as a potential industrial hub, which became known as the "Silk City" and the "Cotton Town of America" for its dominant role in the nineteenth century and, in Williams's time, as a manufacturing metropolis in economic decline. In Williams's epic poem, the city's geographic features, dominated by Passaic Falls, shares focus with history, social issues, and personalities. Insinuated throughout the work is an articulation of Williams's pervasive concern with the debasement of the American language.

The White Mule, Williams's first serious novel, was published in 1937 and was based on his wife's life. That work eventually became part of a trilogy with the publications of *In the Money* and *The Build-Up*, modeled on the lives of his wife's parents. During World War II, he published *The Wedge*, perhaps the finest collection of his poetry. His last book of poetry, *Pictures from Brueghel and Other Poems*, appeared in 1962, less than a year before he died on March 4, 1963.

Williams produced about twenty published poetry collections and thirteen books of prose, including a collection of plays. He became an influence and icon for many of the more recent poets.

In 1928, Williams received the annual award from the *Dial*. In 1948, he was awarded the Russell Loines Award by the National Institute of Arts and Letters. In 1950, when US publishers reestablished the National Book Award, Williams won the first award for poetry, in recognition of the third volume of *Paterson* and *Selected Poems*. In 1963, he was posthumously awarded the Pulitzer Prize for *Pictures from Brueghel and Other Poems*, and the Gold Medal for Poetry of the National Institute of Arts and Letters. The Poetry Society of America continues to present, annually, the William Carlos Williams Award for the best book of poetry published by a nonprofit or a university press. Williams was inducted into the New Jersey Hall of Fame, and his Rutherford home has been included on the National Register of Historic Places. His papers reside in the library of the State University of New York at Buffalo.

Williams is unique in that he can be assessed as having been eminently successful in his lifelong attention to two disparate roles: that of a dedicated and uncompromising physician and that of a consummate modernist poet.

SOURCES

Baldwin, Neil. *To All Gentleness: William Carlos Williams, The Doctor-Poet.* New York: Atheneum, 1984.

Leibowitz, Herbert. *"Something Urgent I Have to Say to You": The Life and Works of William Carlos Williams.* New York: Farrar, Strauss, and Giroux, 2011.

Williams, William Carlos. *The Autobiography of William Carlos Williams.* New York: Random House, 1948.

34

FRANCIS BRETT YOUNG

Closure of the Locks for Medicine Opened the Floodgates for Literature

An assessment of the life and contributions of Francis Brett Young is a combination of two small narratives, one written by an adoring and generally inseparable wife of more than four decades, and the other written by an individual who shared a birthplace with his subject and held office in a society dedicated to preserving Young's literary legacy. During a period that encompassed the two World Wars, Young was one of Great Britain's most prolific and popular authors, but, currently, his name and works are covered by a veil of obscurity.

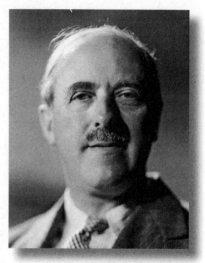

Photo © National Portrait Gallery, London.

Young was born on June 29, 1884, at Hales Owen in Worcestershire, in the West Midlands of England, where his father, a practicing physician, held the position of medical officer and public vaccinator for Romsley District and Bromsgrove Union. When Francis was seven years old, he was sent to a small preparatory school, Iona Cottage High School, in Sutton Coldfield; after four unpleasant years at that school, he entered Epsom College at Epsom Downs in Surrey with a scholarship. While there, he first demonstrated his literary interest by editing two publications: a self-published periodical called the *Laurels Magazine* and the commercially produced *Epsomian*.

Young's early ambition was to become a professional writer, and he hoped to obtain a scholarship at Balliol College, Oxford, to further his goal. But he submitted to his father's insistence that he prepare himself for a career in medicine with the intention that he join his father's practice. In 1901, Francis entered the University of Birmingham School of Medicine one year after it had received its charter. He lived at home and traveled to school daily on the train. His academic performance was excellent, and he was among the best of his thirty-six classmates.

After Young qualified to practice medicine in 1906, he elected to allow himself a period of rest and diversion by signing on as a ship's surgeon for a merchant ship bound for Asia. The round-trip voyage that began on January 5, 1907, and lasted 125 days was marked by no unusual incidents for the young physician. Shortly after his return from the voyage and a brief walking holiday, Young spent two months as a locum tenens (substitute) physician in the Midlands.

In the fall of 1907, he established himself as a practitioner in Brixham, a small fishing town in Devon in southwest England. His success led him to open a second office in nearby Galmpton. During his time at Brixham, Young, a self-taught pianist, produced several compositions, to which he set the poetry of Alfred Edward Housman, Percy Bysshe Shelley, and contemporary poets to music. For a brief period, Young contemplated a career in music.

He began to pursue a literary presence while conducting his practice. His first published work was a short story, "Furze Bloom," set in the Mendips, where his ancestors had lived, south of Bristol and Bath. Several short stories appeared in print in various magazines, and he began work on the novels *The Young Physician* and *The Iron Age*, set in the Midlands, as well as *Undergrowth* and *The Dark Tower*, which take place in the English-Welsh borderlands.

In 1913, the novel *Undergrowth*, coauthored with Francis's younger brother, Eric, was published. One review stated that it was "a remarkable story inspired by the mysticism of the Celtic temperament and vivid with flashes of something like genius in the subtle influences of locality and pagan tradition."

Deep Sea, Young's first solo novel to appear in print, was published in 1914 and captures the atmosphere and personalities of Brixham. Like most of Young's fiction, it drew significantly from individuals he had encountered as well as actual events. That same year, his *Robert Bridges: A Critical Study* assessed the work of the contemporary poet laureate. The *Saturday Review* said it was "the best book of criticism we have opened for a long time." Also, he completed *The Dark Tower* in less than two months. The demands of Young's literary endeavors necessitated his adding a partner for his medical practice.

After Great Britain entered World War I, his days at Brixham ended when he accepted a commission in the Royal Army Medical Corps on January 1, 1916, and immediately left for training. Three months later, he sailed to serve under Lieutenant General Jan Christian Smuts of Boer War fame in the German East African Campaign. After a brief stay in Cape Town, he proceeded by ship to Mombasa and then by land to Nairobi, Kenya, where he was appointed medical officer to the Second Rhodesian Regiment and was deployed to the front.

Less than three months after arriving in East Africa, while he attended troops at the battle front, Young became a victim of dysentery and malaria, which required hospitalization. During his recovery, he wrote the first half of a chronicle of his experiences, *Marching on Tanga*, and shipped it to the publisher. It was lost at sea and required a rewrite. The book was published in 1917. Passages that had been censored from the book were later used covertly in his novel *Jim Redlake*.

When Young's one-year military commitment had ended and he was awaiting discharge, he sustained a fracture/dislocation of the radius and ulna at the elbow. He returned to England for treatment and was subsequently appointed registrar at the Military Hospital at Tidworth in Wiltshire. Shortly after his return, his first collection of poetry, *Five Degrees South*, dedicated to his wife, was published. The *New Statesman's* review of the work stated that it "engages the mind by the earnestness and sincerity of its thought." In 1918, *The Crescent Moon*, which dealt with the conflict between savagery and civilization and had as its setting German East Africa, where Young was stationed, was published.

In 1919 came the publication of *The Young Physician*, which Young dedicated to his father. In a letter to his father, he wrote that "it is only fitting seeing that but for you I should never have been able to write about the life of a medical student (or—for that matter—any life at all)." The work exemplifies the author's liberal extrapolations from places, individuals, and events that he had experienced.

About a year after World War I ended, Young decided that his malaria and injured arm limited his ability to conduct an active medical practice. This provided a stimulus for him to realize his desire and devote his energies to maintaining himself as a professional writer. The consequent need to reduce expenses coupled with the benefit of a more favorable climate, in which he would better tolerate recurrent malarial attacks, led to his move to the island of Capri. For the next fifteen years, Young and his wife spent winters at Capri and summers in England.

Shortly after the Youngs established a permanent residence on Capri, *The Tragic Bride* appeared in print. The novel includes episodes based on experiences Young had while he convalesced for a brief period in Ireland after his discharge from the army. The Dublin described in the novel is where the Youngs met the poet and painter "Æ" and members of Sinn Fein. *Metropolitan Magazine* bought the rights for serialization of the work in America.

During his time on Capri, Young worked on thirteen novels. Most have their settings in Young's native Black Country of the English West Midlands and Welsh Borders, and are referred to as his Mercian novels. These include *The Black Diamond, Cold Harbour, My Brother Jonathan, Jim Redlake, Mr. & Mrs. Pennington, The House under the Water,* and *This Little World.* The remaining novels produced on Capri were *The Red Knight, Woodsmoke, Sea Horses, Black Roses,* and *The Key of Life.*

Pilgrim's Rest, which appeared in 1922, is a narrative of events occurring at an African gold-mining town of the same name that Young had visited during a trip the year prior to the publication of *Woodsmoke,* which also afforded the readership a view of South Africa. The experiences of Young's voyage to Asia as a ship's surgeon provided material for *Sea Horses.* The ship's surgeon in the novel received the same pay as the author and, similarly, suffered from seasickness. The real and fictional ship's stewards bore the same Asian name.

In 1927, *Portrait of Clare,* a romantic family saga set in the West Midlands, was awarded the James Tait Black Memorial Prize as the best novel of the year. It was published in America with the title *Love Is Enough.* The next year witnessed the publication of two novels: *The Key of Life,* which stemmed from Young's visit to Egypt, and *My Brother Jonathan,* with a general practitioner as its hero. The latter incorporates fictional similarities with Young's medical toils and anxieties, including traveling long distances in a dogcart and an unreliable secondhand automobile. His experience of performing a successful tracheotomy in Brixham on a young child with diphtheria was also incorporated in the novel. Young's patient, eighty years after the event, unveiled two plaques on Young's two homes in Brixham.

Between 1930 and 1932, three of Young's most notable Mercian novels, *Jim Redlake, Mr. & Mrs. Pennington,* and *The House under the Water,* were published. One reviewer of *Jim Redlake* encapsulated the general critique of Young's work: "While admitting the competent writing and general technique of Francis Brett Young in this book, one wonders that he should have produced a work so lacking in originality." The novel has many autobiographical elements, including medical schooling and participation in war in Africa, for which General Jan Smuts loaned Young his personal war diaries.

Mr. & Mrs. Pennington, set in contemporary Hales Owen, is the story of a man blindly devoted to his wife, who is at times selfish, conniving, and inappropriate. Although the novel is set in the town in which Young was born, according to the author, "*Mr. & Mrs. Pennington* is a true story, but the events took place in Italy. It cost me over £100 to defend the unfortunate youth and I gave evidence of his character at the trial."

The House under the Water deals with the construction of pipelines and dams and how the rerouting of water adversely affects the lives of inhabitants who are remote and indifferent to the beneficiaries. This novel, which was published in 1932, was followed by seven novels in the ensuing seven years. *White Ladies*, consisting of almost seven hundred pages, is about a ruthless obsession that consumes the lives of members of families involved in Black Country industry over generations. *Far Forest* also focuses on the difficulty of life in the industrial Midlands, whereas, *They Seek a Country* and *City of Gold* have South African settings. The latter is a sequel to the former and follows a family through the annexation of the Transvaal, the development of the diamond industry, and the evolution of the city of Johannesburg. The novel *Portrait of a Village*, which was also serialized in *Good Housekeeping*, is a social history of an unidentified Worcestershire village. Jonathan, from *My Brother Jonathan*, reappears in *Dr. Bradley Remembers*, which is based on the life and times of the author's physician father.

The 1940s opened with the publication of *Cotswald Honey*, which collects several short stories that take place in East African waters and are narrated by the tramp steamer's surgeon. *Mr. Lucton's Freedom*, also published in 1940, was the last of the Mercian novels. It was a lighthearted novel about a wealthy English accountant who adopts a new identity that permits him to expand his encounters and find contentment, albeit short-lived; Young indicated he was not pleased with the work. The next novel, *A Man about the House*, was, by Young's admission, a "pot boiler" and takes place in two venues familiar to the author: the areas of Birmingham and Capri.

At that time of his life, he was concentrating on the production of his epic poem *The Island*, a testimonial to his patriotism for his native land, presented as a history of Britain from the Bronze Age to the Battle of Britain in verse. Young regarded the poem as his greatest work. The public agreed, and the first edition sold out within weeks of its publication in 1944. Six months later, Young immigrated to South Africa. He returned to England on several occasions, once to receive an honorary DLitt degree from the University of Birmingham at the Golden Jubilee celebration. Young died in Cape Town on March 28, 1954, and his ashes were interred in the Worcester Cathedral. His last novel, *Wistanslow*, is obviously autobiographical and was posthumously published in its incomplete form in 1956.

Young, in his prime, was a literary giant and a preferred author of Prime Minister Stanley Baldwin. Young's literary productivity, which includes thirty novels and four collections of short stories, sold more than a half million copies and appeared in more than two hundred editions and in eleven languages. His canon also includes three nonfiction books, three published plays, three volumes of poetry, and a very popular epic poem.

Currently, his name and works have been relegated to obscurity. Most of his works are out of print, and when one seeks recent reviews of his works in electronic platforms, it is rare that more than one is available. His literary obscurity has been appropriately explained by Michael Hall, his sympathetic biographer: "The traditional values which he represented and the lyrical style in which he wrote, were no longer popular. His novels were over-long, repetitious and humourless. He had contrived pale and sentimental characters, smug and comfortable plots. Not a truly creative writer, he only wrote of events and places he knew, and only described people from his own perspective."

SOURCES

Hall, Michael. *Francis Brett Young*. Bridgend, Wales: Poetry Wales Press, 1997.
Young, Jessica Brett. *Francis Brett Young: A Biography*. London: William Heinemann, 1962.

35

RUDOLPH JOHN CHAUNCEY FISHER

The Renaissance Man of the Harlem Renaissance

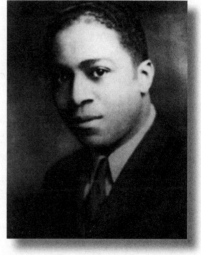

T he combination of physician, researcher, radiologist, medical administrator, orator, musician, musical arranger, and a literary figure who was innovative and contributed to multiple genres certainly merits recognition as a "Renaissance man." And all his accomplishments were achieved during a short life that spanned less than four decades.

Rudolph John Chauncey Fisher was born in Washington, DC, on May 9, 1897, and grew up in Providence, Rhode Island, where his father served as a Baptist minister. Rudolph graduated from Classical High School with high honors in 1915 and entered Brown University. In his freshman year, he won the Caesar Misch Premium in German language study. As a sophomore, he received the Carpenter Prize in public speaking, and the following year he was awarded the Dunn Premium for the student with the highest standing in rhetoric at Brown. In 1917, representing Brown, he won first place at an intercollegiate speaking contest at Harvard University.

Fisher graduated from Brown University in 1919 with a bachelor of arts degree, majoring in English and biology, for which he was awarded honors. While at Brown, he was elected to Phi Beta Kappa, and he spoke at the commencement ceremony. A year later, he received a master of arts degree from Brown.

In July 1919, he participated in a program in New York City titled "Four Negro Commencement Speakers," where he presented the award-winning speech that he had given at Brown, "The Emancipation of Science." In that speech, Fisher stated, "As thinking Christians, we strive not to bring men to heaven, but to bring heaven to men, and with that the aim of science is identical. It is the oneness of purpose that brings science and religion into harmony—a harmony which permits to devote its energies not to self-protection but to making of life worth living. Devoutly revering its supreme ruler, which is law; persistently upholding the principles of its savior, which is evolution; and constantly comforted by its holy spirit, which is truth, science is at least free to serve mankind."

One of the other speakers was the 1919 Rutgers graduate Paul Robeson, who would become a professional football player, lawyer, actor, singer, and political activist. Fisher and Robeson maintained a friendship. That summer, with Robeson singing arrangements by Fisher, who accompanied on the piano, they raised money for graduate school. Later, Fisher created a number of vocal arrangements for Robeson's first New York concert.

Fisher proceeded with his education by attending Howard University Medical School and graduated with highest honor in 1924. He was the recipient of a fellowship of the National Research Council and, for two years, conducted research at Columbia University's College of Physicians and Surgeons. He published two papers in distinguished, peer-reviewed journals on the treatment of bacteriophage and filterable viruses with ultraviolet light.

In 1927, he embarked on a private medical practice, initially on Long Island, and administered a private diagnostic radiology facility. In 1930, he assumed the positions of superintendent and chair of the Department of Roentgenology at the International Hospital, a privately owned hospital in Harlem. The facility went bankrupt in 1931, and Fisher returned to private practice. He died on December 26, 1934, after an operation for intestinal cancer, which may have been related to his extensive exposure to radiation.

Fisher's first published work, a short story titled "City of Refuge," appeared in the February 1925 edition of the *Atlantic Monthly* while he was conducting medical research. The story chronicled an initial optimism, replaced by the harsh reality, experienced by migrants in Harlem, which the author called "city of Satan." The story is interspersed with humor, affirming Langston Hughes's assessment: "The wittiest of these New Negroes of Harlem, whose tongue was flavored with the sharpest and wittiest humor, was Rudolph Fisher." The compendium *The New Negro*, which was published that year, included the story.

RUDOLPH JOHN CHAUNCEY FISHER

In 1926, Fisher received *Crisis* magazine's Amy Springarn Prize for fiction for his short story "High Yaller," which was published the previous year and addresses racial tensions between whites and blacks and within the African American community itself. The intra-racial conflicts between light-skinned and dark-skinned subsets, and the consequences, with legal and social ramifications, of a courtship between members of the two groups being misinterpreted as miscegenation are brought into focus.

"Ringtail" and "The South Lingers On" were also published in 1925, in the *Atlantic Monthly* and *Survey Graphic* respectively. Both short stories dramatize the travails and hopes of the newcomer to Harlem. "The South Lingers On" consists of five sketches that highlight the difficulties of communication between different, native urban Northerners and transplanted rural Southerners, and also between devoted parishioners and their detractors. In "Backslider," "Blades of Steel," and "Common Meter," melodramatic rifts within the Harlem community are brought into focus, against a background of the cabaret dance scene. In "Common Meter," the author dissects orchestrated jazz and the spiritual aspect of the blues.

"The Promised Land," "Guardian of the Law," and the last of Fisher's short stories to be published while he was alive, "Miss Cynthie," are concerned with transition and, at the same time, a desire to maintain an integrity with the heritage of the rural past. "John Archer's Nose" was published in *Metropolitan* magazine a month after Fisher died. In an essay, "The Caucasian Storms Harlem," Fisher notes that, toward the end of the 1920s, many of the Harlem cabarets and clubs were catering to a largely white clientele. In that work, he also laments the "Negro invasion of Broadway" and the tenor of African American stage productions.

The first of Fisher's two novels, *The Walls of Jericho*, was published in 1928 and presents a cross section of life in Harlem, which includes the white visitors. Nearly every class of society is profiled. The novel is satirical and sympathetically treats both the upper and lower classes of the ghetto, providing a sense of hope for black citizens in the urban North. The work is "a social novel with an upbeat ending in which the best elements of Harlem's upper crust ('dickties'), in the end, combine efforts with the lower strata ('rats') to combat organized crime and improve the community."

W. E. B. Du Bois, the African American sociologist and Pan-Africanist, criticized the work for presenting upper-class blacks as snobbish and lacking social concern. By contrast, Nathan Huggins, the W. E. B. Du Bois Professor of History and of Afro-American Studies at Harvard, stated that it "was the only novel in the decade to expose class antagonism among Harlem blacks."

Fisher's other novel, *The Conjure-Man Dies*, has been credited by Henry Louis Gates Jr. in *The Norton Anthology of African American Literature* as the first African American detective story with a black detective and an all-black cast of characters. This had recently been refuted by Stephen F. Soitos in *The Blues Detective: A Study of African American Detective Fiction*. That work contends that others have credited J. E. Bruce's *Black Sleuth*, which was serialized in *McGirt's Magazine* in 1907–1909, as the first detective novel written by an African American. Soitos provides evidence that *Hagar's Daughters* by Pauline Hopkins, published in the *Colored American Magazine* in 1901–1902, can claim primacy as the earliest known literature written by an African American and containing a black detective. Certainly, Fisher can be credited as the first African American author to have a detective novel published as a book.

Fisher uses his medical knowledge in his novel and incorporates black humor (a humorous way of looking at or treating something that is serious or sad). He emphasizes the capacity of individuals to laugh at themselves and at life in general, which is presented as the key to survival and social triumph. Just prior to his terminal illness, Fisher was converting *The Conjure-Man Dies* into a play. It was produced posthumously as part of the Federal Theater Project at Harlem's Lafayette Theater in 1936. Arthur P. Davis, an African American literary scholar, wrote in his review of the novel that it was "not merely a good 'Negro detective story,' but rather 'is a good detective story.'"

Considered to be one of the most talented writers of the Harlem Renaissance, Rudolph Fisher presented portraits and landscapes of African American encounters with urban issues. During a 1933 radio interview, he commented, "But, if I should be fortunate enough to become known as Harlem's interpreter, I should be very happy."

SOURCES

Encyclopedia.com, s.v. "Fisher, Rudolph 1897–1934." *Contemporary Black Biography*. Farmington Hills, MI: Thomson Gale, 2005. http://www.encyclopedia.com/topic/Rudolph_Fisher.aspx (accessed April 5, 2018).

Fisher, Rudolph, and John McCluskey. *The City of Refuge: The Collected Stories of Rudolph Fisher*. Columbia, MO: University of Missouri Press, 2008.

Gates, Henry Louis, and Valerie Smith. *The Norton Anthology of African American Literature*. New York: W. W. Norton, 2014.

Soitos, Stephen F. *The Blues Detective: A Study of African American Detective Fiction*. Amherst: University of Massachusetts Press, 1996.

36

MIKHAIL BULGAKOV

Prohibition from Print Transforms into Posthumous Adulation

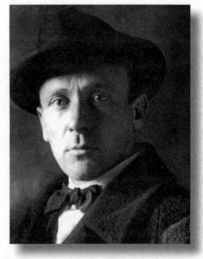

I n a consideration of modern Russian literature, the name of Mikhail Bulgakov has been placed by several critics at the same level as Nobel laureates Boris Pasternak and Aleksandr Solzhenitsyn. Bulgakov shared with those literary giants the restraints imposed on his publications by the Soviet censors. But unlike the others, Bulgakov, who created his masterpiece at a time that his works were banned, did not gain full recognition until twenty-six years after his death.

Bulgakov was born in Kiev, at the time part of the Russian empire, on May 15, 1891(Gregorian calendar). His father, Afanasy Bulgakov, was an assistant professor of comparative religion at the Kiev Theological Academy. Afanasy died of a kidney disease, nephrosclerosis, at age forty-eight when Mikhail was just fifteen years old. The same congenital disorder would claim Mikhail's life at about the same age as his father. After preliminary education at the First Kiev Gymnasium, despite an early interest in literature, Mikhail entered the medical school of the Saint Vladimir Imperial University of Kiev in 1909.

His attraction to medicine as a career may have come from his two maternal uncles, who were physicians. Mikhail's younger brother, Nikolai, became a renowned bacteriologist. Bulgakov's performance at medical school was compromised by his literary endeavors and his romantic involvement with a young lady, whom he married in 1913 after his second attempt to pass his second-year examinations succeeded (he failed his first attempt). In 1914, after World War I began, while still a student, he aided in treating the wounded at a Red Cross hospital at Saratov, a major port on the Volga River.

A year later, he received his degree of "doctor with honors" and was deployed to run several small hospitals near the front in Smolensk. His wife went along to aid him. While there, Bulgakov had to take an antidiphtheritic injection, which caused pain that he treated with morphine, a drug he became addicted to for one year. In September 1917, Bulgakov was transferred to Vyazma, where he was placed in charge of the infectious and venereal disease department.

In 1918, he was released from duties and returned home to Kiev, where he specialized in treating venereal diseases. A year later, the Soviet army captured Kiev. Bulgakov was mobilized and stationed in the small town of Vladikavkaz in the northern Caucasus. He immediately became acquainted with the local literary society there. At that location, his first published work, presenting a poor outlook for the country under Bolshevik rule, appeared in a newspaper. At a time that the Soviet Red Army was advancing on the town, Bulgakov contracted typhus and became seriously ill. This provided an excuse for him to end his medical career and devote himself to writing. While recovering from his illness, control of the town was taken over from the White Army by the Bolsheviks.

Bulgakov was given the position as "head of the literary section of the Arts Sub-department of the Revolutionary Committee." He opened the First Soviet Theatre of Vladikavkaz with a performance of Schnitzler's *The Green Parrot*, a play about the storming of the Bastille. Bulgakov became the head of the theater section of the department. He wrote several short plays, which were performed locally, and he wrote many feuilletons for newspapers in the Caucasus. Without any forewarning, all members of Bulgakov's Arts Department were fired, and he was forced to write and produce plays to generate an income.

None of the plays produced in Vladikavkaz gained permanence. Between 1920 and 1922, he wrote five plays, ranging from comedies to historical dramas. *The Turnbin Brothers* and *The Sons of the Mullah* were staged in Vladikavkaz. Both are family dramas that take place on the eve of the revolution and focus on the clash between cultures and generations. In 1923, after he had settled in Moscow, Bulgakov burned the manuscripts of all five plays.

He arrived in Moscow in the fall of 1921 and gained employment as secretary of LITO, the Literary and Publishing Section under the People's Commissariat of Enlightenment. That position was short-lived, and he moved on to work for a small newspaper. His writings were sporadically accepted by count-less diverse newspapers and magazines. His fame gradually grew based on those contributions. In 1923, he began to work for the periodical *Gudok*, and in the ensuing three years he contributed about one hundred feuilletons and rewrites.

Part 1 of an early Bulgakov work, "Notes on the Cuff," was published in the periodical *Nakanune*'s literary supplements in 1922. The work was autobio-graphical and dealt with the obstacles associated with literary apprenticeship. It was initially censored, removing references to typhus, famine, and political clashes, and was subsequently banned. His novel *Black Snow: A Theatrical Novel* is a continuance of the life of the same writer, from his early days to his theatrical debut. Bulgakov's feuilletons, which included some stories with medical themes, but, more often, a consideration of the negative aspects of bureaucracy, were not highly regarded. A collection of his stories titled *Diaboliad (Deviltries)*, which were critical of the Soviet Communist society, was published in 1925.

Bulgakov had started to work on a series of stories known collectively as *Notes of a Young Doctor* in 1919. They were not published until 1925–1927 when they were included in *The Medical Worker*. The underlying theme is nature versus civilization and his ambivalent attitude toward the Russian Revolution. They include a description of the gradual evolution of a young doctor.

Medicine pervades many of his works. Hospital and operating tables crop up repeatedly. Violence and disease are present. Syphilis and venereal disease are the most commonly presented physical diseases, but mental disease is more prominent. Doctors recur from his earlier writings, such as *Notes of a Young Doctor*, and continue through *The Master and Margarita*.

Bulgakov's most famous novella, *The Fatal Eggs*, first appeared in print in 1925. It is a satirical tale of a scientific experiment that goes awry in the future Soviet Republic of 1928. Among the targets of the prose are the journalists who reported on the experiments. Bulgakov respected science but was skep-tical about the societal consequences. There is, in this work, a Faustian theme of interference with the natural process. The theme of the misuse of science is amplified in *Heart of a Dog*, which contains a doctor hero and is an allegory about the dangers of societal revolution. Given the target of the satire, it is not surprising that the work was never published in the Soviet Union. *Heart of a Dog* was completed the same year and has been recognized as the best satirical novel of the Soviet period. An operation, which consists of the transplantation of the pituitary gland and testis of a recently deceased man to a mongrel dog, is central to the story.

The 1925 collection of stories *Diaboliad*, which included "Diaboliad," "No. 13. The Elpit-Rabkommun Building," "The Fatal Egg," "A Chinese Tale," and "The Adventures of Chichikov," was the sole bound volume containing Bulgakov's work to be published during his lifetime. Although the printing was only five thousand copies, it established the author's reputation as a talented modern writer.

The first parts of Bulgakov's novel *White Guard* were published in issues of the journal *Russia* in 1925. The last third of the work was never published, and the publication of the first parts contributed to the closing of the journal by the government. The partial publication was a sensation, and a complete Russian edition was published in Paris in 1929. *White Guard* is a historical novel about the civil war between the White and the Red Armies as it played out in Kiev, and was provocatively sympathetic to the White heroes. It is obviously autobiographical and includes as a central figure a former army doctor who is a venereologist. To Bulgakov, history is sequentially accidental, and all political change is ephemeral.

Bulgakov's reputation expanded from recognition to fame in 1926 when two of his plays, *Days of the Turbins* (a dramatization of the *White Guard*) and *Zoya's Apartment* premiered in Moscow. *Days of the Turbins* was an overwhelming success and was referred to as "the new *Seagull*," calling to mind Chekhov's triumphant drama. The play became one of the Moscow Art Theater's all-time moneymakers, and it was performed almost one thousand times between 1926 and 1941 despite many years of bans. A *New York Times* correspondent wrote, "The real interest for the audience lies in the fact that this is the first time since the revolution that the revolutionary period has been presented, so to speak, 'without prejudice' and as it really occurred."

Countering the successes of *Days of the Turbins* and *Zoya's Apartment* in 1927, that year and the following year were marked by an increasing number of political attacks on his works. Bulgakov was labeled a White Guardist by the ruling proletarians. The contract for the dramatization of *Heart of a Dog* was canceled, and his new play, *Flight*, was banned before its premiere. The play was never produced during Bulgakov's lifetime.

In 1928, *The Crimson Island*, Bulgakov's most spectacular play, appeared on the Russian stage. It was an expansion of a short story that the author had published in a periodical in 1924 and was a parody of the revolution. After a sensational premiere, it was criticized by Stalin for its political message, and banned in 1929. The work is a play about a play and shows how a work is censored and eventually banned in the Soviet Union.

In 1928, the political leaders in the Soviet Union adopted their first five-year plan, and this had a direct limiting effect on the world of Russian literature. All of Bulgakov's plays were banned, and the apolitical All-Russian Union of Writers, of which Bulgakov was a member, was disbanded. However, Stalin personally arranged for Bulgakov's appointment as an assistant director at the Moscow Art Theater and as a literary consultant for the Theater for the Working Youth; both were inconsequential positions but would provide an income for the destitute author.

In 1931, Bulgakov requested permission to temporarily leave Russia, but did not gain approval. He also failed to have his play *Adam and Eve* published or produced on the stage. It was created to make the point that all wars are wrong and to espouse pacifism. The play foresaw that the Fascists of Germany would become the major enemy of Russia. In 1932, the ban on *Days of the Turbins* was lifted after the play was changed to make it less provocative. To some extent, Stalin revived Bulgakov's career.

In 1933, Bulgakov signed a contract with the Leningrad Music Hall for a three-act play. His first offering was a revision of *Bliss*, which he had worked on years previously, and when that was deemed unpassable by the censors, he shifted to a new play, *Vasilievich*. Both plays used Jules Verne's vehicle of a time machine: in the case of *Bliss*, into the future, and for *Vasilievich*, into the past. Both plays were weak, and neither was performed on the Russian stage.

The play to which Bulgakov devoted much of his effort from its inception in 1929 was initially named *The Cabal of Hypocrites*, but was renamed *Molière* before the general public finally viewed it on February 21, 1936. It received a damning review in the major Soviet newspaper *Pravda*, and performances were terminated on March 9. Bulgakov, in protest, resigned from his position at the Moscow Art Theater in September.

As a consequence, he began work on the autobiographical narrative *Black Snow: A Theatrical Novel*. The work is essentially an in-joke about the literary and theatrical world in the Soviet Union in the 1920s and 1930s. Unfortunately, it was never completed. In 1934, Bulgakov began to draft a play about Russia's greatest poet, Alexander Pushkin, in anticipation of the one hundredth anniversary of the poet's death. The play was to have been staged in 1937 in Kiev, but, after the adverse comments about *Molière*, it was not shown until after Bulgakov died, at which time it appeared at the Moscow Art Theater, bearing the title *Last Days*.

In the latter half of the last decade of his life, Bulgakov was multitasking.

His income came from his position as a librettist for the Bolshoi Theater. That involved working on *Minin and Pozharsky* and starting the libretto for *Rachel*. In 1938, he worked on his play *Don Quixote*, which premiered in March 1941 after he died. In 1939, Bulgakov's main project was a play about Stalin and the beginning of his revolutionary activity. It bore the title *Batum*, for the city where the Russian leader set up a base for his activities in 1901. After plans were made for its premiere in Leningrad, the play was dropped. Throughout the final decade of his life, Bulgakov continued to work on *The Master and Margarita*.

In 1940, Bulgakov's kidney failure rapidly increased and he died on March 10. A guard of honor was established at the Union of Writers building. Groups from the literary world and the theater took shifts standing alongside the casket. A representative of the theater stated, "But the Art Theater knows that art is stronger than death—and for us Mikhail Afasasievich [Bulgakov] is a genuine knight of art."

The Master and Margarita is the major work responsible for Bulgakov's literary immortality. It has been listed as one of the best novels of the twentieth century and the greatest of the modern Russian satires. The first version of the novel was completed in 1928. That version was distinctly different from the final product and was destroyed by the author in 1930. Multiple versions ensued until Bulgakov's final days. In 1966, it was first published in censored form in the journal *Moskova*, and the first full text novel appeared as a book in the Soviet Union in 1973.

The novel presents two seemingly disparate but actually similar venues—contemporary Moscow and Pontius Pilate's Judea—in juxtaposition as a vehicle to critique the Soviet Union and its literary policies.

Bulgakov is memorialized by museums established in his residences in Moscow and Kiev. *The Master and Margarita* was an inspiration for Salman Rushdie's *The Satanic Verses* and the Rolling Stones' song "Sympathy for the Devil." As Bulgakov wrote in his masterpiece, "Manuscripts don't burn."

SOURCES

Encyclopaedia Britannica, s.v. "Mikhail Afanasyevich Bulgakov." Last updated March 3, 2018. http://www.britannica.com/EBchecked/topic/84062/ Mikhail-Afanasyevich-Bulgakov (accessed April 5, 2018).
Proffer, Ellendea. *Mikhail Bulgakov: Life and Works 1984*. Ann Arbor, MI: Ardis, 1984.

37

ARCHIBALD JOSEPH CRONIN
Profitable Prose with Social Consequence

T he medical background of A. J. Cronin, who was among the most widely read literary figures in the first half of the twentieth century, was integral to several of his most popular works. In addition to drawing from medicine to create literature, he uniquely produced literature that contributed to a radical change in the delivery of healthcare throughout Great Britain. From a youth characterized by "unbelievable hardship," Cronin achieved success as a physician before he abandoned medicine for an even more prominent and profitable literary career.

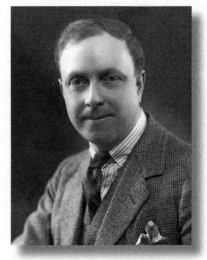

Photo by Bassano Ltd, courtesy of the National Portrait Gallery, London.

Archibald Joseph Cronin was born on July 19, 1896, in Cardross on the northern shore of the Firth of Clyde, about fifteen miles northwest of Glasgow, Scotland. His father was a Catholic mercantile agent, and his mother was a Protestant who converted to Catholicism. According to Alan Davies, one of Cronin's only two biographers, "To most neighbours and relatives in the relatively small, strictly moral and sternly Protestant town of Cardross, Jessie's [Cronin's mother] marriage and conversion were considered a disgrace, and upon her son they inflicted the inevitable ridicule and persecution."

Cronin, an only child, was eight years old when his father died of tuberculosis, and he, with his mother, moved to live with her poverty-stricken parents in Dumbarton. He attended Dumbarton Academy, where he excelled academically, particularly in literature. At age thirteen, he won the Gold Medal in a nationwide (Scotland) contest for the best historical novel. In 1912, Cronin entered St. Aloysius' Catholic School, and he continued to perform well. In 1914, he obtained a Carnegie Foundation Scholarship to study medicine at Glasgow University. Later in life, Cronin stated, "The Scottish view is very practical . . . there is always a choice, you can have medicine or you can have divinity! I chose the lesser evil."

Cronin interrupted his medical education in 1916 to join the Royal Navy Volunteer Reserves and served as a surgeon sublieutenant aboard a destroyer at Harwich. After one year of service, he returned to medical school and graduated with an MB ChB with honors in 1919. That year, he made a trip to India as a ship's surgeon. While at medical school, he met his future wife. The couple married in 1921.

That year, the newlyweds moved to the mining region of Rhondda Valley in Wales. Six months later, they left for a larger colliery town in the neighboring valley of Tredegar. While there, Cronin traveled weekly to Cardiff to prepare for additional graduate medical degrees. In 1923, he was awarded a diploma in public health; in 1924, a membership in the Royal College of Physicians; and, in 1925, an MD from the University of Glasgow for a dissertation titled "The History of Aneurysm." In 1924, he secured a governmental appointment as medical inspector of mines and proceeded to inspect miners throughout Great Britain. As a consequence, he published two significant papers: "Report on Dust Inhalation in Haematite Mines" and "Investigations in First-Aid Organizations in Great Britain."

In 1926, dissatisfied with his position as inspector of mines, Cronin purchased ownership of a medical practice in London. Over the ensuing four years, the practice flourished and provided a significant improvement in Cronin's financial status. In 1930, he developed a gastric ulcer, for which he required prolonged rest. Cronin wrote that "enforced rest would eat into my savings, and the prospect of returning to a profession I disliked would not hasten my recovery." He proceeded to sell his practice, made a permanent break from medicine, and was determined to become a successful author. The family initially rented Dalchenma Farm near Inverary in the Scottish Highlands, and, within three months, Cronin produced *Hatter's Castle*. While awaiting publication, Cronin moved once again, this time to Sussex.

His first novel was a sensational success. It received critical acclaim, as evidenced by Hugh Walpole's assessment in the *New York Herald Tribune* that it was "the finest novel since the war." It became a worldwide best seller and has been translated into many languages, and millions of copies have been sold. In 1942, it appeared as a motion picture. The novel's successful formula was a combination of action, tragedy, and treachery, played out by intriguing characters. From the first of his novels throughout the many that followed, Cronin brings doctors into the plot, and he reveals his broad knowledge of medicine. In *Hatter's Castle*, Dr. Laurie's lack of feeling and interest in financial gain is contrasted with Dr. Renwick's concern for his patients and his idealism.

Cronin's second novel, *Three Loves*, was published just one year after the first novel had appeared. The title refers to the tragic heroine's overly possessive love for her husband, her son, and her religion. The heroine is, arguably, Cronin's most memorable female character. The book generally received encouraging reviews and was thought to be more sophisticated than its predecessor.

Cronin's third novel, *Grand Canary*, which also took less than a year to produce, has been grouped with the first two to define the author's period of literary apprenticeship. During that time, Cronin wrote with the object of achieving popularity and attracting a readership. The drama, which relates the interplay of eight characters aboard a banana boat during a cruise to the Canary Islands, has as its protagonist an idealistic medical researcher in a state of despair. The work provided a vehicle for Cronin to express some of his own resentments against the medical world and its practices. *Grand Canary* was the first of many of Cronin's novels to be adapted to the screen.

The next of Cronin's novels, *The Stars Look Down*, is the most ambitious and intricate of his works and, as his first great literary triumph, initiated the author's best literary phase. The narrative drew from experiences that Cronin had encountered as a physician in the Welsh mining towns. It documents the hazards, including occupational diseases, to which miners are exposed.

The most popular of Cronin's novels, and the one to which social consequences have been assigned, is *The Citadel*. The "Citadel" refers to the medical competency and integrity that should characterize the medical profession. The book had particular appeal in the United States, where it won the National Book Award for Fiction in 1937, and, in 1939, a Gallup poll voted it the most interesting book readers had ever read. In 1938, it appeared as a motion picture, and, forty-five years later, it was aired as a serial dramatization by the BBC.

The tale of a well-trained, intelligent, and idealistic young doctor in a Welsh mining town traces his course, including his exposure to ignorance, medical incompetence, and indifference. He temporarily morphs into a financially driven practitioner, only to become purified, detaching himself from materialistic reward and returning to his original idealism. Both the American Medical Association and the British Medical Association issued statements that the novel presented an unfair representation of the profession and that it was akin to "mudslinging."

On the other hand, the press called for an immediate government inquiry and a reorganization of the medical services in Great Britain. Dr. Hugh Cabot of the Mayo Clinic wrote, "The book appears to be so important that I should be glad to believe that it would be at the disposal of every medical student and practitioner under thirty-five in this country."

Through the voice of his medical hero, Cronin calls for compulsory graduate courses for all medical practitioners, and for the encouragement of all practitioners toward research. He further encourages the development of group practices with specialization, more widespread accessibility of X-ray equipment, the establishment of rural hospitals, and decent hours and pay for nurses. He also champions the eradication of fee splitting (paying a referring physician for a referral), inappropriate large fees, unnecessary operations, needless medical interventions, and the touting of bogus health foods and therapies. The concerns found in *The Citadel* have been credited with playing a role in the creation of Britain's National Health System and also in the Labour Party's 1945 landslide victory.

Cronin's next novel, *The Keys of the Kingdom*, which was written while the author was residing in the United States and first published there in 1941, is a presentation of his concept of religion. Cronin, an observant Catholic, describes the expressions of faith of a saintly priest as contrasted with the dogma of the church. A poll conducted by the Book-of-the-Month Club listed the novel as the outstanding work of fiction of the year. The book set a record by appearing in the number one position on its first inclusion on the *New York Herald Tribune* best-seller chart. Although there was negative criticism by some members of the church, others strongly recommended it to both clergymen and parishioners. Literary critics considered it to be the summit of Cronin's productions. A contemporary review referred to the work as "a more appealing and more memorable book than any the author has written heretofore." In 1944, a motion picture that closely followed the narrative appeared. It had a successful reception and catapulted the career of a young Gregory Peck.

Cronin's next two novels, *The Green Years* and *Shannon's Way*, represent a continuum. *The Green Years* encompassed the ten years, from age eight to eighteen, of a Catholic orphan being brought up by his grandparents in a staunchly Protestant area of Scotland. The main character in this semiautobiographical novel is the object of ridicule and intolerance, and must contend with disappointment before emerging as a more mature young man, with renewed faith, about to enter medical school. The book broke all records for Little, Brown novels published up until 1944. It was a Premium Selection Book of the Book-of-the-Month Club.

In *Shannon's Way*, the man who was being considered at the end of *The Green Years* appears as a physician with a passion for research. He is thwarted by the academic establishment, by staff politics, and by an avaricious colleague. At the end, a promising future is made available for the protagonist's research and his life, in general. It is a tale of desperate struggles that are overcome by energetic perseverance and ingenuity.

Cronin's next novel, *The Spanish Gardner*, was published in 1950 and did not receive critical acclaim or attract a readership equivalent to his previous work. It did, however, follow the pattern of being adapted to the big screen.

Cronin's next publication, *Adventures in Two Worlds*, is often listed as a biography, but it is actually a series of reminiscences and reflections divided into four parts. The first two segments focus on the medical aspects of his life, student days in Scotland, and experiences at the mental hospital and the Rotunda Hospital in Dublin, where he studied obstetrics. The narrative continues to cover the mining communities in Wales. In the last two chapters, Cronin advocates for religion, promoting a "Supreme Intelligence," and offers philosophical considerations.

In 1939, Cronin had moved to America and considered it to be his residence until 1955, when he moved to Switzerland where he spent the last twenty-five years of his life. The last of his novels to be published while he lived in the United States was *Beyond This Place*. The work is a detective story that includes a depiction of legal and political corruption, and a hero's triumph over adversities. But Cronin did not recapture acclaim from literary critics until *A Thing of Beauty*, also published as *Crusader's Tomb*, appeared in 1956. This tale of a dedicated man who sacrifices everything else for art was, according to *Kirkus Reviews*, "the best thing Cronin has done since *Shannon's Way*."

The Northern Light, published in 1958, revolves around the newspaper publishing business and the competition for circulation. It was well received by the public, but critics were less enthusiastic than they had been for the immediately prior work. Similarly, in 1961, there was a lack of enthusiasm for *The Judas*

Tree, the story of a self-indulgent doctor. That work has been coupled with *A Song of Sixpence, A Pocketful of Rye* (sequel of the former), and *The Minstrel Boy* (*Desmonde*) in a consideration of Cronin's *Later Phase: Minor Fiction*. A reviewer of this group of novels, writing for the *New York Herald Tribune*, stated, "It is all too easy to deride the mountains of clichés, the stilted dialogue, the cardboard characters and the simple, uncomplicated emotions that have characterized the [later] novels. The fact remains that he is an immensely successful popular storyteller, whose novels are somehow immensely readable."

More recent audiences best relate to Cronin as "the Man Who Created Dr. Finlay." The long-running BBC radio and television series *Dr. Finlay's Casebook* was based on Cronin's stories that appeared in *Adventures in Two Worlds*, *Doctor Finlay of Tannochbrae*, and *Dr. Finlay's Casebook*. The popularity that Cronin enjoyed during his lifetime is attested to by the sale of over twenty million copies of his books. He was regarded as a major literary figure, who received DLitt degrees from Bowdoin College and Lafayette College. He died in Glion, Switzerland, on January 6, 1981, and was buried in Montreux. The headstone offers the simple inscription "Author of the *Keys of the Kingdom*."

SOURCES

Davies, Alan. *A. J. Cronin: The Man Who Created Dr. Finlay*. Richmond, London: Alma Books, 2011.

Review of *A Thing of Beauty*, by A. J. Cronin. *Kirkus Reviews*. 1956. https://www .kirkusreviews.com/book-reviews/a-j-cronin-2/a-thing-of-beauty/ (accessed May 4, 2018).

Salwak, Dale. *A. J. Cronin*. Boston: Twayne Publishers, 1985.

38

AUSTIN MERRILL MOORE

Respected Psychiatrist and Persistent Poet

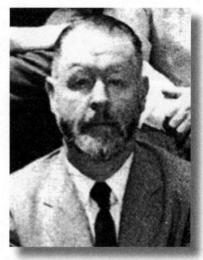

It is highly probable that Merrill Moore's (as he was usually known) poetic productivity is unmatched by any physician, and it is certain that no psychiatrist can lay claim to an equivalent number of published sonnets. William Carlos Williams (see chapter 33), Moore's contemporary poet and physician, unlike most critics, commended Moore's verse. The predominantly negative criticism of Moore's poetry is to be contrasted with the unqualified positive reputation he enjoyed as a psychiatrist.

Austin Merrill Moore was born on September 11, 1903, in Columbia, Tennessee. His father, John Trotwood Moore, was a licensed lawyer who never practiced, but he was one of the leading literary figures in Tennessee. John was a prominent regional novelist, historian, poet, journalist, and magazine editor. From 1949 until his death in 1957, he served as state librarian for Tennessee, and, during his later years, he was that state's poet laureate.

Merrill Moore attended the Montgomery Bell Academy for boys in grades seven through twelve in Nashville. That institution, after which the school in the film *Dead Poets Society* was patterned, does not list Moore as one of its distinguished alumni, but, while a student at the academy, Moore first demonstrated his aptitude for composing sonnets.

He continued his education at Vanderbilt University and received his bachelor's degree in 1924. At Vanderbilt, Moore was an active participant in the Fugitives, a group of poets and literary scholars who took their name from the literary journal *The Fugitive,* to which they contributed. The journal is regarded as being one of the most influential forces in the American literary world. Its contributors included John Crowe Ransom, Allen Tate, Donald Davidson, William Ridley Wills, Walter Clyde Cutty, Laura Riding, and Robert Penn Warren, in addition to Moore.

Moore published sixty-two poetic pieces, mostly sonnets, under the pseudonym "Dendric," in the journal. He remarked of his fellow Fugitives, "We all influenced each other; we all rubbed the edges off each other and knocked sparks out of each other in a peculiar way." Moore was among the younger members of the group, and his style never resembled any other member.

In spite of his father's urging that he become a journalist, Moore opted for a career in medicine, graduating from Vanderbilt University in 1928 with a degree in medicine. After graduating, he spent a year as a rotating intern at St. Thomas Hospital in Nashville. In 1929, he renounced the Southern social and attitudinal standards, developed an estrangement from the Fugitives, and moved to Boston, where he remained for the rest of his life, with the exception of time spent in military service in World War II.

In Boston, he was a resident in neurology at the Boston City Hospital prior to 1932 when he entered psychiatric training as a house officer at the Boston Psychiatric Hospital. Subsequently, he was appointed Commonwealth Fellow in Psychiatry at Harvard Medical School. In 1935, he entered private practice in Boston. During his practice, he cared for Robert Frost and advised Frost on medical care for two of Frost's troubled children. Frost described Moore as a "serious physician." While maintaining an active practice, Moore served as professor of neurology at the Boston City Hospital, where he conducted research on alcoholism, drug addiction, and suicide.

Moore was among the first to attribute a psychological basis to alcoholism. He was a frequent contributor to the *American Journal of Psychiatry.* His bibliography lists 143 medical articles published in peer-reviewed journals. Among the diverse subjects of his publications were alcoholism, the significance of alcoholism in criminals, treatment of schizophrenia, electroconvulsive therapy, "Multiple Therapy in Private Psychiatric Practice," psychosurgery, issues about the psychopathic personality, "American Literature and the Dream," "Some Psychiatric Considerations Concerning Creative Writing and Criticism," "Insanity, Art, and Culture," and "Shell Collecting as Occupational Therapy for Psychiatric Patients."

During World War II, Moore served in the Pacific theater, earning a bronze star and an Army Commendation Medal. While in service, he was also a personal physician to China's General Chiang Kai-Shek. After the war, Moore played a significant role in the concerted efforts of literary men and women that resulted in Ezra Pound avoiding a treason trial for propaganda in support of Fascism.

Moore's first published poem was titled "Dendric," the pen name that he used early in his literary career. It celebrates the art of the black African. During his six years of literary activity in Nashville, he was considered to be a rebel among his group of fellow "Fugitives." The first collection of his poems to be published, *The Noise That Time Makes*, appeared in 1929.

Six years later, after the second book of Moore's sonnets, *Six Sides to a Man*, was published, an article titled "Books: Doctor's Output" appeared in *Time* magazine. It began, "When Poet-Critic Louis Untermeyer went through Dr. Merrill Moore's filing cabinet, he counted approximately 25,000 idiomatic, hybrid or 'American' sonnets. Some were bad, some good; some had been printed in Walter Winchell's column, some had appeared in the Boston Evening Transcript [an afternoon newspaper], some in Harriet Monroe's *Poetry: A Magazine of Verse*. To conceive of the tremendous industry that could turn out 25,000 sonnets," says Mr. Untermeyer, "one must think of the author as a pundit, an immured octogenarian, devoting all his hours to fashioning and perfecting his inflexible models." Nothing could be further from the truth.

Untermeyer's categorizing of Moore's sonnets as idiomatic or hybrid relates to Moore's creation of a distinct sonnet form, one that differs from the traditional sonnets of Plutarch or Shakespeare. The standard fourteen-line form was altered by Moore to feature loose, conversational rhythms and syncopated rhymes.

In 1938, consequent to the publication of Moore's third volume of sonnets, *M: One Thousand Autobiographical Sonnets*, the *New Yorker* magazine featured an article, "Annoyingly Fertile." The article reads,

Talk story about Dr. Merrill Moore, the most prolific sonnet writer who ever lived. The score is 50,000; Tasso [the greatest Italian poet of the late Renaissance], 1000-odd. Harcourt Brace has just published a selection of Dr. M's sonnets. The book is called "M" because the letter is both the Roman numeral for one thousand and his initial. Dr. Moore lectures in neurology at the Harvard Medical School and also has a private practice. He says sonnet-writing is an outlet. One rainy day in '35 he wrote 98. He carries a pocket full of filing cards and jots down sonnets in shorthand as fast as they occur. Almost never corrects them. The shorthand are read into a dictaphone and his secretary transcribes them. His wife indexes and files them away in cabinets. The Doctor has 12 cases so far.

On the occasion of the publication of a brief biography of Moore in 1955, it was pointed out that no other member of the American Psychiatric Association had had a book-length biography written about him or her during his or her life. His sole biographer, Henry Wells, profiles Moore as "an urbane pantheist, a reasonable mystic, a civilized Walt Whitman, a humane artist, and a sympathetic physician."

Moore's sonnets, which number between fifty thousand and a half million, are of unequal merit. Some of the best contain weak lines, while some of the worst have sparks that are exciting. The sonnets are rarely included in modern anthologies because they are more objective than subjective. His works do analyze the mind, soul, and heart, but usually in an indistinct manner. He studies hope, fear, passion, depression, childhood, old age, morbidity, and death, but with little depth or transparency.

Moore was singularly productive, but the productivity was offset by a lack of his personal, careful refinement of the lines he produced. And the publicity, which he or his publishers continually generated, focused on volume produced rather than the messages promulgated. He is regarded as having been a highly unusual poet whose reputation is compromised by the disputable quality of his verse.

Considering what some have described as his "fecundity," Moore wrote, "If I don't write to empty my mind, I go mad. As to that regular, uninterrupted love of writing . . . I do not understand it. I feel it as a torture, which I must get rid of, but never as a pleasure. On the contrary, I think composition a great pain."

SOURCES

Wells, Henry W. *Poet & Physician: Merrill Moore.* New York: Privately printed at the Dolmen Press, 1955.

39

FRANK GILL SLAUGHTER

Short on Surgery, Long on Literature

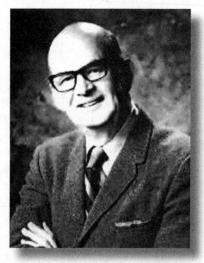

The only best-selling novelist who could claim what are currently regarded to be complete qualifications for surgery used those qualifications for a brief medical career. But his medical background and knowledge are infused throughout much of his literary output.

The widely read novelist, who wrote mainly as Frank G. Slaughter and occasionally as C. V. Terry, was born Frank Gill Slaughter on February 25, 1908, in Washington, DC. Before he was six years old, his family moved to a farm near Berea, North Carolina, where his father worked the farm and delivered the rural mail. Frank was educated in the local schools before entering Trinity College, which became the undergraduate school for men within Duke University when the latter was established in 1924.

Slaughter earned a bachelor's degree when he was seventeen. Further evidence of his scholasticism was election to the honorary society Phi Beta Kappa. He continued his education at Johns Hopkins University, where he earned a doctor of medicine degree in 1930, and then on to surgical training at the Jefferson Hospital in Roanoke, Virginia. In 1934, Slaughter and his family moved to Jacksonville, Florida, where he lived for the remainder of his long life, with the exception of military service during World War II.

Between 1935 and 1942, Slaughter served as a surgeon on the staff of St. Vincent's Riverside Hospital. In 1938, he became a fellow in the American College of Surgeons, and, two years later, he passed the examinations that allowed him to be certified by the American Board of Surgery. The unusual, reversed sequence of those memberships is related to the fact that the American Board of Surgery was not officially organized until 1937.

In 1935, while carrying out his commitments as a staff surgeon, Slaughter purchased a sixty-dollar typewriter on an installment plan for five dollars a month so that he could pursue an interest in writing. For five years, he wrote about one hundred thousand words per year and sold only one short story to the *Chicago Daily News* for twelve dollars. After four rejections and five rewrites, his first novel, *That None Should Die*, was published in 1941. In that work, a young idealistic surgeon comes to grips with personal tragedy, medical quackery, and political intrigue. Congress passes a law to bring medicine and physicians under central control, and the young surgeon finds himself in the middle of a national medical scandal.

The book was a moderate success in the United States, but a best seller in the Scandinavian countries, particularly Denmark. By the 1970s, it had been translated into fifteen languages and had undergone nine paperback printings. One reviewer stated, "It is a story no layman could have told—that no layman, for that matter, would have been justified in trying to tell."

Thirty-one years later, at a time when Frank G. Slaughter had ceased practicing medicine and become a popular novelist with many books to his credit, he presented a paper as part of a *Conference on Ambulatory Care Services*, held by the Committee of Public Health of the New York Academy of Medicine. It was titled "A Functional Model for Improving the Medical Care System," the concept of which had been appended to *That None Should Die* and was integral to the novel.

Slaughter's paper proposed that doctors organize themselves into group clinics with competent diagnosticians and specialists, subject to standards set by the American Medical Association. All treatment required referral to the clinics with the exception of tuberculosis and the mentally ill. The internists in the clinics were to be family doctors in the sense that they would make outside calls when necessary. In sparsely populated areas, dispensaries would be maintained.

The population was to be divided into three groups. The Low-Income Group would be cared for by the state and local governments that would require more expenditure of tax money. Their medical care was to be equivalent to all others, but the Low-Income Group members are required to attend the clinic in their district at certain specified times, except in the case of an emergency. The Medium-Income Group would be covered by a system of health insurance collected from their income that was turned over to a state insurance commission. The clinics would be reimbursed for service by the state insurance fund. Patients in this category could attend any clinic in the state or, by special arrangement, in another state. Patients in the High-Income Group could go anywhere since they provided for their own medical care. They could arrange for their own insurance coverage.

When the novel containing the plan was published in 1941, it was denounced as medical heresy by organized medicine, and the author was declared a "medical Bolshevik." Over the years, Slaughter maintained the practicality of the plan with the one modification of substituting "capitation" for "fee-for-service." He also predicted that the plan would provide for the development of preventive medicine.

During the war, Slaughter served in the US Army Medical Corps, enlisting as a major in 1942 and attaining the rank of lieutenant colonel. He sailed for Manila as chief surgeon aboard the hospital ship *Emily H. M. Weder*. Before he was discharged, four more of his novels were published. After his discharge, Slaughter returned to Jacksonville and ended his surgical career in order to devote his time to literary activity.

Most of Slaughter's fifty-eight books are related to medicine, in some manner. In *The Road to Bithynia*, he deals with Luke, physician to Paul and the patron saint of medicine, and describes the medical training that was carried out during Jesus's time. In *The Galileans*, he depicts the medical school and the great library of Alexandria in the first century AD, and describes the plastic surgical techniques imported from ancient India and the treatment of goiter with seaweed, which were used at that time. In *Divine Mistress*, centered around Andreas Vesalius, the story of the author of *De Humani Corporis Fabrica* in 1543 and the father of modern anatomy is told.

Sangaree, which was published in 1946 and appeared on the motion picture screen in 1953, is a historical romance that takes place on a Georgia plantation in the post–American Revolutionary years, and contains several medical incidents, including the advent of a bubonic plague. Medically related books range from *Doctor's Wives*, which considers the problems and consequences associated with physicians' inattention to their spouses, to *Surgeon's Choice: A Novel of Tomorrow*, which deals with the problems physicians encounter in the modern practice of medicine.

Slaughter published several biblically or historically based novels, often assisted by playwright, novelist, and editor William DuBois. *The Song of Ruth* and *Constantine: The Miracle of the Flaming Cross* are considered to be among the best in this category. Slaughter explained his approach to historical fiction this way: "First, I contract with the reader to tell a moving and absorbing story. Second, I write about real people whenever possible, depicting them exactly as my research, which must be extensive, shows them to have been. Third, I portray historical events exactly as they happened according to available information. This technique of what might be called truth-in-fiction requires much more work than is usually put in the average historical novel, but I long ago decided not to settle for less."

Five of Slaughter's novels—*Buccaneer Surgeon, Darien Venture, Buccaneer Doctor, The Golden Ones,* and *The Deadly Lady of Madagascar*—were published under his pseudonym "C. V. Terry." In addition, Slaughter authored three works of nonfiction: *Immortal Magyar: Semmelweis, the Conqueror of Childbed Fever; The New Science of Surgery;* and *Medicine for Moderns: The New Science of Psychosomatic Medicine.*

The New Science of Surgery covers the use of new anesthetics, war surgery, gas gangrene, peritonitis, embolism, neurosurgery, psychosurgery, plastic and burn surgery, cancer, plasma to conquer shock, and new antibiotics to treat infection. *Medicine for Moderns*, written for the laity, considers how emotions induce physical change, how childhood conflicts affect later life, the effect of emotional factors on heart disease, intestinal disorders, diabetes, asthma, migraine, and allergies. New therapies are included.

Frank G. Slaughter, to whom the quote "Seek truth and you will find a path" has been ascribed, died on May 17, 2001, after a prolonged illness. His last novel, *Transplant*, was published in 1987. His popularity is confirmed by sales that exceed fifty million copies and by the fact that most of his novels remain in print.

SOURCES

"A Functional Model for Improving the Medical Care System." *Bulletin of the New York Academy of Medicine* 49, no.5 (May 1973): 361–75.

Lewis, Paul. "Frank Slaughter, Novelist of Medicine, Is Dead at 93." *New York Times,* May 23, 2001.

40

LEWIS THOMAS
Dual Distinction

The name Thomas is the Greek form of an Aramaic name that means "twin." It is a most appropriate surname for Lewis Thomas, who gained equivalent distinction in medicine and in literature. In medicine, Thomas was the triple threat who progressed from basic research, to leadership as a clinician, to apices of leadership of two medical schools and a distinguished medical institute. In literature, he won two National Book Awards.

Lewis Thomas, the son of a general practitioner and a nurse, was born in Flushing, New York, on November 25, 1913. At the age of fifteen he matriculated at Princeton University, where his aca-

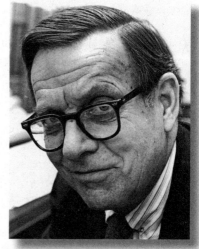

Photo courtesy of Yale University, Harvey Cushing / John Hay Whitney Medical Library.

demic performance was mediocre. In 1986, his alma mater named a biomedical laboratory for him. Thomas graduated from Harvard Medical School in 1937 and interned at the Boston City Hospital. During his internship, he published several poems, mainly about medical experiences, in the *Atlantic Monthly*, *Harper's Bazaar*, and the *Saturday Evening Post*. He proceeded to complete a residency in neurology at the Columbia Presbyterian Medical Center in 1941.

Thomas was appointed the first Tilney Fellow in Neurology at Columbia with the understanding that he would spend a year at the Thorndike Memorial Laboratories of the Boston City Hospital, working on the treatment of meningococcal meningitis, and return to New York as the chief resident at the Neurological Institute. He never returned to the Neurological Institute but was mobilized in 1942 after the United States entered World War II as part of a naval research unit at the Rockefeller Institute Hospital, where he studied streptococcal infection and rheumatic fever, in addition to other infectious diseases. For a year, beginning in December 1944, his unit was stationed on Guam and Okinawa, where he worked on a malignant form of encephalitis and conducted experiments to demonstrate an association between streptococci and the development of rheumatic heart disease.

The next segment of Thomas's life characterizes him as an upwardly mobile academician on a fast track. His first appointment was at the Johns Hopkins Hospital in the infectious disease section of the Department of Pediatrics. In 1948, he took charge of the new research division of microbiology and immunology in the Department of Medicine at Tulane University in New Orleans. From 1950 until 1954, he was chair of pediatrics and medicine at the Heart Hospital attached to the University of Minnesota.

His tenure at the New York University School of Medicine began with an appointment as chair of the Department of Pathology in 1954. Four years later, after transforming that department to one that was recognized for fundamental research, he shifted to the chair of medicine and became the director of the New York University medical division in Bellevue Hospital. In 1956, he had been appointed to the New York City Board of Health, on which he served for fifteen years. From 1966 through 1969, he served as dean of the New York University School of Medicine.

In 1971, Thomas became chair of pathology at Yale Medical School, and, a year later, he was named dean of that school. In 1973, he became the president of the Memorial Sloan-Kettering Cancer Center in New York. Over the course of his medical career, he was held in high regard for his research, which formed the basis of over two hundred scientific publications. He was honored with membership in the American Academy of Arts and Sciences and the National Academy of Science. At a symposium held in his honor, he was referred to as the "father of modern immunology and experimental pathology."

In 1971, Thomas began writing a monthly essay under the heading "Notes of a Biology Watcher" in the *New England Journal of Medicine*. In 1974, twenty-nine of those essays were compiled and published in a volume titled *The Lives of a Cell: Notes of a Biology Watcher*. The first essay, which provided the volume's title, draws an analogy between the cell with its components and planet earth and its occupants. As John Updike wrote in a 1974 essay in the *New Yorker*, "Dr. Thomas has the mystic's urge toward total unity." The book was also reviewed by Joyce Carol Oates, who was effusive in her praise and used the essays as examples of laudable structure and style. The book was translated into eleven languages and sold over a quarter of a million copies. In 1975, it was awarded the National Book Award for arts and letters, after it had also been considered in the category of science.

Four years later, Thomas's second collection of essays, *The Medusa and the Snail: More Notes of a Biology Watcher*, was published. It also contained twenty-nine essays that had appeared in the *New England Journal of Medicine*. The title essay uses the symbiotic relationship between a jellyfish (the medusa) and a sea slug (the snail) to discuss the concept of "the self" and "the other."

One review stated, "He [Thomas] has this facility for taking the darker sides of human existence—whether they be death, disease, fear, worry, or just plain warts—and turning them to the light." Noted biologist Stephen Jay Gould, writing in the *New York Times*, critiqued, "Dr. Thomas's musings radiate with two features, both rare and worth treasuring. He has a vision—a kind and humane vision—and visions are in dreadfully short supply in an intellectual world of intense specialization and cynicism. More important, he maintains an undiminished sense of wonder before nature—the ultimate antidote to human folly."

The Medusa and the Snail won the Christopher Award, given by the Christophers, a Christian organization, for works that "affirm the highest values of the human spirit," and the American Book Award "for outstanding literary achievement."

In *Late Night Thoughts on Listening to Mahler's Ninth Symphony*, a collection of twenty-four essays, Thomas expresses his concern for the fate of the planet. The essays include concerns regarding nuclear warfare and worldwide tensions that interfere with the pleasures of listening to classical music. Various essays also address the state of psychiatry, scientific research, and language.

Published the same year in 1983, *The Youngest Science: Notes of a Medicine Worker* is a selective autobiography of Thomas's life. Stephen Jay Gould, in the *New York Review of Books*, wrote, "Thomas's essays are unsurpassed for their uncanny knack of starting with a simple fact, a bit of home-grown Yankee wisdom, and slyly developing its implications until some profound truth slips through before you hardly notice."

Et Cetera, Et Cetera: Notes of a Word-Watcher is a collection of forty essays in which Thomas traces over seven hundred English words to their etymological roots. He muses on the development of a universal language.

Thomas's last publication, *The Fragile Species*, is kaleidoscopic. It brings to readers' attention evolutionary biology, the time of the plague, the phenomenon of aging, the fear of dying, and some of the medical problems with which we are currently confronted. Historian of molecular biology Horace Freeland Judson indicated, "But this is Lewis Thomas with a difference, for his passionate concern with the state of the species and the biosphere has deepened." The *New England Journal of Medicine Review* concluded, "*Fragile Species* is required reading. It belongs in the book bag of every medical student and on the night table of every physician."

Thomas died on December 3, 1993, of a rare non-Hodgkin lymphoma. An obituary referred to him as "the poet-philosopher of medicine . . . whose essays clarified the mysteries of biology." He is memorialized by the Lewis Thomas Prize, awarded annually by the Rockefeller University to a scientist for artistic achievement.

SOURCES

Berger, Marilyn. "Lewis Thomas, Whose Essays Clarified the Mysteries of Biology, Is Dead at 80." *New York Times*, December 4, 1993. http://www.nytimes.com/1993/12/04/obituaries/lewis-thomas-whose-essays-clarified-the-mysteries-of-biology-is-dead-at-80.html?pagewanted=all- (accessed April 5, 2018).

Thomas, Lewis. *The Youngest Science: Notes of a Medicine-Watcher*. New York: Viking, 1983.

Woodlief, Ann. "Lewis Thomas (25 November 1913–3 December 1993)." *Twentieth-Century American Nature Writers: Prose*, vol. 275, *Dictionary of Literary Biography* (Farmington Hills, MI: Gale Group, 2003). https://www.vcu.edu/engweb/LewisThomas.htm (accessed April 5, 2018).

41

WALKER PERCY

Northern Cure Transforms Career of Southern Writer

Walker Percy followed the pattern of the previously considered John Keats, Robert Bridges, Francis Brett Young, and A. J. Cronin for whom illness played a role in the termination of their abbreviated medical careers, thereby allowing their energies to be devoted to literary contributions. In the case of Percy, it was during a two-year period, when his tuberculosis was treated at the Trudeau Institute in the Adirondack Mountains in northern New York State, that enforced leisure and consequent reading and reflection redirected the young physician to an interest in philosophy and semiotics. These interests found expression in highly regarded diverse contributions to literature.

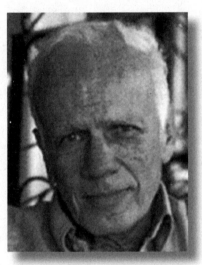

Photo by Rhoda K. Faust, Maple Street Book Shop, New Orleans, LA.

Percy was born in 1916 in Birmingham, Alabama, and was given the name of his paternal grandfather, a distinguished citizen of the community who committed suicide by shooting himself within a year of his grandson's birth. In 1929, while Percy and one of his younger brothers were at camp in Wisconsin, they received word that their forty-year-old father, who was a successful lawyer, had shot himself and died. Walker's mother and her three sons moved to Athens, Georgia, and settled in her family home. After spending one year as a student at

Athens High School, Walker moved with his mother and two brothers to Greenville, Mississippi, at the invitation of their bachelor second cousin, William Alexander Percy, known as "Uncle Will," who was revered as the son of a US senator, a decorated officer in World War I, and a poet.

Walker would credit Uncle Will with providing the major influence during the period of his youth. Almost immediately upon his arrival, Walker established what would become a lifelong friendship with historian Shelby Foote. As a high school student, Percy was exposed to Carl Sandburg, Stephen Vincent Benét, and Vachel Lindsay, all of whom stayed at the Percy house in Greenville. Walker's first published work, a short story, appeared in his school newspaper, *The Pica*, in 1930. His second published article, "The Passage of Arthur," also written as a high school student, would later provide the title for his fourth novel, *Lancelot*.

In March 1932, tragedy once again struck the young Percy. His mother, with his youngest brother as a passenger, plunged her car from a wooden bridge into a creek. Percy's mother died while his ten-year-old brother survived after attempting to save his mother. Throughout his life, Percy believed that his mother committed suicide. Uncle Will formally adopted the three boys. During his senior year at high school, Percy was awarded first- and fourth-place honors for his poetry by the Mississippi High School Press Association.

In 1933, Percy entered the University of North Carolina. Four years later, he received a bachelor of arts degree. His academic performance was excellent as evidenced by his election to Phi Beta Kappa. He chose to enter medical school after rejecting further studies for a career as a lawyer or in the clergy. As he later stated in an interview, "Medicine was left as the obvious last resort." From 1937 through 1941, Percy resided at Bard Hall, while he studied medicine at Columbia University College of Physicians and Surgeons. During his studies, he developed an interest in pathology. While a student, he underwent two years of Freudian psychoanalysis with a psychiatrist, mainly related to the feelings generated by his father's suicide and what Walker considered to be the suicidal death of his mother. Percy graduated twenty-fifth in a class of 104 students.

He placed first in a competitive examination for an internship on the Columbia division of Bellevue Hospital in New York City. The internship began in January 1944, and in the interval between graduation and that time, Percy worked as a physician at a clinic in Greenville. During that experience, he met his future wife, who was studying to become a medical technician. Between January and March, Percy, as an intern, performed about 125 autopsies on patients with tuberculosis and also cared for patients with the disease. The practice throughout the country, at the time, was that the examinations and autopsies were performed without the use of masks and rubber gloves. This resulted in the frequent contraction of tuberculosis by medical personnel and an eventual mandate for personnel to wear masks and gloves when performing autopsies.

Percy was one of many physicians in training when he was diagnosed, just six months after beginning his internship, as having contracted tuberculosis. He was initially admitted to Bellevue Hospital and treated with a pneumothorax to rest the involved lung. In September, he moved to the Trudeau sanatorium to complete a cure. At the time, before the advent of specific antibiotic therapy, treatment consisted of rest, good nutrition, and exposure to clean, cool, dry air. As Walker later wrote, "I was in bed so much, alone so much, that I had nothing to do but read and think. . . . I gradually began to realize that as a scientist—a doctor, a pathologist—I knew so very much about man, but had little idea what man is."

He delved into European existentialism through the works of Dostoevsky, Tolstoy, Kierkegaard, Heidegger, Marcel, Sartre, Mann, and Camus. Walker left Trudeau for New York City in the fall of 1944, but the cure for his tuberculosis was not complete. In 1945, he spent 136 days at the Gaylord Farm Sanatorium in Connecticut. Decades after his cure was complete, Percy would remark, "I was the happiest man ever to contract tuberculosis, because it enabled me to get out of Bellevue and quit medicine."

He initially returned to Greenville in 1946, but after marrying in November and vacationing in August 1947, he moved to New Orleans, where he and his wife started taking religious instruction. In December, the couple was baptized as Catholics. Shortly after Percy settled in New Orleans, he began work on his first novel, *The Charterhouse*, which was submitted for publication in 1953, but was never accepted. An editor referred to that novel as an uneven work of Catholic fiction showing flashes of great talent coupled with serious weaknesses.

Percy's second novel, *The Gramercy Winner*, which replicated Thomas Mann's *The Magic Mountain* by its depiction of a young man recovering from tuberculosis, was rejected by all the publishers to whom it was submitted. At the same time, several of Percy's essays appeared in print. In the periodical *Thought*, he reviewed Susanne Langer's *Feeling and Form*, in which the general thesis is that the peculiar human response is one of symbolic transformation, and that the art symbol conveys its own meaning. According to Percy, symbolization was the essential act of the mind.

His first philosophical essay, "Symbol as Hermeneutic in Existentialism," appeared in the journal *Philosophy and Phenomenological Research*. He contends that symbolization was a universal and unique human response that provided a bridge between empiricism and existentialism. In another essay, "Stoicism in the South," which appeared in *Commonwealth*, Percy argues that the former relationship between blacks and whites in the South, which was based on mutual respect, had disappeared. He opines that blacks had a "sacred right" to be treated as equals.

In "The Coming Crisis in Psychiatry," Percy considers, "Is psychiatry a biological science in which man is treated as an organism, with instinctive drives and needs not utterly or qualitatively different from those of other organisms? Or is psychiatry a humanistic discipline which must take into account of man as possessing a unique destiny by which he is oriented in a wholly different direction?" In "Semiotic and a Theory of Knowledge," Percy describes the processes of understanding words, and relating a certain word to a certain object. He states that "unless a person says that a certain word is a certain object, that person will never know the word or the object." In "The Southern Moderate," he offers proposals concerning segregation, contending there was no quick solution and that the solution should be based on sociological analysis.

In the spring of 1959, Percy submitted a novel titled *Confessions of a Movie-Goer* to a well-known literary agent, who, in turn, sent it to a publishing house, which had published works by Percy's uncle Will. Multiple and extensive revisions were carried out by the author over the ensuing year and a half, during which several of Percy's essays were published. "The Culture Crisis" offered evidence that the state of the world was very unfavorable and that the situation was not being appropriately discussed. "The Message in the Bottle" is a dialogue between an island castaway and a scientist, focusing on the relationship between faith and knowledge. "Naming and Being," a contribution to the field of semiotics, stresses the importance of the copula (the linguistic term for the word that creates a pairing between the subject of a sentence with a predicate, i.e., subject complement).

In May 1961, bearing the new title of *The Moviegoer*, Percy's first successful effort in the realm of fiction was published. The existentialist tale of despair, but with hope, takes place in post–Korean War New Orleans. "It is a novel about a young New Orleans war veteran of good family, now in a good job, disenchanted with life, who goes to the movies as one might take a drug to deaden the realities of life. . . . The novel is the story, principally, of how he and a girl—his cousin, who is unhappy and maladjusted for other reasons—finally come together and how he gives up his drifting and goes to medical school."

The novel won the National Book Award in 1962. It was later included in *Time* magazine's one hundred best English-language novels from 1923 to 2005. The Modern Library would rank *The Moviegoer* sixtieth on its list of the hundred best English-language novels of the twentieth century.

Percy continued to divide his literary efforts between fiction and nonfiction. In the 1965 issue of *Harper's*, he published an article titled "Mississippi: The Fallen Paradise," in which he extolls the heroic contributions of James Meredith and Medgar Evers to the civil rights movement. In 1966, Percy's novel *The Last Gentleman* appeared in print.

In that work, the pattern of *The Moviegoer* is replicated, in that the protagonist is a young, aimless man from an old Southern family. In this case, he has moved north and suffers from both amnesic spells as well as episodes of déjà vu. A chance viewing through a telescope brings the young dislocated man into the complicated structure of a New York family. The work was nominated for the National Book Award and received praise from Joyce Carol Oates, who wrote that it "is one no critic should want to swipe at, for it is rare to encounter a work engaging in nearly every line."

While the main character of *Love in the Ruins: The Adventures of a Bad Catholic at a Time Near the End of the World*, Percy's third novel, is similar to those in his previous novels, in that the protagonist evidences alienation and existential doubt, the book is somewhat of a departure in that it contains elements of science fiction. In the novel, Dr. Thomas More, a descendant of Sir Thomas More, the author of *Utopia*, is a psychiatrist in the small town of Paradise, Louisiana, who is exposed to a highly fragmented community in a nation that has become significantly polarized between left and right, black and white, and in religious and social issues. Dr. More, who is a lapsed Catholic, an alcoholic, and a womanizer, has invented a device that can diagnose and treat the mental disintegration that fostered society's woes. His goal is to correct the situation and avoid the villainous use of the device by adversaries.

A collection of Percy's essays on semiotics was published in 1975 with the title *The Message in the Bottle*. It constitutes an attempt to reconcile the Judeo-Christian ethic, which allows for individual freedom and responsibility, and the rationalism of science that considers humans as organisms in society stripped of individual freedom. The work also probes the ill-defined issue of language use. The reviews were widely divergent, ranging from "a Copernican break-through" to "amateur crackpot."

Percy's fourth novel, *Lancelot*, in 1977, was a main selection offered by the Book-of-the-Month Club. It consists of a monologue by a failed Southern lawyer, for whom there were great expectations, told to a silent physician priest in a prison hospital cell. The narrative is a tale of evil resulting in despair. The decadence of the time was emphasized by the author's assignment of char-acters' names from the age of King Arthur's Camelot. During the time span, contemporary moral depravity and evils are unveiled. The novel begins with the character Lancelot Lamar's realization that his youngest daughter had been fathered by another man and extends to both Lancelot murdering one of his wife's lovers and the destruction of his New Orleans plantation mansion.

The Second Coming, a sequel to *The Last Gentleman*, was nominated for the National Book Critics Circle Award in 1980. The book explores the same theme that pervades Percy's novels—a search for a meaningful way to live in a world in which "isms" have failed. The central character, a suicidal middle-aged widower, develops a relationship with a young woman who has escaped from an insane asylum. Together they move to a resolution of each other's despair.

Percy's next publication, *Lost in the Cosmos*, a humorous nonfictional satire on self-help books, eventually outsold his other books. The thesis is formu-lated as follows: "The problem is that in an age of acute self-consciousness and an age of the objective scientific knowledge of things, the relationship of the knower to himself is that he cannot know the first thing about himself." Percy believed that the gap between the reliability of one's knowledge of the world and the lack of reliability of knowledge of one's self was continually increasing.

The sixth and last of Percy's novels, *The Thanatos Syndrome*, was published in 1987. Dr. Thomas More from *Love in the Ruins* returns to his psychiatric prac-tice in the late 1990s after spending two years in prison for illegally peddling drugs. He determines that the aberrant behavior of his family and previous patients is caused by the radioactivity of the sodium isotope, which had been deliberately released into the water supply to improve social welfare. The work also includes a consideration of the future of Catholicism.

During his life, Percy was regarded as a significant modern Catholic writer. He was the recipient of an award from the Catholic Book Club and was invited to be a member of the Pontifical Council for Culture in Rome. At the same time, he was labeled a "Southern writer of the New South." He received many honors. He was elected a fellow of the American Academy of Arts and Sciences. He received the Jefferson Award, one of the highest intellectual honors the US government can bestow; the PEN/Faulkner award and many honorary degrees. Percy died on May 10, 1990, of metastatic prostatic cancer.

Among the many quotes attributed to the "Dostoyevsky of the Bayou" are "We love those who know the worst of us and don't turn their faces away," "You live in a deranged age, more deranged than usual, because despite great scientific and technological advances, man has not the faintest ideas of who he is or what he is doing," "Since grief only aggravates your loss, grieve not for what is past," and, apropos the theme of this book, "Nevertheless, the physician, insofar as he is a novelist, is in the business of diagnosis, not therapy." And "I would not recommend to young writers that they serve an apprenticeship in medicine or to physicians that they take up novel writing."

SOURCES

Allen, William Rodney. *Walker Percy: A Southern Wayfarer*. Jackson: University Press of Mississippi, 1986.

Samway, S. J., Patrick H. *Walker Percy: A Life*. New York: Farrar, Straus, and Giroux, 1997.

Tolson, Jay. *Pilgrim in the Ruins: A Life of Walker Percy*. New York: Simon & Schuster, 1992.

42

GORDON STANLEY OSTLERE
(RICHARD GORDON)

The Monocle Bespeaks Medical Mirth

T he attraction of readers to doctors as subject matter has been and continues to be apparent. One physician who lived for more than nine decades had to his credit sixteen novels with the word *Doctor* in their titles.

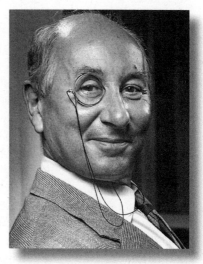

Gordon Stanley Ostlere was an English surgeon and anesthesiologist, who wrote using the pseudonym "Richard Gordon" during the second half of the twentieth century. He was born on September 15, 1921, educated at Cambridge, and received his medical training at St. Bartholomew's Hospital and the London School of Medicine and Dentistry. He qualified as a physician in 1945 and initially worked as an anesthetist at the institute where he had trained.

In the 1940s, he contributed to the medical literature with several single-authored articles on the effects of the drug curare in poor-risk patients, trichlorethylene used in general anesthesia, anesthesia in cardiac surgery, and epidural analgesia in the treatment of hypertension due to toxemia of pregnancy. He published three medical textbooks—*Anaesthetics and the Patient, Trichlorethylene Anaesthesia*, and *Anaesthetics for Medical Students*—all of which reappeared in 1989 as *Ostlere and Bryce-Smith's Anaesthetics for Medical Students*. Ostlere, also, held the position of assistant editor of the *British Medical Journal* with responsibility for the obituaries. He joked that he learned to write editing physicians' obituaries.

FROM MEDICINE TO MANUSCRIPT

In the early 1950s, he left his medical practice in order to devote to writing full-time. In 1951, he had married an anesthesiologist who supported him during his transition. The two remained married for over sixty-five years when he died. After completing the manuscript of his first novel, he spent a short period as a ship's surgeon, during which he wrote *Doctor at Sea* (1953). While engaged as a ship's surgeon, his first work of fiction, *Doctor in the House* (1952), was published and enjoyed great success.

"Richard Gordon" made his first literary appearance as the author of a humorous "exposé" of the training and extracurricular activities of a medical student, Simon Sparrow, at the mythical St. Swithin's Hospital in London. In that work the reader is also introduced to Sir Lancelot Spratt, the short-tempered demagogic chief of surgery who is a recurring character in many of Gordon's subsequent novels. The motion picture adaptation of *Doctor in the House* had the greatest attendance for a film in Great Britain in 1954. It became a popular television series that ran in 1969–1970.

Many of the salient characters who were introduced in Gordon's first novel reappear in eighteen subsequent novels, as do other distinctive characters. The readers of the "Doctor" series of books, published between 1952 and 1999, were exposed to development, maturation, and aging of characters who became distinctly familiar to the audience. The public's familiarity with the characters was enhanced by multiple motion picture and television adaptations. The film adaptation of Gordon's second novel, *Doctor at Sea*, cemented star status for the British actor Dirk Borgarde, who had been introduced to the public as Simon Sparrow in *Doctor in the House*. That film also provided the first English-speaking role for the popular French star Brigitte Bardot.

The Doctor series was sustained, sequentially, with *Doctor at Large* (1955), *Doctor in Love* (1957), *Doctor and Son* (1959), *Doctor in Clover* (1960), *Doctor on Toast* (1961), *Doctor in the Swim* (1962), *The Summer of Sir Lancelot* (1965), *Love and Sir Lancelot* (1965), *Doctor on the Boil* (1970), *Doctor on the Brain* (1972), *Doctor in the Nude* (1973), *Doctor on the Job* (1976), *Doctor in the Nest* (1979), *Doctor's Daughters* (1981), *Doctor on the Ball* (1985), *Doctor in the Soup* (1986), and *The Last of Sir Lancelot* (1989). The British National Health System comes under criticism in *Doctor in Nest*, and in *The Last of Sir Lancelot*, in which the second coming of Florence Nightingale focuses on her attempt to reconstruct the dysfunctional health system.

The Doctor series was representative of British farce that was prevalent at that time in literature and in the theater. As *Kirkus Reviews* commented about

GORDON STANLEY OSTLERE (RICHARD GORDON)

The Summer of Sir Lancelot, it is "like measles, endemic, low-grade, infectious, and—yes—spotty." Gordon's lightheartedness and, at times, irreverence pervaded his other publications.

The Captain's Table (1954) is a nautical misadventure replete with farcical mayhem. *Nuts in May* (1964) details a romp in which a financially successful father leads his prodigal son, who had been dismissed from Oxford and ended an engagement to a financially attractive fiancée. *The Facemaker* (1967) focuses on the recently introduced topic of plastic and reconstructive surgery and the criticisms the procedures evoked from orthodox medicine. *Surgeon at Arms* (1968) is a continuance of the life of the plastic surgeon who was the central figure in *The Facemaker*. In *Surgeon at Arms*, the protagonist is deeply involved in the care of soldiers with burns and damaged limbs during World War II.

The Facts of Life (1969) is a novel about the birth control pill. *The Medical Witness* (1971) is a tale of a conceited forensic pathologist and his downfall brought about by the destruction of his perceived certainties. *The Sleep of Life* (1975) is a historical novel replete with facts concerning the discovery of anesthesia. The tale incorporates the history of the introduction of nitrous oxide, ether, and chloroform as anesthetic agents. Arguments between proponents and an antagonistic medical establishment concerning the appropriateness of their use are highlighted.

The Invisible Victory (1977) weaves together the early use of sulphonamides and the discovery and production of penicillin with the activities of a young English chemist who is developing germ warfare during World War II. The novel culminates at the Nuremberg trials, during which the hero participates in determining who deserves credit for discoveries concerning the antibiotics. Three historical novels—*The Private Life of Florence Nightingale, The Private Life of Jack the Ripper*, and *The Private Life of Doctor Crispen*—were published in sequence from 1978 to1981. *The Private Life of Jack the Ripper* was described as "a masterly evocation of medicine in 1888" and "a dark and disrobing medical mystery."

The most recent of Richard Gordon's publications could be classified as "compendia cum comedy." In *Great Medical Disasters* (1983), the author explores several bizarre medical happenings. *Great Medical Mysteries* (1984) is a hilarious collection of medical mysteries, including those related to George Washington, Napoleon, and Adolf Hitler. The last chapter of the book bears the title "Why Do So Many Doctors Write Books?"

In that chapter, Gordon considers many of the individuals who are considered in this book. Gordon writes, "[Medicine] is an occupation as different from an author's as anchorman to anchorite," and "The privilege of educated compassion for the infinite, fascinating fancies and frailties of human beings explains why some of us write books as well."

The Alarming History of Medicine (1983), according to *Kirkus Reviews*, is "idio-syncratic, crotchety—and very funny." In this work, Gordon concludes that the history of medicine is "largely the substitution of ignorance by fallacies," and "the seventeenth-century physician was useless but decorative," in addi-tion to "Victorian physicians were brilliant at identifying the disease that they had no idea how to cure."

The Literary Companion to Medicine: An Anthology of Prose and Poetry (1993) offers selections from literary touchstones that provide a window to the medi-cine of the times. Each short segment is introduced by witty and succinct com-ments by Gordon. *An Alarming History of Famous and Difficult Patients*, which was published in 1997, was the last of Gordon's major literary contributions. The work consists of thirty-one generally humorous and, at times, satiric anec-dotes about medical issues related to famous individuals or fictional characters. Washington's false teeth, Hitler's missing right testicle, Boswell's gonorrhea, Elizabeth Barrett Browning's anorexia, and Florence Nightingale's sexual ori-entation share equal billing. Throughout Gordon's compendia, history is inoc-ulated with humor.

When Gordon was interviewed on radio in 1986, he indicated that when he was a youth, he aspired to become a comic writer. When asked why he became an anesthetist, he responded, "I wanted a seat in the operating theatre." Gordon Stanley Ostlere died on August 11, 2017, one month before his ninety-sixth birthday.

SOURCES

Barker, Dennis. "Richard Gordon Obituary." *Guardian*, August 15, 2017, https://www.theguardian.com/books/2017/aug/15/richard-gordon-obituary (accessed April 5, 2018).

Internet Movie Database, s.v. "Richard Gordon." http://www.imdb.com/name/nm0330546/?ref_=nv_sr_1 (accessed April 5, 2018).

World Book Online Encyclopedia, s.v. "Richard Gordon." http://www.worldbookonline.com/wb/Article?id=ar734780&st=Doctor+Light+Comics.

43

JOHN BENIGNUS LYONS

The "Doctor Who Found His Forte in Writing"

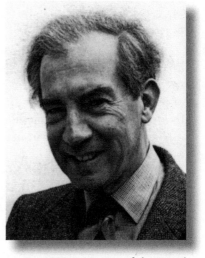

Image courtesy of the Royal College of Surgeons in Ireland.

As the caption that headlined Professor J. B. Lyons's obituary in the *Irish Times* indicated, he was a notable physician and medical historian, best recognized as "one of the greatest Irish medical writers of the twentieth century." That designation was based on the recognition that he was "a gracious man and caring physician, his published work was marked by a depth of knowledge, sophistication and culture."

John Benignus Lyons, better known as J. B. Lyons, the son of a dispensary doctor, was born on July 22, 1922, in Kilkelly, County Mayo, Ireland. After beginning his studies at the local national school, he completed precollegiate studies at Castlenock College near Dublin. There, he developed an interest in literature and Anglo-Irish history. He won the Bodkin Memorial prize for an essay. Despite those attractions, he decided to prepare himself for a career in medicine.

Lyons studied medicine at the University College Dublin and graduated in 1945. After completing internships at the Mater Hospital and the County Hospital in Castlebar, he moved to England to continue his training. In 1949, he became a member of the Royal College of Physicians of Ireland and was awarded an MD degree by the National University of Ireland. That year, stimulated by James Johnston Abraham's (see chapter 30) *The Surgeon's Log*, Lyons elected to spend a sabbatical year as a ship's surgeon aboard the *MV Soudan*, which took him to Japan, Singapore, Hong Kong, Bombay, Alexandria, and Tangier. That voyage was followed by another to South America as the ship's surgeon to the Royal Mail's *Highland Monarch*.

After the year of travel, Lyons became a medical registrar at the Crumpsall Hospital in Manchester, England, followed by work at the Manchester Royal Infirmary. During that period, he developed an interest in neurology. In 1955, he returned to Ireland when he was appointed consultant physician at the St. Michael's Hospital in Dún Laoghaire, a seaside town 7.5 miles southeast of central Dublin. In 1959, he became a fellow of the Royal College of Physicians of Ireland, and, in 1965, he joined the staff of Mercer's Hospital in Dublin.

Lyons's first literary contribution was a novel, *A Question of Surgery*, which he wrote shortly after returning to Dublin and published in 1960. The narrative describes the trials and tribulations of a young, capable surgeon in quest of an appointment to the staff of a hospital, and the frustrations brought about by social, political, and professional issues. The author examines the problem of encouraging excellence in an environment of a national health system. The book was translated into Dutch and German.

Two novels, *South Downs General Hospital* and *When Doctors Differ*, were published during the next two years. A reviewer, commenting on the author's style, wrote, "the author has acquired that essential part of the novelist's trade: the ability to string words together so that the reader wants to turn the page and read on." All three novels written by Lyons bear the pseudonym "Michael Fitzwilliam," a name derived from the hospital where he worked, St. Michael's, and Fitzwilliam Square, where he had his office.

Lyons's interest in neurology led to his being awarded a scholarship by the World Health Organization to visit neurological centers in four major cities in the United States. On his return, he wrote *A Primer of Neurology*, which was published in 1974 and enjoyed popularity among students. In 1975, he was appointed professor of the history of medicine in the Royal College of Surgeons in Ireland, a position he would hold for twenty-five years. Lyons divided his time between medical practice and writing until 1987, when he formally resigned his medical posts and stated, "I can now become a full-time writer."

Lyons's literary forte was nonfiction, particularly biography. His first biography to be published was *The Citizen Surgeon*, which appeared in 1966. Lyons chronicled the life of Sir Victor Horsley, a pioneer of neurological surgery, who also directed his efforts toward temperance, the suffrage of women, medical reform, and free healthcare for the working class. In 1978, Lyons published a small illustrated book that consisted of brief descriptions and vignettes under the title *Brief Lives of Irish Doctors*. Lyons's second major biography, *Oliver St. John Gogarty, the Man of Many Talents*, was published in 1980. Lyons found a kindred soul in Gogarty, who combined a medical career with literary contributions.

Lyons considered *The Enigma of Tom Kettle*, published in 1983, to be his best biography. It detailed and evaluated the life of an Irish economist, journalist, lawyer, writer, poet, soldier, and home rule politician that spanned the end of the nineteenth century and into the early twentieth century. Lyons's other published biography, *Surgeon-Major Parke's African Journey*, is a profile of one of the best-known Irishmen of his time, hailed as "the man who saved Stanley" and "the first Irishman to cross Africa."

Lyons was a respected James Joycean scholar. His book *James Joyce and Medicine*, published in 1973, offers a unique approach to Joyce's life. The work considers Joyce's episodes of physical and emotional ill health, his failed attempt to study medicine, his relationship with Oliver St. John Gogarty, the use of medical jargon, and descriptions of anatomy and illnesses in Joyce's writings. There is a detailed description of Joyce's stomach disorder that eventually required surgery and led to his death.

Lyons also published a collection of essays titled *Thrust Syphilis Down to Hell and Other Rejoyceana*, *The Quality of Mercers: The Story of Mercer's Hospital, 1734–1991*, and *What Did I Die of?: The Deaths of Parnell, Wilde, Synge and Other Literary Pathologies*. Related to his position in the Royal College of Surgeons in Ireland, he published *An Assembly of Irish Surgeons: Lives of Presidents of the Royal College of Surgeons in Ireland in the 20th Century*, *A Pride of Professors of Medicine at the Royal College of Surgeons in Ireland, 1813–1985*, and he coauthored *A Portrait of Irish Medicine: An Illustrated History of Medicine in Ireland*.

In 1994, Lyons produced an engaging biography of *William Henry Drummond: Poet in Patois* for the Canadian Medical Lives series. Lyons contributed fifteen brief biographies for the 2004 edition of the *Oxford Dictionary of National Biography*. Two years previously, to mark Lyons's eightieth birthday, several of his colleagues provided contributions and arranged for the publication of *Borderlands: Essays on Literature and Medicine*. The publication took its title from the designation that Lyons had assigned to his articles on medical historical topics. The introduction to the publication referred to Lyons's "innate literary talent, enquiring mind, devout professionalism in medicine and loyalty to his muses," and concluded that "posterity may well award Jack [J. B. Lyons] the accolade of one of the most significant Irish medical historians of the last century."

SOURCES

Coakley, D. "J. B. Lyons (1922–2007)." *Irish Journal of Medical Science* 177, no. 2 (2008): 179–80.

"Doctor Who Found His Forte in Writing." *Irish Times*, November 10, 2007, http://www.irishtimes.com/news/doctor-who-found-his-forte-in-writing -1.981123? (accessed February 26, 2018).

44

FERROL AUBREY SAMS JR.

Georgia-Georgia

errol Sams Jr., known as Sambo by his family, friends, and patients, is the only physician listed among the "Notable Alumni" in the category of "Arts, Education, Media and Industry" on the 2017 website for Mercer University, the oldest private university in the state of Georgia, located in Macon. He is recognized by his alma mater as a "widely read Southern author."

His ancestry, birth, education, medical practice, and the settings for his novels are all located within the boundaries of Georgia. He was born in rural Fayette County in 1922, when the census was about eleven thousand. During his youth, he lived in a house that had been

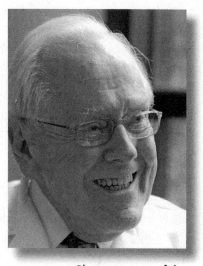

Photo courtesy of the Sams family.

built by his great-grandfather in 1848 on a farm seven miles from the nearest town. Sambo, whose father was the school superintendent of Fayette County, traced his lineage back six generations, to 1820, when James Sams settled in Fayette County.

Ferrol enrolled at Mercer University, less than seventy-five miles from his home. His most memorable and consequential experience as an undergraduate occurred during his freshman year in 1939. During a mandatory two-semester course in rhetoric and writing, his professor, who had a reputation of being hypercritical and exacting, suggested that Sams had the talent to consider a career as a writer.

Sams, however, planned for a life as a doctor in rural Georgia and continued to fulfill the requirements for entrance into medical school. After completing the first semester at Emory University School of Medicine, about twenty-five miles from his home, he deliberately flunked out to join the US Army Medical Corps. He initially taught anatomy to medics before transferring to a field hospital. The personnel in his unit landed on a Normandy beach after D-day in World War II and followed General George Patton's army across France. At the end of the war, Sams returned and completed his medical studies at Emory in 1949. Before graduating in1949, he met Helen Fletcher, a Phi Beta Kappa honor graduate from the former Florida State College for Women.

Prior to his graduation, Sams married Helen, who would graduate with Alpha Omega Alpha (medical school honor society) recognition for academic excellence, a year behind her husband, in July 1950. In 1951, the couple began their medical practice in Fayette County. They practiced together for fifty-five years, retiring within weeks of each other. Ferrol Sams Jr. died in his home on January 2013. Less than four weeks later, the longest period they had been apart in more than sixty-four years of marriage, his wife died.

The "Sams" imprint on the medical care in Fayette County continues with the activities of their oldest child, Ellen Sams Nichol—a medical practice administrator—and two sons, Ferrol Aubrey Sams III and James Sams, who are both physicians in Fayetteville, currently reporting a census of 110,000, as an extension of Atlanta. The youngest son, William Fletcher Sams, is a Superior Court judge in Fayette County.

Sams, at the age of fifty-eight, realizing that the demands of general practice had prevented a latent desire to write, decided that it was time to become a writer. He was spurred on by his remembrance of the encouragement of his English professor. As Sams later indicated in an interview related to his election to the Georgia Writers Hall of Fame, he followed the pattern of his youth on a farm, when he'd done chores in the early morning before beginning his school day. From 4:00 a.m. to 6:00 a.m. every day, before discharging his medical obligations, he wrote prose to develop a style.

Using pen and ink on lined paper, he drew on personal experiences of growing up in the rural South during the Great Depression and wrote about the local characters he encountered. He emphasized, on the occasion of a book signing for his last work, *Down Town*, that the characters actually provided a distinctiveness to the small town. He wrote with the style of a Southern storyteller, incorporating humor and folklore in an engaging, easy-flowing prose.

Sams published eight books. The first novel, *Run with the Horsemen*, was published in 1982. It is the coming of age of a sensitive, picaresque young boy, Porter Osborne Jr., growing up on a farm in rural Georgia. The book was a *New York Times* best seller and became the first in a trilogy in which Porter Osborne Jr. is featured.

The second book, *The Whisper of the River*, published in 1984, follows Porter's adventures at a Baptist college where he reexamines his beliefs and moral issues, and comes of age. Sams later indicated in an interview that the hero of the novel was the fictional Baptist college, which transformed a typical rural Southern boy. For the past quarter century, students who have been accepted for matriculation as freshmen at Mercer are encouraged to read the book during the summer prior to their arrival on campus.

The final book of the trilogy, *When All the World Was Young*, was not published until 1991. After completing the first year of medical school, Porter Osborne elects to interrupt his studies to serve in the army as a surgical technician. He participates in the invasion of Normandy, and, during his three years of service, he wrestles with issues of faith, family, and integrity while continuing as a happy prankster evoking happiness and mirth. The hero returns home to complete his medical studies, a wiser and happier man. The novel won the Townsend Prize for Fiction, which is awarded biennially by the Georgia Center for the Book for work produced by a writer living in Georgia.

During the interval between completion of the second book of the trilogy and beginning the composition of the third book, Sams published three unrelated works: *The Passing: Perspectives of Rural America* (1988), *The Widow's Mite* (1989), and *Christmas Gift!* (1989). In *The Passing*, the essays of Sams and the illustration of Jim Harrison provide a poignant remembrance of the charms of the rural American landscape, which had become a victim of urban sprawl and modernization.

The eight essays in *The Widow's Mite* offer a microcosm of the social problems, eccentricities, and characters that provide a literary portrait of the fading rural South. In *Christmas Gift!* the author relates one rural Southern family's celebration of Christmas, thereby offering a more detailed description of Southern hospitality and traditions, and the disappearing distinctive characteristics of rural Southerners.

Sams's next published work appeared three years after the third book of the trilogy. *Epiphany* presents within its binding three philosophical novellas with the common theme of the effect of sudden revelation on individuals. The title story considers injustice, racism, and the harassment of an old-time small-town general practitioner by a pompous, impersonal medical bureaucracy. *Harmony Ain't Easy*, the title of the second story, is the tale of Sams and Helen's long love and marriage. It maintains the homespun style that characterizes the author's narratives.

The final publication (2001) of Sams's, *Down Town*, maintains the consistency of the author's folksy voice in a humorous novel. It offers a description of the emotional bond, extending from the end of the Civil War through the twentieth century, between the citizens of Fayette County, Georgia, and the rural South.

In 2000, the Georgia Writers Hall of Fame was established at the Hargett Rare Book Room and Manuscript Library of the University of Georgia, "Honoring Georgia's Deep Literary Legacy." The individuals recognized were Georgia writers whose work reflects the character of the state—its land and people. Among the fifty-seven writers whose portraits are on display, the novelist Ferrol Sams Jr. and the poet John Stone were physicians.

Most of the honored novelists are more recognizable because of a broader readership, e.g., Erskine Caldwell (*Tobacco Road*), Pat Conroy (*Prince of Tides*), Margaret Mitchell (*Gone with the Wind*), Alfred Uhry (*Driving Miss Daisy*), and Frank Yerby (*Foxes of Harrow*). None are more distinctively "rural South" than Sams. Among the honorees, only Ferrol Sams Jr. can lay claim to a constancy in his literary contributions that is expressed in the title of the song "Georgia on My Mind."

SOURCES

Kerley, Gary. "Ferrol Sams (1922–2013)." In *New Georgia Encyclopedia*. University of Georgia Press. Article published March 4, 2004. Last edited by NGE Staff on November 25, 2013. http://www.georgiaencyclopedia.org/articles/arts-culture/ferrol-sams-1922-2013. (accessed April 5, 2018).

Yardley, William. "Ferrol Sams, Doctor Turned Novelist, Dies at 90." *New York Times Books*, February 1, 2013. http://www.nytimes.com/2013/02/02/books/ferrol-sams-doctor-turned-novelist-dies-at-90.html (accessed April 5, 2018).

45

RICHARD SELZER

Surgeon and a Short Story Stylist

A self-described epiphany transformed a respected and successful general surgeon into, arguably, the most highly regarded modern author of medical short stories. As expressed in a 1982 *New York Times* book review, "His marvelous insight and potent imagery make his tales of surgery and medicine both works of art and splendid tools of instruction."

Richard Selzer was born in Troy, New York, on June 24, 1928. His father was a general practitioner who died when Richard was twelve years old. This left the family in dire financial straits and necessitated Richard commuting daily to attend Union College, from which he graduated with a bachelor of science degree in 1948. He received his doctor of medicine degree

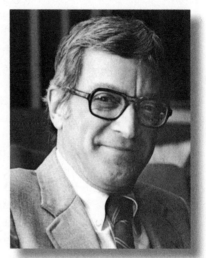

Photo courtesy of Yale University, Harvey Cushing / John Hay Whitney Medical Library.

from Albany Medical College in 1953 and proceeded to the Yale Medical School surgical residency at the Grace New Haven Hospital two years before Sherwin Nuland (see chapter 46).

When the Korean War broke out, Selzer was drafted during the second year of his residency. He served for two years as a medical officer in the US Army, initially in charge of a unit in a remote part of Korea. He contracted malaria toward the end of his first year of assignment and was transferred to Japan for his second year of service. He returned to his training and was eventually selected, in a highly competitive pyramidal system, to be the chief surgical resident. Upon completion of the surgical residency, he joined the clinical surgical faculty at the Yale Medical School and remained affiliated with that institute until his retirement in 1986.

Conversations with his medical contemporaries and surgical colleagues reveal that Selzer was a respected general surgeon who sustained a busy practice before he retired to devote himself to a literary career. A computer-generated search of the peer-reviewed surgical literature failed to reveal his name on a scientific article. But, throughout his surgical career, he was an active participant in the education of medical students and surgical residents at Yale.

When Selzer was forty years old, he deliberately embarked on a personally directed regimen to develop his literary skills. His first publications were horror stories that appeared in the *Ellery Queen Magazine*. He would continue to publish articles in magazines, such as *Esquire* and *Harper's*.

His first book of short stories, *Rituals of Surgery*, was published in 1974. In that work, Selzer fuses the occasional horrors and devastating aspects of surgery with the compassion of those who participate in the dramas. As he would later express in "Five-Finger Exercises," which appeared in the *Writer* in 1999, "The pen is the writing instrument most genial to my hand. It has the same heft as the scalpel. . . . Ply either one and something is shed. From the scalpel, blood, from the pen, ink."

In his second book of short stories, *Mortal Lessons: Notes on the Art of Surgery* (1976), the essays are diverse, ranging from descriptions of internal organs to ethical issues such as abortion and smoking to reminiscences of his youth in Troy. The descriptions of the workings and the disruptions of functions of the human body are presented with empathy and humor. The work established Selzer's reputation as a writer, and *Kirkus Reviews* considered it "an impressive display of knowledge, and art, magic, and mystery."

Confessions of a Knife (1979) incorporates largely autobiographical essays that merge art, religion, and science. It offers a glimpse into medicine and thought-provoking reflections on health, illness, and mortality. In the *New York Times* review of Selzer's *Letters to a Young Doctor* (1982), it was stated that "Richard Selzer does for medicine what Jacques Cousteau does for the sea. He transports the reader to a world that most of us never see, a world that is vivid and powerful."

Selzer's objectivity and elegant style continue to be displayed in *Taking the World in for Repairs* (1986) as he brings to the reader's attention "the singular details of a single human life." The book contains twelve essays, including a boy's love for a girl dying of tuberculosis, the life cycle of a worm that resides in a man's intestine, a stay with monks at an island monastery, and the work of surgeons who visit Peru to correct birth defects of native children. *Imagine a Woman* (1990) is made up of six tales that deal with the pathology that affects human beings, its physical and psychological consequences, and the cures. The tales are brought to life by the author's compassion coupled with a precise and impeccable style.

Down from Troy: A Doctor Comes of Age (1992) is a departure from his previous publications in that it is a memoir of Selzer's youth in Troy, New York, during the Great Depression. The essays present the influence of his father, who was a physician, and his mother, who was a singer. Selzer traces his life through his youth, his medical training, his surgical activities, and his literary career.

In *Raising the Dead: A Doctor's Encounter with His Own Mortality* (1993), Selzer relates the "declared dead" coma he experienced as a consequence of Legionnaires' disease. *What One Man Said to Another* (1998) is a series of conversations between Selzer and a friend, the writer and artist Peter Josyph. The work, which is a spoken autobiography of Selzer, was selected as one of the *New York Times Book Review*'s notable books of 1993. Only two of the twenty-seven tales that make up Selzer's *Doctor Stories* (1998) are new, but the author's lengthy introduction provides a significant addition to his appealing prose.

Five new essays are added to several of his previously published writings in *The Exact Location of the Soul* (2001). Two of the five new pieces consider diseases that surgeons cannot cure and the spread of AIDS in Haiti. *The Whistler's Room* (2004) is a revision and translation of a German novel, which had been published in 1929. It is a tale of four soldiers with tracheal damage, which requires tracheostomy, and their communications with one another. A compassionate surgeon cares for them and is able to restore the voice of two of his patients.

Selzer's only original novel, *Knife Song, Korea*, was published in 2009 and was named one of the *California Literary Review*'s critic picks for best books of 2009. One reviewer compared the small novel with Hemingway's *The Old Man and the Sea* and Steinbeck's *Of Mice and Men*. It was also an award-winning finalist in Fiction & Literature in 2010 sponsored by USA Book News. The story stems from an unpublished novel, "The Bronze Gong," originally written by Selzer, drawing from his own experience in Korea. It tells of the hardships and loneliness of a young American army physician stationed in a remote Korean village during the war.

The last of Selzer's major publications, *Diary* (2010), is a chronological extension of his memoir *Down from Troy*, covering the years 1999 through 2008. It focuses on the author's inner life as he frequents the Yale libraries and park benches. In 2010, the *Abaton*, a medical humanities journal, initiated the Selzer Prize for Writing to be awarded annually for the best essay by a medical student. This was appropriate because after Selzer ceased teaching surgery and anatomy, he shifted his energies to teaching medical students, residents, and nurses how to write. During his literary career, Selzer was the recipient of a Guggenheim Fellowship, an American Medical Writers Award, and a National Magazine Award.

Selzer died in Connecticut on June 15, 2016. His papers are archived in the Truman G. Blocker Jr. History of Medicine Collections, Moody Medical Library, University of Texas Medical Branch in Galveston. Among Selzer's notable quotes are "You cannot separate passion from pathology any more than you can separate a person's spirit from his body," and "There are no 'great' subjects for the creative writer; there are only the singular details of a single human life." In 2001, Susan Balée wrote in the *Philadelphia Inquirer*, "Selzer has a grace all his own, both as a prose stylist and as a surgeon."

SOURCES

Mullan, Fitzhugh. "Medical Meditations." Review of *Letters to a Young Doctor*, by Richard Selzer. *New York Times*. August 29, 1982. https://www.nytimes .com/1982/08/29/books/medical-meditations.html (accessed May 4, 2018).

Review of *Down from Troy: A Doctor Comes of Age*, by Richard Selzer. *Publishers Weekly*. June 29, 1992. https://www.publishersweekly.com/978-0-688 -09715-8 (accessed May 5, 2018).

Review of *Mortal Lessons: Notes on the Art of Surgery*, by Richard Selzer. *Kirkus Reviews*, 1976. https://www.kirkusreviews.com/book-reviews/richard -selzer-2/mortal-lessons-notes-on-the-art-of-surgery/ (accessed May 4, 2018).

Watts, Geoff. "Allen Richard Selzer." *Lancet* 388 (August 6, 2016): p. 558.

46

SHERWIN BERNARD NULAND

From Electricity to Eloquence—
Shock Breeds Success

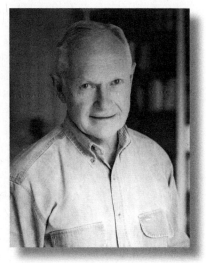

Sherwin Nuland's biography, in large part, combines an autobiographical publication of the complexities of the environment of his youth with a moving video in which he personally details his profound depression and electric shock therapy, and the criticism of his literary contributions. All of his writings are categorized as nonfiction, but the poignancy of his prose emanates from a surgeon whose own life could form the nucleus of a captivating novel.

Sherwin Bernard Nuland was born in the Bronx, New York, on December 8, 1930, and given the name Shepsel Ber Nudelman. When he went to kindergarten, he adopted the first and middle names Sherwin Bernard, and, on October 17, 1947, when he was a high school senior, his name was legally changed to its current form.

Nuland grew up in a small first-floor flat fronting the street in a lower-middle-class, sparsely settled area of the South Bronx. Living in the apartment were Sherwin and his older brother, their Russian immigrant parents, Sherwin's widowed maternal grandmother, and his mother's unmarried sister. Yiddish was the language of the household. Nuland's father, who was born in a Besarabian shtetl (a rural grouping of simple homes) and worked at a sewing machine in a garment sweatshop in New York, was an overly domineering parent. After he had become a highly regarded author, Nuland indicated in *Lost in America: A Journey with My Father*, which was published in 2003, that the lingering power his father had over him had been a powerful contributing cause of his depression. The narrative states, "For too many years—while he lived and after his death—I have been consumed with the futile effort of trying to rid myself of Meyer Nudelman."

Nuland's studies, from kindergarten through eighth grade, took place in a Bronx public school. He completed his high school education at the academically prestigious Bronx High School of Science. Later, he was awarded a bachelor's degree from New York University in 1951, after spending four years at the Bronx campus in preparation for entering medical school. He conducted his medical studies at the Yale School of Medicine. Four years later, he began surgical training as one of thirteen interns in the Yale program. He bested the competition and was one of two men from that group to complete the training in 1960.

Nuland joined the surgical department of the Yale–New Haven Hospital as a member of the surgical faculty, a position he held until his death. In the early 1970s, he published four articles on the role of surgery as adjunctive therapy and assessment in the treatment of Hodgkin's disease. His other medical publications relate to medical history or the care of patients and do not represent scientific contributions.

Within a few years of Nuland's appointment to the surgical faculty, he developed depression, which would consume the latter half of his thirties and his early forties. In February 2001, after Nuland had gained recognition for his literary contributions, he recounted his depression and successful electroshock therapy in a poignant TED (technology, education, design) talk, which can be captured on YouTube. The moving articulation of his suffering and relief has had over one million "hits."

At the age of forty-three, unable to sustain a surgical practice, dissatisfied with his first marriage and family relationships, and unable to cope with life, he was admitted to the Institute for Living in Hartford, Connecticut. After three months as an inpatient without evidence of improvement, in January 1974, he began a series of electroshock therapy treatments that extended over twenty sessions.

With the paralyzing depression cured, or at least under control, Nuland joined a surgical practice in a small Connecticut city and, within three years, returned to his position on the surgical faculty in New Haven. He devoted an increasing amount of time to writing, and in 1992 he ceased doing surgery and devoted the remainder of his life to writing and bioethics.

The first bound publication of Nuland's writing was *The Origins of Anesthesia*, consisting of fifteen monographs and presented in 1983 as a volume in the Classics of Medicine Library. Nuland's first independently published book is *Doctors: The Biography of Medicine* (1988). The work incorporates fifteen segments, which span twenty-four centuries, from the fourth century before the Common Era to the twentieth century. Nuland's approach is to use the biographies of several heroic figures as a nucleus for discussion of significant advances in medicine. Progressing through history in chronologic order: Hippocrates, Galen, Ambroise Paré, Andreas Vesalius, William Harvey, Giovanni Battista Morgagni, John Hunter, René Laennec, Ignaz Semmelweis, to those involved in the discovery of inhalation anesthesia, and continuing with Rudolf Virchow, Joseph Lister, William Stewart Halsted, Helen Taussig, and the doctors who brought about organ transplantation. This compendium was recommended by the *New York Times*, in which it was stated, "Nuland succeeds in bringing his subjects vividly to life, and he leaves you with a much better understanding of what they achieved."

The second of Nuland's books, *Medicine: The Art of Healing* (1992), is a compilation of forty-eight works of art that are related to medicine, presented chronologically and accompanied by an informational and cultural essay. Art is considered an insight into contemporary issues of medical knowledge and practice. The thesis is that art and medicine belong together.

In 1994, Nuland gained literary acclaim with the publication of *How We Die: Reflections of Life's Final Chapter*, which won the National Book Award for nonfiction and was a finalist for the Pulitzer Prize. It remained on the bestseller list of the *New York Times* for thirty-four weeks and sold over a half million copies. The work emphasizes the personal aspects of dying, the diverse causes of death, the variety of scenarios of dying, the potential for critical decisions (beginning to be made by the moribund individual or health proxy), and the ripple effect that may follow an individual death.

As Nuland indicates in the introduction, his participation on the bioethics committee at the Yale–New Haven Hospital "sharpened my comprehension of critical issues faced not only by patients and health professionals but at one time or other by all of us." The author's intent is to demystify death and to make readers more knowledgeable so they can take control of their own destiny. Nuland writes, "The good death has increasingly become a myth. . . . The greatest dignity to be found in death is the dignity of the life that preceded it."

Nuland's subsequent publications, with the exception of the autobiographical *Lost in America* (2003), maintain a consistent medical focus. *The Wisdom of the Body*, published also as *How We Live* (1997), describes biological concepts in a manner that makes them understandable to a general readership. Using the bases of anatomy, physiology, and pathophysiology to achieve an appreciation of clinical circumstances and their medical and surgical treatments, the author enables the audience to become educated regarding health and disease.

The Doctor's Plague: Germs, Childbed Fever, and the Strange Story of Ignác Semmelweis (2003) is a testament to the heroic contributions and consequent tragedy of one man. It also profiles how obstinacy, politics, and personal pride can interfere with medical progress and the well-being of the public. In *The Art of Aging: A Doctor's Prescription for Well-Being* (2007), Nuland sets out to provide a formula to make the later years of life better and more satisfying.

The Uncertain Art: Thoughts on a Life in Medicine (2008) is a collection of articles, most of which previously appeared in the *American Scholar* magazine. The book emphasizes the extraordinary outcomes that occur in medicine in an attempt to restore the doctor-patient relationship in a technologically dependent medical environment. Nuland writes, "To become comfortable with uncertainty is one of the primary goals in the training of a physician." In the last of his published books, *The Soul of Medicine: Tales from the Bedside* (2009), Nuland presents a series of tales, narrated by physicians, to once again create a focus on the doctor-patient relationship. This book did not enjoy the favorable reviews that Nuland's previous publications received.

As part of the Penguin Lives series, Nuland produced a small biography, *Leonardo da Vinci* (2000), in which he completes a twenty-year quest to understand his subject, a complex, multifaceted artist and a questionable genius. Nuland devotes much of his brief narrative to da Vinci's pioneering contributions to anatomy. The reviews were mixed. On one hand, the reviewer in *Time* magazine wrote, "Nuland's ability to distill one of the greatest minds ever into its pure essence is truly awe-inspiring." By contrast, the *New York Times* review challenged Nuland's conclusion that da Vinci was a transcendent genius. "Nuland's one-sided view of science leads to some very doubtful claims. . . . In the end it does a disservice to Leonardo to portray him as some savant with a mystical access to the truth."

Nuland's other biography, *Maimonides* (2005), was published as part of a series titled "Jewish Encounters." Nuland writes as one Jewish doctor considering, perhaps, the most extraordinary of Jewish doctors. The book is a sympathetic guide to an appreciation of the life and contributions of an intellectual giant and, at the same time, an assessment of Jewish ethics.

Nuland also contributed articles to the *New Yorker*, the *New York Times*, and the *New Republic*. He produced a series of lectures for the Teaching Company's Great Courses on the History of Western Medicine. In 2011, he was awarded the Jonathan Rhoads Gold Medal, by the American Philosophical Society, for Distinguished Service to Medicine. He died on March 3, 2014, of prostate cancer.

SOURCES

Gellene, Denise. "Sherwin B. Nuland, Author of 'How We Die,' Is Dead at 83." *New York Times*, March 5, 2014.

Gross, John. "The Stories of Medicine's Heroes." Review of *Doctors: The Biography of Medicine*, by Sherwin B. Nuland. *New York Times*. June 14, 1988. Books of the Times. https://www.nytimes.com/1988/06/14/books/books-of-the-times-the-stories-of-medicine-s-heroes.html (accessed May 5, 2018).

Nuland, Sherwin. "How Electroshock Therapy Changed Me." Filmed February 2001. TED video, 22:15. https://www.ted.com/talks/sherwin_nuland_on_electroshock_therapy.

Nuland, Sherwin B. *Lost in America: A Journey with My Father*. New York: Knopf, 2003.

Papineau, David. "Behind the Smile." Review of *Leonardo da Vinci*, by Sherwin B. Nuland. *New York Times*. November 26, 2000. https://archive.nytimes.com/www.nytimes.com/books/00/11/26/reviews/001126.26papinet.html?scp=8&sq=david+papineau&st=cse (accessed May 7, 2018).

47

VASILY PAVLOVICH AKSYONOV

Practice Medicine to Increase Personal Survival of Gulag Incarceration!

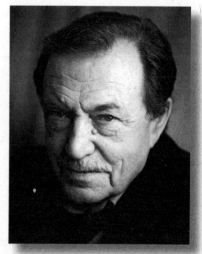

Vasily Aksyonov, one of the most admired Russian writers of the second half of the twentieth century, is unique among "Physicians with a Literary Legacy" in that he deliberately qualified as a physician in order to gain a privileged status in the event he was subjected to a long period of incarceration in a Soviet forced labor camp (a gulag).

Aksyonov was born on August 20, 1932, in Kazan, the capital city of the Tatarstan republic, about five hundred miles east of Moscow, to a prominent Communist father, Pavel, and mother, Yevgenia Ginzburg, who was a journalist and educator. In 1937, both of his parents were objects of a Stalinist purge for alleged connections with Trotskyites and exiled to a gulag for eighteen years. Initially, Vasily's care was assumed by his grandmother and uncle. In 1947, he joined his mother in the Magadan Prison area, where he graduated from high school. He intended to become a writer, but his parents decided that he should acquire a medical degree, which would make him a more valued person in case he was confined to a labor camp in the future. He graduated from the First Pavlov State Medical University of St. Petersburg in 1956 and served as a medical resident at the Quarantine Station of the Leningrad port. He then worked as a physician in the village of Voznesenie, Onega, in northern Russia before moving to Moscow, where he practiced from 1958 till 1960, when he ended his medical career.

When his parents were released from prison, Vasily's mother returned to Moscow for "rehabilitation" in 1955. In 1967, she published her magnum opus, *Journey into the Whirlwind*, focusing on the era of Stalin's repression. *Within the Whirlwind* was published in 1981 as the continuation of Ginzburg's Gulag memoirs from her time in the frozen prison camps.

In the beginning of the 1960s, Vasily Aksyonov became a frequent contributor to *Yunost* (*Youth*), a liberal magazine. Aksyonov, quickly, became a favorite of the Soviet 1960s generation, which objected to the cultural restrictions and somberness of the general ambiance associated with the Communist Party in the Soviet Union at the time. The youth group, bearing the name "Sestidesyatniki" ("the 60s generation") presented themselves as "hip," if their dress, attendance at bars and dance halls, and being devotees of American jazz and rock 'n' roll were any indication. Published in 1960, Aksyonov's first novel, *Colleagues*, was based on his medical experiences. The work was well received, and, coupled with his next novel, *Ticket to the Stars*, which was set among the contemporary Soviet "hipsters" and published about a year later, Aksyonov was raised to immediate fame that never left him.

Aksyonov's stylish, colloquial, subversive flaunting of the Soviet Union's state-imposed standards established him as the leader of a literary cult. His novels were awaited with great anticipation and generated large sales throughout all regions of the nation. The next publication, *Oranges from Morocco*, occurred in 1963. Although the plot was inconsequential—several men in love with two women, one of whom is married to one of the suitors' bosses—the arrival of a shipment of rare oranges at a far eastern Russian fishing town served as an unusual attraction for the characters, who deviated from the Soviet average traits and expressions.

Between 1964 and 1980, eight minor novels were published by Aksyonov in Russian. In 1979, Aksyonov contributed dissident writings to the recently created magazine *Metropol*. This led to confrontation with the authorities. There is general agreement that *The Burn*, a novel that was completed in Russian in 1975, is the author's magnum opus. His most read novel by an English-speaking audience was smuggled out of Russia and printed in Italy in 1980. This novel brought into focus the frustration experienced by intellectuals restricted by Communism. The action of his next published novel, *The Island of Crimea*, assumed that Crimea was geographically insular rather than a peninsula. This physical advantage contributed to the defeat of the Bolsheviks and the creation of an outpost for democracy near Russia.

In 1980, Aksyonov was invited to visit the United States, and, at the same time, the Soviet government revoked his citizenship. His wife, Maya, moved with him, and for the next twenty-four years he resided in Washington, DC, and Virginia, where he taught Russian literature at George Mason University. In 1989, on the occasion of the publication of his novel *Say Cheese*, he was interviewed on C-SPAN. In 1994, *Generations of Winter*, a Tolstoyan novel, was released. It chronicled Soviet life during three generations between the early period after World War I and the mid-1940s, at the height of Stalin's rule. The novel became a successful Russian television miniseries consisting of twenty-two episodes.

Throughout the narrative, real historic figures mingle with fictional characters, over whom Dr. Boris Nikitovich Gradov, a distinguished Moscow surgeon, maintains the status of benign patriarch. The surgeon's three children—Kirill, a Communist activist and ideologue; Nikita, a military man without political conviction; and the youngest, Nina, a cynic and bohemian poet—are swept up in Stalin's world of mandated conformance, the violation of which leads to prolonged and dire incarceration.

After more than two decades of residence in the United States, Aksyonov and his wife were allowed to return to Russia as citizens. In 2004, he received the Russian Booker Prize for his historical novel *Voltairian Men and Women*, using the second half of the eighteenth-century correspondence between the acerbic French philosopher and Catherine the Great, the empress of Russia, as the backdrop. Aksyonov subsequently spent most of his time in Moscow and Biarritz, a seaside town on France's southwestern Basque Coast. In 2006, he published "Moscow-Ow-Ow" in a Russian magazine. The story, an eerie love triangle, plays out in 1952, the last year of Stalin's rule, mainly in a typical Moscow high-rise apartment.

Aksyonov suffered a stroke while driving his car in January 2008 in Moscow. He died on July 6, 2009. According to Natalia Ivanova, the deputy editor of Russia's *Znamya* magazine, Aksyonov was loved by generations of Russian readers. The charm of his novels and the pleasure afforded the reader made Aksyonov a favorite of many of his audience. The publication of twenty-two novels satisfied the interest of his avid readership. In a telegram of condolence, President Dmitri A. Medvedev of Russia referred to Vasily Aksyonov as the literary embodiment of the 1960s period of hope.

Internationally recognized Russian author Aleksandr Solzhenitsyn, who was born almost fourteen years before Aksyonov, was more widely read by an

American audience. While Solzhenitsyn's writings focus on imprisonment and trying to get out, Aksyonov brings to the forefront hope of freedom, light, and forced frivolity.

SOURCES

Russiapedia, s.v. "Prominent Russians: Vasily Aksenov." https://russiapedia
.rt.com/prominent-russians/literature/vasily-aksenov/ (accessed April 5,
2018).
Yoffe, Mark. "Vasily Aksyonov: Libertarian Russian Writer and Leading Light in
'Youth Prose,' He Fell Foul of the KGB." *Guardian*, July 15, 2009. https://
www.theguardian.com/books/2009/jul/16/vasily-aksyonov-obituary
(accessed April 5, 2009).

48

OLIVER WOOD SACKS

Stories Stem from Synaptic Struggles

O n August 30, 2015, Oliver Wood Sacks moved from the roster of physicians who are currently adding to literature for the general public to the larger list of deceased doctors who are remembered for their literary contributions. A featured obituary, "Oliver Sacks, Neurologist Who Wrote about the Brain's Quirks," appeared in the *New York Times*, the newspaper that had previously referred to him as a "poet laureate of contemporary medicine."

Sacks, who was also referred to as the "Scheherazade of brain disorder," could have laid claim to a unique distinction of relationships with two of the most highly regarded comedians of modern time. Wes

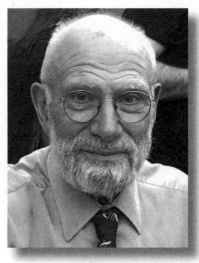

Photo © Luigi Novi / Wikimedia Commons.

Anderson—the author, director, and producer of the classic movie *The Royal Tenenbaums*—patterned the character Raleigh St. Clair, played by Bill Murray, after Sacks. In the motion picture *Awakenings*, based on Sacks's memoir, the role of the fictionalized neurologist was portrayed by another comedic genius, Robin Williams.

Sacks's own life contains elements of aberration, drama, and intrigue. He was born on July 9, 1933, in northwest London and inherited a notable genetic pool. His father, an orthodox Jew, was a busy general practitioner. His mother, Muriel Elsie Landau, was a graduate of the London School of Medicine for Women. In 1920, she qualified as a fellow of the Royal College of Surgeons, and, the following year, she was awarded an MD in obstetrics and gynecology, and conducted an active private practice in that discipline. She served on the staff of the Elizabeth Garrett Anderson Hospital for forty years and also on the staffs of the London Jewish Hospital and Madame Curie Hospital for Women. In 1965–66, she was president of the Medical Women's Federation of Great Britain.

Oliver was one of four sons, three of whom became doctors. He had three distinguished first cousins: Israeli diplomat Abba Eban; Nobel laureate economist Robert Aumann; and film director, producer, and writer Jonathan Lynn.

After receiving his early education during World War II in an English boarding school, Sacks attended St. Paul's School in London. He entered Queens College, Oxford, in 1951, at which he received a BA in physiology and biology in 1954, a BM BCh and MA in 1958, and an MD in 1960. Feeling oppressed and stifled by the medical culture in Great Britain, Sacks opted to develop a medical career in the United States. He left London, arrived in Canada, and crossed its vast expanse on a motorcycle to begin training in neurology at Mt. Zion Hospital in San Francisco, where he developed a friendship with poet Thomas Gunn and became exposed to drugs and a bohemian lifestyle.

After completing a residency at Mt. Zion Hospital, Sacks extended his training for two years at UCLA, where he was engaged in a fellowship in neurology and psychiatry. While in California, he experimented with drugs, including LSD and amphetamines. He motor biked back and forth to work and rode recreationally as part of a motorcycle gang. He distinguished himself at Muscle Beach by setting a California state weightlifting record, earning the appellation "Dr. Squat." Sacks wrote about his "lost years" in California in "Altered States," an article that appeared in the *New Yorker* in 2012 and in his book *Hallucinations*, which was published the same year.

According to Sacks's recollection, he was thirty-two years old and had reached the depths of dissipation and dependence on drugs when he deliberately transformed himself. He moved to New York City, began to care for patients with neurological disorders, ceased taking mind-altering drugs, and began Freudian psychoanalysis, which he continued throughout the remainder of his life.

Sacks's first institutional appointment was at the Beth Abraham Hospital in the Bronx, where he cared for patients with postencephalitic "sleeping sickness," employing levadopa (L-DOPA) as therapy. Initially, he incorporated clinical research into his practice. His first scientific publication, on hereditary photomyoclonus (a rare cerebellar ataxia in individuals extremely sensitive to photic stimuli), appeared in the journal *Neurology* in 1964. In the 1960s, he also published a review of axonal dystrophies, on the rare Hallervorder-Spatz dystonia and dementia, and on retroperitoneal fibrosis associated with methysergide therapy (formation of excessive fibrous tissue from taking methysergide for headaches). In the 1970s, Sacks published several articles on the use of L-DOPA in patients with Parkinsonism and dementia.

Shortly after his arrival in New York, Sacks identified himself as a physician interested in the care of individual patients rather than a research scientist. In 1966, he began a long-term association with nursing homes run by the Little Sisters of the Poor that he considered particularly gratifying. The same year and extending to 1991, he held an appointment as consulting neurologist at the Bronx Psychiatric Center. From 1966 to 2007, he rose from the academic rank of instructor to clinical professor of neurology at the Albert Einstein College of Medicine. From 1992 to 2007, he also held an appointment at New York University School of Medicine. In 2007, he was appointed professor of neurology and psychiatry at Columbia University Medical Center. Concomitantly, he was designated "Columbia University Artist" as part of a newly established effort to bridge the arts and sciences. In 2012, Sacks returned to the faculty of New York University School of Medicine as a consulting neurologist at the epilepsy center.

Sacks was best known in the literary world as a nonfiction storyteller whose stories had medical bases and were referred to as "pathographies" or "neurological novels." His first book, *Migraine*, was written in 1967 and published in 1970. The work reviews the subject for the lay population, using case histories, particularly those associated with visual aura. Sacks also suffered from migraines, having experienced his first episode when he was three or four years old. The book evoked little in the way of literary excitement and had modest sales.

Sacks's second and most famous book, *Awakenings*, also had unimpressive initial sales when it was published in 1973. W. H. Auden, the famous Anglo-American poet, thought it was "a masterpiece." The work details the experience of catatonic patients with "sleeping sickness," consequent to encephalitis lethargica, who are treated with the drug L-DOPA, which effects dramatic improvement followed by dismal relapse. In 1990, the motion picture adaption *Awakenings*, starring Robin Williams and Robert De Niro, was a critical success and rejuvenated interest in Sacks's writings.

Sacks's next book, *A Leg to Stand On*, was based on his personal experience of becoming psychologically disassociated from his leg, which was healing in a cast after surgery for a ruptured quadricep muscle sustained while he was running from a bull on a Norwegian mountain. Sacks's broad popularity was established in 1985 with the publication of *The Man Who Mistook His Wife for a Hat*. The book consists of twenty-four essays, assembled in four sections, each dealing with a specific aspect of brain function. The title story became the basis of an opera of the same name that premiered in 1986.

The success of *The Man Who Mistook His Wife for a Hat* was transformative for Sacks. A fifty-two-year-old man, who had been a "complete recluse," "in a kind of rictus of shyness" and spent hours swimming alone in Long Island Sound, became a public figure, who was profiled in *People* magazine in 1986. For the remaining three decades of his life, Sacks thrived as a writer with a devoted audience, which continued to be enchanted by tales of neurological disorders and their dramatic, improbable manifestations. Sacks did maintain a presence as a physician, continuing to care for a few private patients and participating in the neurologic clinics of the medical schools with which he was associated.

In *Seeing Voices: A Journey into the World of the Deaf* (1989), Sacks considered language perception by the deaf. The book consists of three long chapters that sequentially offer expositions of the history of the deaf, including their struggle for acceptance, the rich and beautifully expressive language of the deaf, and the issues that provoked a strike at Gallaudet University when a "hearing" candidate was chosen as president of the university rather than one of the two other candidates who were deaf.

An Anthropologist on Mars: Seven Paradoxical Tales (1995) depicts autistic savants and other patients with neurological disorders who not only subsist but thrive. The title story, which appeared in the *New Yorker* and won a Polk Award for magazine writing, includes the improbable circumstances of "The Case of the Colorblind Painter" and "A Surgeon's Life," in which an individual with Tourette's syndrome (multiple motor tics and at least one vocal tic that may be obscene or scatological) succeeds both as a surgeon and an amateur pilot.

The Island of the Colorblind (1997) brings into focus the Micronesian atoll of Pingelap, where many occupants have total colorblindness, impaired visual acuity, and profound photophobia. The second half of the book considers lytico-bodig disease (amyotrophic lateral sclerosis, Parkinsonism, dementia), which was prevalent among the Chamorro people of Guam. Sacks suggested that the consumption of the fruit bat exposed the natives to a neurotoxin, which was part of the bats' diet.

Sacks's own childhood attraction to chemistry formed the basis for *Uncle Tungsten: Memories of a Chemical Boyhood* (2001). The autobiographical narrative offers an introduction to the history and science of chemistry and the author's personal interest in the subject. Included in the book are descriptions of the abuses endured by young Sacks at boarding school. His attraction to chemistry persisted, as evidenced by his reflection on the occasion of approaching the age of eighty. In "The Joy of Old Age (No Kidding)," which appeared in the *New York Times* in 2013, he indicated that he recently dreamed of the liquid metal mercury because its atomic number in the periodic table of elements is eighty.

Sacks's next two publications stemmed from his hobbies. The first, *Oaxaca Journal*, published in 2002, was generated by his lifelong interest in ferns, scientifically referred to as pteridology. In the book, the author presents his personal journal of the New York Botanical Gardens' scientific travels in the province of Oaxaca in Mexico to identify species of ferns. In the narrative, Sacks diverts from the scientific discoveries to relate how both modern and pre-Hispanic Mexico impressed him. He writes, "The power and grandeur of what I have seen shocked me, and altered my view of what it means to be human."

Sacks, who was a proficient pianist, expressed his devotion to music coupled with an interest in the relationship between music and the mind in *Musicophilia: Tales of Music and the Brain* (2007). In the book he focuses on "musical misalignments," both disorders and powers that affect musicians and others. A case is made for the benefits of music therapy for individuals with aphasia, Parkinsonism, and dementia. As is characteristic of all his writings, Sacks enforces his concepts and theories with dramatic and poignant individual examples.

In *The Mind's Eye* (2010), Sacks relates case studies of people whose daily activities and specific occupational needs have been compromised by neurologic pathology. The author includes his own lifelong inability to recognize faces and his recent experience with unilateral loss of vision as a result of radiation of an ocular melanoma in 2006. *Hallucinations* (2012) is a casebook of unusual disorders, including hallucinations, in sane individuals. It incorporates Sacks's personal experiences with hallucinations accompanying migraines during his childhood, and hallucinations induced by his use of LSD, mescaline, amphetamines, and morphine. The undertone of the narrative is a destigmatization of what should be regarded as a clinical manifestation. Sacks also considers the possibility that hallucinations might be contributory to life stories and artistic inspiration.

Sacks's last book, *On the Move: A Life*, was published in 2015. The narrative underscores the author's belief that patients may know more about their conditions than those attending them. Sacks stresses that doctors should listen to their patients and incorporate the patients' accounts in the processes of diagnosis and management. In this memoir, Sacks finally reveals to his readers several aspects of his life that he previously had not expressed. This includes his motorcycling, his extreme bodybuilding, his reliance on drugs, and his early involvement in the gay world, followed by a long period of celibacy, and, more recently, a relationship with a writer.

In 2015, three months before *On the Move* appeared in bookstores, the same title appeared in his op-ed in the *New York Times*. Sacks wrote about learning that his ocular melanoma had metastasized to the liver and how he faced the realization that he had terminal cancer. On August 14 of that year, in the Sunday Review of the *New York Times*, Sacks, a self-declared "old Jewish atheist," published his poignant thoughts on the Sabbath. Sixteen days later he died.

During his life, Sacks was, arguably, the most famous and adulated neurologist in the world. More than a million copies of his books have appeared in print. He explicitly stated, "In 1961, I declared my intention to become a United States citizen, which may have been a genuine intention, I never got round to it."

In the early 1990s, he received honorary degrees from Georgetown University, Tufts University, New York Medical College, Medical College of Pennsylvania, and Bard College. In 1996, Sacks became a member of the American Academy of Arts and Letters. In 1999, he became an Honorary Fellow of the Queens College, Oxford, and the New York Academy of Sciences. He received the Lewis Thomas (see chapter 40) Award for Writing about Science in 2001. In 2002, he was elected a fellow of the American Academy of Arts and Sciences. In 2005, he received an honorary degree from Gallaudet University and an honorary doctor of civil law from Oxford University. In 2008, he was appointed Commander of the Order of the British Empire.

Sacks wrote, "Every act of perception is, to some degree, an act of creation, and every act of memory is, to some degree, an act of imagination," and "In examining disease, we gain wisdom about anatomy and physiology and biology. In examining the person with disease, we gain wisdom about life."

SOURCES

Cowles, Gregory. "Oliver Sacks, Neurologist Who Wrote about the Brain's Quirks." *New York Times*. August 30, 2015. https://www.nytimes.com/2015/08/31/science/oliver-sacks-dies-at-82-neurologist-and-author-explored-the-brains-quirks.html (accessed May 6, 2018).

Sacks, Oliver. *On the Move: A Life*. New York: Alfred A. Knopf, 2015.

Wallace-Wells, David. "A Brain with a Heart." *New York News and Politics*, November 4, 2012. http://nymag.com/news/features/oliver-sacks-2012-11/ (accessed April 5, 2018).

49

JOHN STONE III
Iconic and Not Remembered

The discovery of John Stone III's literary legacy and iconic status was serendipitous. It was the consequence of gathering material on Ferrol Sams (see chapter 44). It is ironic that my discovery was an individual with whom I had the closest proximity and shared "Resident Alumnus" status at the University of Rochester Medical School.

John Stone was born in Jackson, Mississippi, on February 7, 1936, the grandson of a general practitioner. John's father, a production manager, died when John was a high school senior. John showed his propensity for producing poetry and prose before he embarked on his medical studies. He edited his Jackson High School

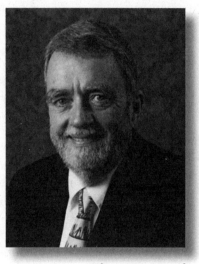

Photo courtesy of
Emory University.

and Millsaps College literary magazines. He continued to hone his literary skills by attending the Bread Loaf Writers Conference in Vermont for three summers between 1969 and 1972 while he was an untenured member of the medical faculty at Emory University in Atlanta.

An interesting association with another physician has not previously been chronicled in accounts of John Stone's life. Hiram C. Polk Jr., one of the most recognizable names in modern American surgery, was born in Jackson, Mississippi, one month before John Stone. They were friends throughout their youths and graduated the local high school in the same class. They enrolled at Millsaps College, a private liberal arts college, located in their hometown and affiliated with the United Methodist Church. Currently, the college, where Stone and Polk were fraternity brothers, reports a student body of 910 undergraduates. Polk went on to Harvard Medical School, while Stone graduated from Washington University, where Polk completed a surgical residency. John Stone received the Distinguished Alumnus Award from Millsaps College in 1997; Hiram C. Polk Jr. followed his friend in receiving the same honor in 2005.

From July 1962 until June 1964, Stone was an intern and resident in medicine at the University of Rochester, where he and I, an untenured member of the surgical faculty at the time, doubtless crossed paths. I have no personal recollection of his presence, nor do any of his other medical contemporaries at Rochester.

Over the ensuing five years, Stone completed his training in medicine and cardiology at Emory University. In the introduction to *In the Country of Hearts* (1990), Stone's collection of essays, he indicates that the early death of his father was a strong personal motivation to choose cardiology as a career. Stone's diverse contributions to the Emory University School of Medicine over four decades added significantly to its reputation. Initially, he concentrated his efforts at Grady Memorial Hospital, Atlanta's inner-city teaching hospital and an integral element in Emory's clinical training. Stone founded an emergency medical residency program that eventually became an independent clinical department. With George R. Schwartz and Peter Safar, Stone coedited *Principles and Practice of Emergency Medicine* (1979), the first textbook in that specialty.

In his last nineteen years on the faculty, Stone served as associate dean for admissions. He was voted best clinical professor for the Emory University School of Medicine three times, and in 1973, he received the Thomas Jefferson Award, the school's top award for service, leadership, and achievement. He was elected to the prestigious status of master of the American College of Physicians, which bestowed upon him the Nicholas E. Davis Memorial Award for Scholarly Activities in the Humanities and History of Medicine in 1996. Stone created one of the first medical school courses, focusing on the humanities in medicine. His charismatic personality attracted students to his Atlanta classroom and to the Emory Summer Studies Program at Oxford University, in which he participated annually.

The first line in Stone's *In the Country of Hearts* is "Each of us is born with two hearts." As a cardiologist, Stone was concerned with the "literal heart" the complex pump required to sustain life. The humanist Stone produced poetry and prose that considered and targeted the "metaphysical heart." Stone indicated that he "wore the double harness of medicine and literature" easily because both are concerned with the human condition, be it of the body or the spirit.

Stone first gained broad recognition when *The Smell of Matches*, a seventy-seven-page collection of his poems, was published by the Rutgers University Press in 1972. His work received the annual Georgia Writers Association Award, the first of four such awards Stone would receive during his life. In 1980, *In All This Rain*, an anthology of fifty-one of Stone's recent poems, was published by the Louisiana State Press. A reviewer in *Annals of Internal Medicine* wrote, "Not a brilliant poet, John Stone is a good one, getting better."

Renaming the Streets (1985), the third volume of Stone's poetry, features eight poems collectively referred to as "the Pigeon Sonnets," and also addresses the art of Edward Hopper and Leonardo da Vinci. The anthology won the literature award from the Mississippi Institute of Arts and Letters. *In the County of Hearts*, his collection of twenty-three essays in which the author reflected on his career in medicine, was published in 1990 and earned Stone his fourth Georgia Writers Association, Writer of the Year Award. *Where Water Begins*, an addition to Stone's poetry and prose, expressing his fascination with the mysteries and miracles of life, was published in 1998.

Music from Apartment 8 (2004) was Stone's final published work. It included a sampling from his previous four books along with twenty-two new poems divided into three sections, adventures with his ninety-five-year-old mother in her nursing home, his memories of travels in the Middle East, and his experiences growing up in Mississippi and Texas. The collection of poems covers a span of thirty years, thereby offering evidence of Stone's evolving interests and changes in literary style.

In order to emphasize the integral role for the humanities in providing evidence-based medical care, *On Doctoring: Stories, Poems, Essays*, coedited by John Stone and Richard Reynolds, dean of the Robert Wood Johnson Medical School, was gifted to all first-year students at US medical schools by the Robert Wood Johnson Foundation. The program was initiated in 1991 and continued for seventeen years. Writings by John Keats, Oliver Wendell Holmes, Sir William Osler, Sir Arthur Conan Doyle, Anton Chekhov, W. Somerset Maugham, William Carlos Williams, Lewis Thomas, Ferrol Sams, Richard Selzer, and John Stone—all of whom are featured in the present volume—are included.

Stone spoke at celebratory events for over 140 institutions in forty states and gave named lectures. He composed the poem "The Spirits of This Lawn" in honor of James Wagner on his inauguration as the tenth president of Emory University on April 2, 2004. Stone joined with music professor William Ransom in a performance titled *The Poet and Pianist* at several Emory University alumni events, including one held at Carnegie Hall. Stone also wrote the libretto for a choral symphony, *Canticles of Time*.

Stone served on the editorial boards of several literary and medical journals, including *Pharos*, the journal of the medical honor society Alpha Omega Alpha. David Bottoms, Georgia's poet laureate, stated that reading Stone's writing "is like getting a house call from an eminent physician of the spirit."

SOURCES

"John Stone," Georgia Writers Hall of Fame, https://georgiawritershalloffame.org/honorees/john-stone (accessed April 5, 2018).

Kerley, Gary. "John Stone (1936–2008)." In *New Georgia Encyclopedia*. Article published December 23, 2002. Last edited by NGE Staff on September 4, 2013. https://www.georgiaencyclopedia.org/articles/arts-culture/john-stone-1936-2008 (accessed April 5, 2018).

Review of *In All This Rain*, by John Stone. *Annals of Internal Medicine*. 94, no. 3 (March 1, 1981): 422.

Wrobel, Sylvia. "Remembering John Stone, Doctor-Poet." *Emory Report*, 61, no. 12 (November 17, 2008). https://www.emory.edu/EMORY_REPORT/erarchive/2008/November/Nov17/JohnStoneTribute.htm (accessed April 5, 2018).

50

MICHAEL STEPHEN PALMER

Therapeutic Thrillers

After Michael Palmer had descended through the depths of despair, as a consequence of addiction, and reached the nadir of his thirty-six years of life, writing became an integral part of his therapy and a road to recovery. Over the ensuing thirty-five years of his life, he produced twenty novels, most of which were medical thrillers, while he remained sober and free of addictive drugs.

Michael Stephen Palmer was born on October 9, 1942, in Springfield, Massachusetts. He graduated with a premed major from Wesleyan University in 1964. Four years later, he received a medical degree from Case Western Reserve University. He was trained in internal medicine at Boston City Hospital and Massachusetts General Hospital, and became certified by the American Board of Internal Medicine.

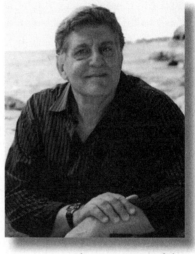

Photo courtesy of the Palmer family.

He engaged in medical practice and was appointed chief of medicine at the Falmouth Hospital on Cape Cod. In the mid-1970s, he became addicted to alcohol and self-prescribed drugs, which were initiated in response to a failed marriage and the pain associated with a series of knee operations. In 1978, he admitted to writing false prescriptions for narcotics and had his hospital privileges suspended. He was placed on two years of probation but did not have his license rescinded.

His initial response was to begin injecting himself with Demerol, and he considered himself to be suicidal. This led him to seek psychiatric help and support systems for addicts. After the two-year suspension ended and he had successfully controlled his addiction, he gradually returned to medicine. He began working as an emergency room physician and as a counselor for physicians with addictions. In the mid-1990s, he ended clinical practice to become the associate director of the Massachusetts Medical Society's Physician Health Services, which assisted doctors with addressing personal mental health problems and recovery from substance abuse.

Shortly after embarking on his road to recovery, Palmer took up writing. According to his own comments, he had recently read the medical thriller *Coma* by his Wesleyan classmate Robin Cook (see chapter 53) and thought that if Cook could write a novel, he could follow suit. After Palmer had achieved literary success, he told writers at the *Boston Globe*, "In retrospect, having a book to write was one of the things that kept me sane," and "I loved the feeling of being in control when my life was not."

Palmer's first publication, *The Sisterhood*, appeared in 1982, three years after it was begun. The plot revolves around a group of well-intentioned nurses who have formed a society that performs selective euthanasia. His second book, *Side Effects* (1985), pits a caring pathologist against a large, unethical pharmaceutical company and includes a connection to Nazi experimenters. Palmer's fourth thriller, *Extreme Measures*, about a young doctor threatened by the hospital elite whose members are engaged in criminal activities, was published in 1991 and was made into a motion picture in1996 under the same name.

In 1994, *Natural Causes*, a tale about a doctor who prescribes alternative medicines that are lethal, was the first of Palmer's books to make the top five of the *New York Times* best-seller list. This was followed by *Silent Treatment* (1995), which presents a villainous physician who is contracted by an insurance cartel for cost containment. In *Critical Judgment* (1996), a small-town doctor takes on a large manufacturing concern that is contaminating her community with a toxic effluent.

The Patient (2000) includes the use of a robotic neurosurgical procedure at a time when it was still in a developmental stage. *The Society* (2004) is a thriller set against a background of outrages associated with a managed care health system. Tess Gerritsen (see chapter 60) wrote about Palmer's next publication, *The Fifth Vial* (2007), "Michael Palmer's 'The Fifth Vial' is a tale set at the very edge of our medical knowledge, and of a thrilling heroine as she confronts a theft that haunts me still."

The First Patient (2008) incorporates presidential politics and nanotechnology in a story that keeps the reader turning pages. *The Second Opinion* (2008) is of interest in that the protagonist, Thea Sperelakis, is a physician with Asperger's syndrome, about which Palmer was knowledgeable because one of his children has that diagnosis. *The Last Surgeon* (2010) pits a doctor suffering from post-traumatic stress disorder against a psychopath who commits murders that are not recognizable as murders.

A Heartbeat Away (2011) deals with the release of a deadly virus in the US Capitol by a terrorist group. This requires the president to quarantine everybody in the building. Every person in line for presidential succession, except the director of homeland security, is trapped inside and exposed to the virus. Although the book received five stars from most of the readers, *Publishers Weekly* stated, "Readers with a low tolerance for the hyperbolic are advised to give this one a pass."

In *Oath of Office* (2012), Dr. Lou Welcome, a doctor with a failed marriage and who has been disciplined for alcohol addiction but is now sober and works for a DC physician wellness office, draws directly from Palmer's personal experiences. For the first time in Palmer's works, his main character, Dr. Lou Welcome, returns in a subsequent novel, *Political Suicide* (2013), and in future works.

On October 30, 2013, Palmer died of a heart attack, which he sustained while going through customs at John F. Kennedy International Airport in New York City. Two of his novels were published posthumously. In *Resistant* (2014), Welcome reappears to counter the evil efforts of a fringe organization that uses a flesh-eating, antibiotic resistant bacterial strain to force the government into ending entitlement programs. *Trauma* (2015), which Michael Palmer had been working on before he died, was completed by his son Daniel.

Michael Palmer stated that he was comfortable with his medical career. He told the *Boston Globe*, "It seemed to me that I was put on earth to take care of people." But Palmer's agent indicated that "Michael really loved the writing process." He also devoted time to the administration and sustenance of the International Thriller Writers Association. Palmer's books frequently made best-seller lists. Approximately five million copies of his works have been sold and have been translated into thirty-five languages.

SOURCES

Marquard, Bryan. "Michael Palmer, 71; Physician Wrote Medical Thrillers."
    Boston Globe. November 3, 2013. https://www.bostonglobe.com/metro/
    2013/11/02/michael-palmer-swampscott-physician-who-wrote-best-seller
    -medical-thrillers/YBhkxwixGWruT5rXsQ5LqI/story.html (accessed April
    5, 2018).
Review of *A Heartbeat Away*, by Michael Palmer. *Publishers Weekly.* December 13,
    2010. https://www.publishersweekly.com/978-0-312-58752-9 (accessed
    May 7, 2018).
Vitello, Paul. "Michael Palmer, Doctor Who Became Top Author, Dies at 71."
    New York Times, November 7, 2013. http://www.nytimes.com/2013/11/08/
    books/michael-palmer-tormented-doctor-who-became-top-author-dies
    -at-71.html (accessed April 5, 2018).

51

JOHN MICHAEL CRICHTON

Uniquely First in Three Media Simultaneously

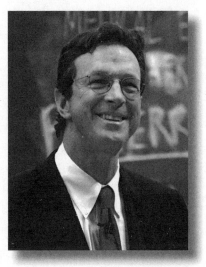

In 1994, Michael Crichton could claim the unique distinction of authoring the most popular book, *Disclosure*; cowriting the most popular motion picture, *Jurassic Park*; and producing the most popular television show, *ER*, concurrently satisfying audiences in written and visual media. Only the combination of talent and indefatigability could achieve that result, and Crichton was an extremely talented workaholic. The roles of a prolific best-selling author, a motion picture and television writer, a film director, and a video-game producer were all encompassed by an individual with a medical degree and a stature of six feet nine inches that merits the declaration that he was "bigger than life."

Photo by Jon Chase / Harvard News Office.

John Michael Crichton was born in Chicago, Illinois, on October 23, 1942. His father was a journalist who became president of the American Association of Advertising Agencies. Michael, as he came to be known, grew up on Long Island in Roslyn, New York. He demonstrated an early interest in writing, and when he was a fourteen-year-old (one source states seventeen-year-old), he was paid for his first publication, the description of a family vacation titled "Climbing up a Cinder Cone," which appeared in the *New York Times*. After graduating high school in Roslyn, Crichton enrolled in Harvard University with the intent of majoring in English to prepare himself for a literary career.

Initially, he was receiving grades of C and C plus for his writing, which was severely criticized by the faculty. To test the system, he submitted an essay by George Orwell, which was pertinent to an assignment, under his own name and received a B minus. This prompted Crichton to change his major to anthropology and take the prerequisite courses for medical school. He graduated in 1964 with a bachelor of arts degree summa cum laude and as a member of Phi Beta Kappa. He spent the next year, during which he was a lecturer in anthropology at Cambridge University, as a Henry Russell Shaw Travelling Fellow.

Crichton entered Harvard Medical School in 1965 and graduated in 1969. The first section of his 1988 publication *Travels* (almost eighty pages) focuses on his medical experiences. During his first year as a medical student, he discussed with a member of the faculty the desire to quit, and his discontent with medicine continued throughout the four years. The finality of his decision to "quit medicine" was expressed when he decided not to apply for an internship. He wrote, "Quitting medicine assured me that I would be forced into all sorts of changes I might not otherwise have made." Crichton spent the year after graduating from medical school as a postdoctoral fellow at the Salk Institute for Biological Studies in La Jolla, California, doing research. This afforded him the opportunity to gain exposure to the motion picture industry.

During the time spent as a medical student, Crichton published several novels under an assortment of pseudonyms. Crichton's first novel, *Odds On*, appeared in 1966 with the author listed as "John Lange," derived from the German word for "long" and relating to the author's height. The work describes a foiled robbery that had been planned with the help of a computer. *Scratch One*, another thriller, was published the following year with the same authorship. In 1968, two more novels, *Easy Go* and *A Case of Need*, were published, the first bearing the name of "John Lange" as its author. *A Case of Need* was a medical thriller in which a pathologist investigates an illegal abortion that results in the patient's death. The work, which was initially published under the authorship of "Jeffrey Hudson," a name that Crichton had taken from a seventeenth-century dwarf, was awarded the 1969 Edgar Award® for the best mystery fiction of the year. Over a five-year period, beginning in 1966, Crichton wrote ten novels on weekends and vacations. In 1970, he published *Dealing*, listing "Michael Douglas" (himself) and his brother, Douglas Crichton, as the authors.

Written during his final year of medical school and published in 1969, *The Andromeda Strain* was the first novel published under his own name, and it gained Crichton immediate fame. The work, which initiated Crichton's association with the genre of science fiction, tells the story of a crashed satellite returning from outer space and exposing people to deadly microbes, and the attempt of scientists to discover a cure and avoid destruction of the entire population. *The Andromeda Strain* appeared as a successful motion picture in 1971.

In 1970, Crichton's first nonfiction book, *Five Patients: The Hospital Explained*, was published. By three decades, it preceded a plethora of books by several authors that directed the public's attention to medical matters. Crichton included a brief history of medicine to provide a background for the medical culture and practice of the time. The work presents five diverse patients whose situations are used to emphasize the need to improve medical care and is a criticism of the contemporary medical establishment.

In 1972, *Binary* was published with "John Lange" as the author. The same year witnessed the publication of the second novel under Crichton's name, *The Terminal Man*. The work, classified as science fiction, tells of scientists' attempt to create smarter human beings and their failure to control their creations. That year, two of his novels, *Dealing* and *A Case of Need* (as *The Carey Treatment*), appeared on the motion picture screen, and, shortly thereafter, Crichton embarked on his career as a director. His first effort was a television adaptation of *Binary*, in 1972, followed by the movie *Westworld* (1973) from his own script. He later directed Robin Cook's *Coma* (1978) and his own *The Great Train Robbery* (1979), along with three additional, relatively inconsequential films.

The Great Train Robbery, unlike previous novels, is an adventure story rather than science fiction. It is set in the mid-1800s and is based on a real crime. The movie received the Edgar Allan Poe Award for Best Motion Picture by the Mystery Writers Association of America. In 1976, Crichton's *Eaters of the Dead* appeared, after which he absented himself from writing fiction and spent four years traveling to exotic places. Several episodes of his travel were later described in *Travels*, and the experiences and encounters influenced his subsequent fiction.

While filming *The Great Train Robbery* in England, Crichton followed the path of another physician with a literary presence, Sir Arthur Conan Doyle, into the realm of spiritualism and psychic experiences. Crichton returned to writing fiction in 1980 with the publication of *Congo*, which was later adapted to a 1995 film. Crichton produced no new fiction for seven years until *Sphere* (1987), a psychological thriller that takes place on the floor of the Pacific Ocean, and it, too, became a motion picture in 1998 with the same title.

Arguably, Crichton is best identified with *Jurassic Park*, which was published in 1990. At the end of the twentieth century, of the twenty million purchased copies of paperbacks authored by Crichton, 8.4 million were of *Jurassic Park*. The book tells the tale of modern humans' encounters with genetically engineered creatures from the age of dinosaurs. Crichton adapted the work for a film that was released by Universal and Steven Spielberg in 1993. The movie set a record for attendance.

In 1992, *Rising Sun*, which uses the Japanese business world within the United States as a platform for detective fiction, was published. As indicated previously, 1994 represented Crichton's banner year. While *Jurassic Park* was setting records in theaters, *Disclosure* was published and reached the top of the *New York Times* best-seller list. In the category of detective fiction, the work uses cutting-edge technology to resolve the issue of guilt in the circumstance of sexual harassment by a female superior. The pilot episode of *ER* also aired on television in 1994. The script of the only episode attributed to Crichton had been written twenty years previously.

In 1995, *The Lost World*, a sequel to *Jurassic Park*, was published, and, two years later, it appeared as a movie. It was Crichton's only sequel, and, although the book sales resulted in it being considered successful, it was not well regarded by critics. The next year, Crichton, once again, changed direction by publishing *Airframe*, which was reviewed in the *New York Times* as a "Thriller Not to Carry on Your Next Plane Trip." It is an entertaining unraveling of the cause of an in-flight accident that results in death and injury to passengers. The interaction between humans and machines is brought into focus.

Three years later, Crichton returned to the science fiction genre for his next novel, *Timeline*, which incorporates time travel back to the Middle Ages in order to gain an appreciation of archeological findings. The narrative was deemed his most enjoyable work since *Jurassic Park* and was produced as a film, under the same title. After another hiatus of three years, *Prey* was published in 2001. It explored the relatively recent field of nanotechnology, genetic engineering, and computer-based artificial life. A reviewer wrote, "Despite its absurd moments, 'Prey' is irresistibly suspenseful."

The last novel to be published during Crichton's lifetime was *State of Fear* (2004), in which ecoterrorists plot mass murder to support their view of climate change. The thriller had an initial print run of 1.5 million copies and reached the number two position on the *New York Times* best-seller list. The work is an expression of Crichton's passionate efforts to counter the theory of global warming. Crichton was a loud and repetitive critic of those who were formulating policy to reduce global warming.

Crichton served on the Board of Overseers of Harvard University and the Board of Trustees of the Los Angeles Museum of Art, as an avid collector of twentieth-century American art. He died of cancer, perhaps lymphoma, on November 4, 2008. One of his completed novels, *Pirate Latitudes*, was published posthumously in 2009, and an unfinished work by Crichton was completed and published with the title *Micro* (2011). In 2015, Crichton's world of prehistoric animals was revisited by a new movie, *Jurassic World*. Although the film did not capture the awe and astonishment of the original, it drew a large audience.

In terms of his literary corpus, Crichton is characterized as a tremendously successful writer of commercial fiction. His work contains little in the way of character development or consideration of the psychological complexities that define the players who participate in his tales that evolve with a rapid pace. Steven Spielberg, the motion picture director/producer, said of Crichton, "He was the greatest at blending science with big theatrical concepts, which is what gave credibility to dinosaurs again walking the earth."

SOURCES

Crichton, Michael. *Travels*. New York: HarperCollins, 1988.

Golla, Robert, ed. *Conversations with Michael Crichton*. Jackson: University of Mississippi Press, 2011.

Holt, Jim. "It's the Little Things." Review of *Prey*, by Michael Crichton. *New York Times*. November 24, 2002. https://www.nytimes.com/2002/11/24/books/it-s-the-little-things.html (accessed May 7, 2018).

Lehmann-Haupt, Christopher. "A Thriller Not to Carry on Your Next Plane Trip." Review of *Airframe*, by Michael Crichton. *New York Times*. December 5, 1996. https://www.nytimes.com/1996/12/05/books/a-thriller-not-to-carry-on-your-next-plane-trip.html (accessed May 7, 2018).

Spielberg, Steven. "Statement from Steven Spielberg on the Passing of Michael Crichton." Business Wire. November 5, 2008. https://www.businesswire.com/news/home/20081105006061/en/Statement-Steven-Spielberg-Passing-Michael-Crichton (accessed May 7, 2018).

Trembley, Elizabeth A. *Michael Crichton: A Critical Companion*. Westport, CT: Greenwood, 1996.

PART II

THE PRESENT

Men and women of the medical profession continue to provide literature created specifically for public consumption. As writers whose personal profile includes a medical career or a medical education and who are alive at the time of the publication of this work come into focus, both consistencies with the past and distinctly new directions become apparent. Works of fiction continue to issue forth from the pens and computer keyboards of physicians and surgeons, but it is difficult to identify one or more literary giants who come close to the notability of Rabelais, Schiller, Keats, Doyle, Chekhov, Maugham, or Percy.

Some novels, particularly those categorized as thrillers, have had extraordinary sales, far exceeding those attained in the past. This is reflective of a markedly expanded readership. As was true in the past, the analytic training to which physicians are exposed continues to find expression in the production of detective fiction. The empathy associated with illness and medical care also continues to pervade recent novels and short stories written by physicians.

The most apparent difference between the literature of the past and that of more modern times, particularly the present, pertains to nonfiction. The public and, consequently, the readership have become more informed and more desirous of remaining informed about more diverse issues related to health and healthcare. This has resulted from the liberalization and expansion of education and the widespread dissemination of information by print, radio, television, and the internet. Included in the information imparted to the masses are medical facts and issues. The public is continually receiving information about medical disorders, pharmaceuticals, surgical procedures, delivery of healthcare, and their political implications. The public has repeatedly been informed about AIDS, cancer, Ebola, radiation effects, virility, women's health issues, palliative care, end-of-life considerations, and the concept of wellness among other topics.

The appetite of readers for medical matters has been whetted as medicine has become ever more popularized in literature. The most widely read newspapers, the most highly regarded magazines, and the major network and cable news outlets incorporate medical professionals on their staffs of reporters. In response to the expanding interest in medicine, knowledgeable physicians have created a new genre of medical nonfiction, which satisfies the desires of readers to penetrate the mystique of medicine and be made more aware of what specific medical issues might potentially affect their lives. Concomitantly, the foibles and dramatic events in the lives of physicians and medical personnel have become a central theme for fiction.

Medicine, with its fascinating scientific advancements, its dramatic emotional implications, and its sociological and political importance, has become a dominant theme for those physicians who continue to satisfy the public's appetite for literature. The number of current doctors who can claim publications, either fiction or nonfiction, addressed to a general readership is large. Those who have been selected for inclusion here are particularly notable or recognizable.

ERIC R. KANDEL

Medical Nobel Laureate Creates Compelling Literature

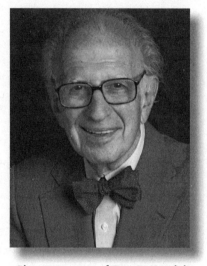

Photo courtesy of Eric R. Kandel.

The Nobel Prize in Physiology or Medicine for 2000 was jointly awarded to Arvid Carlsson, Paul Greengard, and Eric R. Kandel "for their discoveries concerning signal transduction in the nervous system." Within the ensuing twelve years, Kandel published two engaging and compelling literary gems for a broad readership.

The first work details a balanced blend of the dramatic autobiographical maturation of a leading neuroscientist and the development of an understanding of the physiological process of recording, modifying, and preserving memory. *In Search of Memory: The Emergence of the New Science of Mind* (2006) is, in part, a narrative of Kandel's life, beginning with his early memories of Vienna and the threat imposed by the presence of the Nazis. It extends through his youth and his personal development in America. The autobiographical theme dramatically concludes when the seventy-nine-year-old author receives word on Yom Kippur, the highest of Jewish holy days, that he had been awarded a Nobel Prize.

In the narrative of his development as a scientist, Kandel credits the contributions of others while creating a sense of personal excitement as each of an extensive sequence of scientific milestones is identified. Beginning with a series of electrophysiological studies on the sea snail, *Aplysia* (1962), and continuing with the definition of the specific proteins and chemical reactions that are involved in basic learning integral to the process, Kandel's unraveling of the mystery of both short- and long-term memory is captivating.

Sherwin Nuland (see chapter 46), who reviewed Kandel's book in the *New York Times*, indicated that he was not acquainted with any work that excelled over *In Search of Memory* in "demonstrating how biological research is done, or of telling the story of a brilliant scientist's career." The book has been compared with James D. Watson's *The Double Helix: A Personal Account of the Discovery of the Structure of DNA* and was awarded the 2006 Los Angeles Times Book Award for Science and Technology.

Kandel's second, richly illustrated popular book, *The Age of Insight* (2012), is a history of the late-nineteenth-century Vienna, coupled with an exploration of the neuroscience of the appreciation of art. The work identifies the author as a profound intellectual whose interests extend beyond neuroscience and delve deeply into Austrian art and psychoanalysis. Kandel draws from his expertise as a biologist to explore the role of neural transport of visual stimuli to the brain and the interplay of the individual's unconscious on the appreciation of art.

The psychoanalytic theories of Sigmund Freud; the writings of Arthur Schnitzler; and the art of Gustav Klimt, Oskar Kokoschka, and Egon Schiele are invoked in the author's attempt to unify neuroscience and aesthetics. The underlying thesis is that one's personal appreciation of art is dependent on the perceptual and emotional contribution of the viewer. The book presents the concept of the appreciation of art in biological terms.

In accordance with policy, Kandel provided a meticulously detailed autobiography for the archives of the Nobel Prize. His personal history reads like a novel in which the protagonist, girded solely with the armor of his intellect, surmounts life-threatening danger, translocation from his homeland with its attendant need for cultural adjustment, and financial constraints. The explication of his scientific accomplishments is an extensive romantic narrative that details a magnificent quest. The "Holy Grail" is the scientific basis of memory.

Kandel was born in Vienna on November 7, 1929, into a Jewish middle-class family. In March 1938, Hitler triumphantly marched into Vienna and was enthusiastically received by the Viennese people. Kandel was exposed to the anti-Semitic fervor that reached its climax on Kristallnacht, November 9, 1938, when Nazi brown shirts harassed Jews and destroyed their homes and places of business. In April 1939, Eric Kandel and his older brother left for the United States, followed by his parents five months later.

He lived with his maternal grandparents in Brooklyn before his parents arrived, and was tutored by his grandfather in Hebrew so that he could gain a scholarship to the Yeshiva of Flatbush. He graduated the Yeshiva elementary school in 1944 and subsequently completed his high school education at a Brooklyn public school, where he achieved a distinguished academic record that resulted in the award of a scholarship to Harvard University.

At Harvard, he majored in nineteen- and twentieth-century European history and wrote an honors dissertation titled "The Attitude toward National Socialism of Three German Writers: Carl Zuckmayer, Han Carosa, and Ernst Junger." While at Harvard, Kandel became intrigued with psychoanalysis and the biology of conscious and unconscious memory. This led to his completing the courses required for entrance to medical school after he graduated from Harvard, and in 1952, he entered New York University Medical School.

While at medical school, although Kandel initially planned for a career in psychiatry and psychoanalysis, he soon became interested in neural science and the biology of the mind. He spent an elective period in Harry Grundfest's laboratory at Columbia University, where he was exposed to studies on action potential conduction and techniques used to evaluate intracellular electrical activity. After graduating medical school in 1956, he completed an internship at Montefiore Hospital in the Bronx and also worked in Grundfest's lab. In 1957, as an alternative to serving in the military mandated by the physicians' draft, he began a two-year appointment in the US Public Health Service in the Laboratory of Neurophysiology at the National Institutes of Health (NIH).

Most of Kandel's two years at the NIH were devoted to the study of the hippocampus part of the human brain and its ability to store memory. He realized that the basis of learning and memory must reside in the modification of neural interconnections by sensory signals. In 1962, Kandel completed a residency in psychiatry at the Massachusetts Mental Health Hospital, which was affiliated with Harvard. During his residency, he decided to direct his attention to a study of the nervous system of the giant marine snail *Aplysia*, which was capable of learning and memory and had the advantage, for investigators, of a small number of large cells.

After spending sixteen months in a Paris research laboratory, in order to perfect techniques to conduct neural studies on the *Aplysia*, he was able to publish, in 1965, initial findings of presynaptic potentiation that seemed to be associated with a simple form of learning. When he returned to Harvard, he was confronted with the choice of becoming an academic psychiatrist or a neurobiologist. He opted for a position in the Departments of Physiology and Psychiatry, where he formed the Division of Neurobiology and Behavior.

Kandel and his associates demonstrated that the snail's protective gill-withdrawal reflex could be modified by both habituation and sensitization to allow for two forms of learning. The group of investigators showed that repetition of stimuli resulted in long-term memory and identified the neural circuitry and traffic associated with learning. They also defined the biochemical changes that occurred to affect learning and memory storage. In 1974, Kandel moved his lab to Columbia University, where he became the founding director of the Center for Neurobiology and Behavior. While he was at Columbia, his studies determined the exact site of the synaptic change produced by short-term sensitization and defined the chemical transmitters involved.

In 1983, Kandel helped to establish the Howard Hughes Medical Research Institute at Columbia, devoted to the study of molecular neural science. The investigators demonstrated that while short-term memory did not require new protein synthesis, long-term memory did. They identified proteins that were required to convert short-term to long-lasting memory. Studies were extended to vertebrates in which the molecular basis of memory storage in the hippocampus was investigated. While continuously contributing to the research endeavor at Columbia, Kandel taught medical and graduate students, and coauthored the popular textbook *Principles of Neural Science*, which was first published in 1981 and is currently in its fifth edition.

Recognition of Kandel's extraordinary contributions is evidenced in the many accolades that he has received. He was elected to the National Academy of Sciences, the National Science Academies of Germany and France, the American Academy of Arts and Sciences, the American Philosophical Society, the National Institute of Medicine, and the Orden Pour Le Mérite für Wissenschaften und Künste (Order of Merit for Science and Art).

He was awarded the American Association of Medical Colleges Award for Distinguished Research in the Biological Sciences, the Wolf Prize of Israel, the Dr. A. H. Heineken Prize for Medicine from the Royal Netherlands Academy of Arts and Sciences, the Austrian Decoration for Science and Art, and the Benjamin Franklin Medal for Distinguished Achievement in the Sciences of the American Philosophical Society. He also received the Viktor Frankl Award of the City of Vienna, which made him an honorary citizen of that city. He was awarded the Grand Decoration of Honour in Silver with Star for Services to the Republic of Austria, and he became a Foreign Member of the Royal Society of London—and many more.

Kandel, with whom I have been privileged to have dined and conversed, is truly ingratiating. His scientific publications and two popular books are lucid and engaging. He represents the biological analog to theoretical physics and cosmology's Stephen Hawkins. Dr. Assad Meymandi, writing about *In Search of Memory* in the journal *Psychiatry*, stated, "As one who has been doing book reviews for more than 40 years, I have become accustomed to examining the down side of books. It is astounding that I can say nothing negative about this most impressive and seminal work. . . . Dr. Kandel is my kind of saint—the kind of saint who KNOWS, yet lets his knowledge get marinated in the elixir of spirit, faith, and transcendence, giving it the lofty status of being in the presence of God and better yet, dining with God on an infinitely rich, intellectual diet."

SOURCES

"Eric R. Kandel: Biographical." NobelPrize.org. 2000. https://www.nobelprize .org/nobel_prizes/medicine/laureates/2000/kandel-bio.html (accessed April 5, 2018).

Kandel, Eric. "Eric R. Kandel: Interview Transcript." Interview by Adam Smith. NobelPrize.org. June 13, 2008. https://www.nobelprize.org/nobel _prizes/medicine/laureates/2000/kandel-interview-transript.html (accessed April 5, 2018).

Meymandi, Assad. "Eric Kandel: My Kind of Saint." *Psychiatry* 6, no. 11 (November 2009): 48–50.

Pondrom, Sue. "The Biological Mind and Art." *Annals of Neurology* 72, no. 5 (November 2012): A7–8.

53

ROBERT BRIAN "ROBIN" COOK

Primacy and Prolificacy in Medical Thrillers

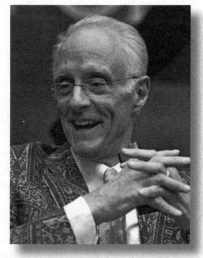

Photo courtesy of Robin Cook.

The publication of *Coma* in 1977 represents the birth of the medical thriller, now regarded to be a sub-genre of fiction. Over the ensuing decades, *Coma*'s author, Robin Cook, has produced an unmatched number of medical thrillers and has maintained his position as the most popular author in that category. His life and the diversity of his interests rival the panoramic scope of his writings.

Robert Brian "Robin" Cook was born on May 4, 1940, in Brooklyn, New York, and spent his early years in Queens. When he was eight years old, he moved with his family to the small town of Leonia, New Jersey. He graduated from a public high school, where he excelled as an athlete and was the class valedictorian. He planned a career in medicine and proceeded to Wesleyan University. In 1964, he continued to distinguish himself academically, graduating summa cum laude with a major in chemistry and a notable performance in government. He gained a medical education at Columbia University College of Physicians and Surgeons.

While at medical school, he worked nights and weekends running a blood/ gas laboratory for the cardiac surgery team. His laboratory experience led to an invitation to spend two medical school summer electives in a similar facility, conducting research at the famous Jacques Cousteau Oceanographic Institute in Monaco. Cook graduated medical school in 1968 and interned in surgery at the Queens Hospital in Honolulu.

The doctors' draft associated with the Vietnam War mandated that he spend two years as a military physician. From 1969 through 1971, Cook served in the US Navy, initially on the flagship of the submarine fleet in the South Pacific, and subsequently at the Navy's Deep Submergence Systems Project (SEALAB), where he trained as an aquanaut medical officer. In that position, his propensity for writing became manifest with his first publication, *A Medical Watch Standard Guide to Saturation Diving* (1971).

He returned to civilian life as a resident in ophthalmology in the Harvard program at the Massachusetts General Hospital. On completing his training, Cook established a practice in general ophthalmology in Marblehead, Massachusetts, and accepted a clinical position at the Massachusetts Eye and Ear Infirmary, where he saw patients and instructed medical students and ophthalmology residents. At the same time, considering the possibility of entering politics or a governmental position of some kind, he enrolled as a full-time student at Harvard's Kennedy School of Government.

He terminated his schooling in politics and government within several months, after *Coma* had a successful launching (1977). He maintained his activities in ophthalmology for about eight years as he increasingly devoted his attention to a literary career.

Cook's literary career can be traced to the underwater environs of his service aboard a nuclear submarine. While at sea, he wrote *The Year of the Intern*, which was published in 1973. The novel brought into focus the dehumanizing experiences of a young physician in training. The book failed to gather a broad readership but anticipated, by five years, the publication of Samuel Shem's *House of God* that addressed the same theme and achieved great success and cult-like status.

Determined to succeed as a popular author, Cook deliberately studied accumulated data to determine what made a best seller. He settled on thrillers that play out against a backdrop of contemporary medical practice and ethical and social issues.

Cook wrote *Coma*, the first medical thriller and a book that would change the public's perception of medicine as a sacrosanct profession, while he was a senior resident in ophthalmology. The novel reached the number six position on the *New York Times* best-seller list of 1977 and was referred to as the "number one thriller of the year." A year later, it appeared as a motion picture directed by Michael Crichton (see chapter 51).

Cook's unmatched productivity as an author of medical thrillers is attested to by his publication of thirty-three books in that category. His latest work, *Host*, was published in 2015. Cook's works of fiction have addressed many of current medicine's most critical problems. The narratives have brought to readers' attention the illicit acquisition of organs for transplantation, in vitro fertilization, genetic engineering, stem cell therapy, cloning, food poisoning, an outbreak of the Ebola virus, bioterrorism, xenotransplantation, medical nanotechnology, malfeasance of pharmaceutical companies and managed care consortia, euthanasia of the elderly, and ambulance-chasing lawyers.

Among the medical thrillers published by Cook are ten works that constitute the Jack Stapleton and Laurie Montgomerie series. In those novels, two forensic pathologists solve diverse medical or biotechnical crimes. Ten of Cook's thrillers have been adapted for either the motion picture screen or television.

Cook, whose book sales have exceeded one hundred million copies, stated, "I think of myself more as a doctor who writes, rather than a writer who happens to be a doctor." He regards his books as instructional vehicles to inform the public about current medical issues and expanding biomedical research.

His work has gained for him several awards, which include a Distinguished Alumnus Award from Wesleyan University in 1982 and the same institution's James McConaughy Award in 2012. In 2004, he was appointed by President George W. Bush to the Board of Trustees of the Woodrow Wilson Center in Washington, DC. In 2014, he was the recipient of the Literary Legend Award from the Florida Heritage Book Festival and the first Robert B. Parker mystery writer's award.

He indicates that he is currently working on a new thriller and is developing a motion picture and video production company, which will showcase his works. During a personal interview, he presented himself as an individual whose mind and body are in constant meaningful motion.

SOURCES

"About Robin Cook." RobinCook.com. 2018. http://robincook.com/about -robin-cook.php (accessed April 5, 2018).

McDonald, Jay. "What a Shock: Robin Cook Fuses Stem Cells with a Suspenseful Tale." BookPage. October 2007. https://web.archive.org/ web/20071016063803/http://www.bookpage.com/0109bp/robin_cook .html (accessed May 8, 2018).

54

PATRICK TAYLOR

From Medical Forefronts to the Irish Countryside

Two of the significant advances in medicine that have occurred in the past half century are transperitoneal minimally invasive surgery and in vitro fertilization. Minimally invasive surgery, which characterizes most modern operative procedures, had its genesis in obstetrics and gynecology, while in vitro fertilization is a by-product of the visualization of the female pelvic organs using a scope inserted through the abdominal wall into the peritoneal cavity.

Patrick James Taylor was in the forefront of laparoscopic evaluation of gynecologic disorders and, as an offshoot, in vitro fertilization. Taylor, who was born

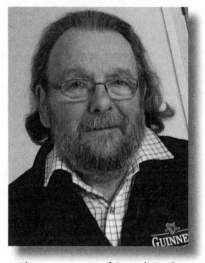

Photo courtesy of Patrick Taylor.

on August 23, 1941, in Blackpool, Lancashire, England, while his Ulsterman physician father was stationed there as a volunteer in the Royal Air Force, would gain recognition for his contributions to obstetrics and gynecology, and also become one of Ireland's most popular authors.

After World War II ended, the Taylors returned to their hometown of Bangor in County Down, Northern Ireland. After completing his early education in Ulster, Patrick attended Campbell College Belfast, a private boys' boarding school, from which he graduated in 1958. In his senior year, he won a prize for an essay written in the style of the sixteenth- and seventeenth-century English philosopher/statesman Francis Bacon, providing an early hint of his later literary capability. From 1958 through 1964, Taylor was a student at Queen's University of Belfast School of Medicine, graduating with MB BCh and BAO degrees. His future interest in viewing gynecologic pathology and operating through endoscopes was manifest by his thesis in1985 titled "The Effects of Hysteroscopically Detected Intra-Uterine Adhesions in Eumenorrhaeic Infertile Women," for which he was granted an MD.

After an internship at the Royal Victoria Hospital Belfast, over the following four years, he completed training in obstetrics and gynecology. In 1969, he gained membership in the Royal College of Obstetrics and Gynecology and was subsequently elected a fellow. In 1969, Taylor spent one month in Oldham General Hospital, Manchester, England, learning laparoscopy from Dr. Patrick Steptoe, a pioneer in its use. During his training, Taylor performed his first recovery of an oocyte (an ovarian cell) while working with the future Nobel laureate Robert Edwards.

Taylor had difficulty establishing a practice in Ulster. This, coupled with raging political strife in Northern Ireland, led him to immigrate to Canada with his wife and daughter. Before leaving Ireland, he performed the first laparoscopy in Belfast. After a brief period of unrewarding practice in Welland, Ontario, he accepted an appointment as an assistant professor of obstetrics and gynecology at the University of Calgary in Alberta. There he established a multidisciplinary infertility clinic, which was responsible for the third in vitro fertilized baby born in Canada. Taylor became president of the Canadian Fertility Society in 1979. When that society merged with the Canadian Andrololology Society in 1980, he was elected the first president of the new organization. Taylor also was active in the American Association of Gynecologic Laparoscopists. He rose to the rank of professor at the University of Calgary in 1981.

In 1987, Taylor was appointed deputy director of the Bourn Hall Fertility Clinic, which had been founded in Cambridgeshire, England, in1980 by Mr. Patrick Steptoe and Professor Robert Edwards, the pioneers of in vitro fertilization. After rising to the position of director, Taylor resigned when the clinic was sold to a pharmaceutical company in 1989.

He returned to Canada as professor and director of human reproduction and fertility at the University of Manitoba, a position he held for two years before moving to the University of British Columbia in 1991. During the ensuing decade, he was a professor at the university and two-term chairman of the Department of Obstetrics and Gynecology at an affiliated hospital, St.

Paul's Hospital in Vancouver. At the same time, he served as editor in chief of the *Journal of the Society of Obstetricians and Gynecologists of Canada* (*SOGC*).

During his academic career, Taylor authored approximately one hundred articles, which appeared in peer-reviewed journals. One of the most intriguing is "Pregnancy and Infertility in the Lowland Gorilla." He coauthored three medical texts: *Laparoscopy and Hysteroscopy in Gynecological Practice* (1988), *Unexplained Infertility* (1993), and *Diagnostic and Operative Laparoscopy* (1995). He was recognized for his medical achievements with the President's Award of Excellence by the International Society for Reproductive Medicine, a Life Time Achievement Award from the Canadian Fertility and Andrology Society, and the President's Award of the Society of Obstetricians and Gynecologists of Canada. Taylor retired from medicine in 2001 so he could spend more time writing.

His literary potential shone through in a monthly humor column, which he contributed to *SOGC*, and a monthly column called "Taylor's Twist" for *Punch Digest for Doctors* (later *Stitches: The Journal of Medical Humor*).

Taylor began writing fiction in 1994 at the suggestion of a novelist friend. His first publication, *Only Wounded: Ulster Stories*, a collection of sixteen short stories, appeared in 1997. It brings into focus the violent conflict surrounding the sovereignty of Northern Ireland, profiling the ordinary people caught up in the partisan brutality.

Continuing with the theme of the Northern Ireland conflict, Taylor published the novel *Pray for Us Sinners* in 1997. *Quill & Quire* in its critique wrote that the thriller offered an explanation rather than an indictment of the mid-1970s violence, and that it was "flawlessly researched, and . . . nails the chips-and-guns-with-everything atmosphere of violence." *Now and in the Hour of Our Death* was published in 2005 as a sequel to *Pray for Us Sinners*. The narrative followed the lives of two young lovers whose lives were torn apart by the conflict in Northern Ireland nine years previously.

Taylor is generally identified by his Irish Country Stories series that he initiated in 2004. Dr. O'Reilly, who is a presence in Taylor's stories for over a decade, first appeared in *Apprenticeship of Doctor Laverty* in 2004. The book was reissued by another publisher in 2007 with a new title, *An Irish Country Doctor*, at which time it made the *New York Times* extended best-seller list.

Set in the fictional village of Ballybucklebo in Northern Ireland, the series follows a young Dr. Laverty as he begins an apprenticeship with Dr. Fingal Fishertie O'Reilly and as his life progresses over the course of time. Two of the novels, *A Dublin Student Doctor* and *Fingal O'Reilly, Irish Doctor* relate events that occurred prior to Dr. Laverty's presence. The sequence of publications was the following: *An Irish Country Doctor* (2007), *An Irish Country Village* (2008), *An Irish Country Christmas* (2008), *An Irish Country Girl* (2010), *An Irish Country Courtship* (2010), *A Dublin Student Doctor* (2011), *An Irish Country Wedding* (2012), *Fingal O'Reilly, Irish Doctor* (2013), *An Irish Doctor in Peace and War* (2014), *An Irish Doctor in Love and at Sea* (2015), *An Irish Love Story* (2016), and *An Irish Country Practice* (2017).

In its review of *An Irish Country Girl*, the *Globe and Mail*, the Canadian national newspaper, remarked, "Patrick Taylor has become the most popular Irish-Canadian writer of all time." A recent survey of interested readers in the United Kingdom rated Taylor as eighth on its list of the twenty most important Irish authors.

Nearly two million copies of Taylor's books have been sold, and they have been translated into thirteen languages. Many have been condensed and published in *Readers Digest*. All twelve of the Irish Country novels have been on the best-seller list of the *Globe and Mail*, and six have been on the *New York Times* best-seller list. When asked to articulate his philosophy of life, Taylor responded, "Life's a carousel. You get one ticket; enjoy the ride. And if you're a writer, take notes."

SOURCES

Brouwer, Adair. Review of *Pray for Us Sinners*, by Patrick Taylor. *Quill & Quire*. 2000. https://quillandquire.com/review/pray-for-us-sinners/ (accessed May 8, 2018).

Kath. "The 20 Greatest Irish Authors of All Time." *For Reading Addicts* (blog). September 12, 2015. http://forreadingaddicts.co.uk/polls-and-discussion/the-20-greatest-irish-authors-of-all-time/4420 (accessed May 8, 2018).

Lederman, Marsha. "Bestselling Novelist Patrick Taylor's Literary Obscurity." *Globe and Mail*. October 23, 2015. https://www.theglobeandmail.com/arts/books-and-media/bestselling-novelist-patrick-taylors-literary-obscurity/article26959412/ (accessed May 8, 2018).

"Patrick Taylor: Irish Country Author." PatrickTaylorAuthor. 2018. http://patricktaylorauthor.com/ (accessed April 5, 2018).

55

STEPHEN J. BERGMAN

The Rhodes to Irreverence

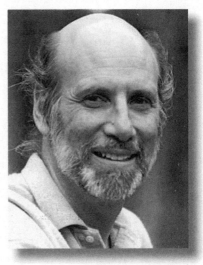

A traumatic internship year transformed a young scholar into a satirical critic of medical training. Like Athena, the goddess of wisdom, who emerged from the skull of Zeus, Samuel Shem was born from the mind of Stephen Bergman. Over the years, the assessment of him by the medical educational establishment has morphed from an "enfant terrible" to one who played a role in generating appropriate change.

Stephen J. Bergman was born in Hudson, New York, on August 6, 1944. He was educated at public schools, graduating in 1962 from high school, where he excelled academically and at basketball and golf. Four years later, he graduated

Photo courtesy of Stephen J. Bergman.

from Harvard University, magna cum laude, with membership in Phi Beta Kappa and a letter in golf. He received a Rhodes scholarship and concentrated on electrophysiology at Balliol College, Oxford, from 1966 to1969. His thesis was titled "Electrophysiological Analysis of Inhibitory and Excitatory Processes in the Nervous System of *Periplaenta American*" (cockroach). That work, which constituted the first report of a common inhibitory motoneuron in insects, was published in the *Journal of Insect Physiology* in 1970. The paper is Bergman's sole scientific publication. Based on that work, he was awarded a DPhil from Oxford in 1971.

In 1969, confronted with the options of embarking on a medical education or being drafted during the Vietnam War, which he vehemently opposed, Bergman entered Harvard Medical School. He graduated, in 1973, with the academic honor of election to Alpha Omega Alpha (medical school honor society). He spent one year as a medical intern at the Beth Israel Hospital in Boston, followed by three years in a psychiatry residency at the MacLean Hospital, also in Boston.

Although he elected not to take the certifying examination for psychiatry, he conducted a private practice for approximately twenty years. He developed a specific interest in caring for patients with alcohol addiction. From 1977 to 2002, Bergman held the position of Clinical Instructor in Psychiatry at Harvard, for which he received no compensation. In 1995, he was the recipient of a Robert Wood Johnson Foundation Award for addiction study at the Harvard Medical School Division on Addiction. In 2014, he was appointed Clinical Professor of Medicine, Division of Medical Humanities, at the New York University Medical School.

Bergman admits to "a life-saving dedication to doing anything creative" and began to experiment with prose while at Oxford, in anticipation of satisfying his basic desire to become a writer. Medicine would provide for sustenance while writing would satisfy his soul.

The House of God, which gained both fame and notoriety for its author, was written during Bergman's psychiatry residency from 1974 to1977, and was published in 1978 with the pseudonym Samuel Shem as the author. The satirical novel is described by the *New York Times* as a "raunchy, troubling and hilarious" tale of one year's dehumanizing experiences encountered during residency training in a distinguished hospital. The novel was repugnant to many faculty members and older clinicians, but it resonated with younger physicians and medical trainees.

In 1999, *Newsweek* listed it as "*the* novel to read about becoming a doctor." In the 2003 edition of the novel, which was published on the occasion of its twenty-fifth anniversary, noted author John Updike wrote an introduction in which he stated that it was "more timely than ever," and compared it to Joseph Heller's immensely popular military satire, *Catch-22*. In the British journal *Lancet*, Bergman's (Shem's) *The House of God* was referred to as "one of the two most significant American medical novels of the 20th century"; the other was *Arrowsmith*. In 2008, in celebration of the thirtieth anniversary of its publication, a symposium, sponsored by the Center of Literature and Medicine at Hiram College, was conducted at the Cleveland Clinic. The discussions focused on the impact that the book had on medical residency programs. The book has sold more than two million copies in thirty languages. In 2016, *Publishers Weekly* listed *The House of God* as one of the ten best satires of all time (along with *Don Quixote* and *Catch-22*).

Samuel Shem's second novel, *Fine*, was published in 1985. It tells of a young Freudian psychoanalyst's transformation into a more complete therapist. Critics referred to it as "funny. . . . Full of dazzling, zany intelligence . . . energetic and exuberant," and "sporadic, chaotic entertainment for those who are somewhat sophisticated (but not too sophisticated about psychoanalysis)."

A sequel to *The House of God*, titled *Mount Misery*, in which the protagonist is engaged in a psychiatry residency and exposed to competing therapeutic approaches and evil members of the staff, was published in 1996. Connecting with the patient is espoused as the keystone for successful therapy. The reviewer for the *Boston Globe* considered the work to be "outrageously funny, a sage and important novel by a healer and a Shakespearean."

In *The Spirit of the Place* (2008), Samuel Shem changes venue from upscale hospitals with training programs he endured to a small, rural, decayed, and depressing community, not unlike the one in which Bergman spent his youth. The plot follows a character-flawed young doctor through fields of human, family, and societal defects to the extent that one reviewer headlined the review "Samuel Shem's New Book May Depress You." By contrast, physician and author Abraham Verghese wrote for the jacket cover, "An incredible and heartfelt story. . . . *The Spirit of the Place* entertains, satisfies, and affirms; it is beautifully conceived and brilliantly executed." The book was the winner of the national Best Novel of the Year Award 2008 from USA Book News, and the IPPY-Independent Publishers Book Award (Silver Medal) for Best Literary Fiction 2009.

Stemming from his position as affiliated scholar at Stone Center, Wellesley College, and codirector of the Gender Relation Research Project at the Wellesley Center for Women, Samuel Shem and his wife, Janet Surrey (a clinical psychologist), published a nonfiction book titled *We Have to Talk: Healing Dialogues between Women and Men* (1999). In 2015, Surrey and Shem published *The Buddha's Wife: The Path of Awakening Together*. This book presents the story of Princess Yasodhara, the wife of the Buddha, abandoned when he left to seek enlightenment. The book is divided into two parts: the first being a historical narrative of her alternative journey to enlightenment by relating to others in contradistinction to the Buddha's solitary meditation, and the second part providing the reader with a program to achieve his/her goals.

Bergman also has a distinct literary presence in drama. Two of Samuel Shem's plays, *Room for One Woman* and *Napoleon's Dinner*, have been published in the Best Short Plays anthologies. Bergman and Surrey wrote *Bill W. and Dr. Bob* about the relationship between the two men who founded Alcoholics Anonymous, and their wives, who created Al-Anon. The first production appeared Off Broadway in 2007 and ran for 132 performances. The play received the 2007 Performing Arts Award by the National Council on Alcohol and Drug Dependence. A revival was presented in 2013 and ran for 251 performances, a record for a modern Off Broadway drama. It was presented in Costa Rica in 2015 and, once again, Off Broadway in 2016.

Bergman has been a prolific speaker and may hold the record for number of medical school commencement addresses, including at Harvard in 2009 and New York University in 2014. In 2008, he delivered the Gold Lecture in Medical Humanities at the American Association of Medical Colleges and the keynote address at the American Society of Bioethics and Humanities. He spoke at the Hemingway Centennial Celebration at the John F. Kennedy Presidential Library.

He has been honored by the Boston Public Library as one of "Boston's Best Authors." He was awarded the Vanderbilt University Medal of Merit, the Surgeon General C. Everett Koop Medal of the Institute at Dartmouth Health Care, the Gold Foundation National Humanism in Medicine Award, the Yale University Bicentennial Professorship in Humanism in Medicine, and a Visiting Artist/Scholar Residency at the American Academy in Rome.

In 2008, the *Harvard Club of New York Bulletin* stated, "Samuel Shem is easily the finest and most important writer ever to focus on the lives of doctors and the world of medicine." In a 2002 article titled "Fiction as Resistance," which appeared in the *Annals of Internal Medicine*, Bergman indicated that he wrote as resistance "to brutality and inhumanity, to isolation and disconnection." In an interview in the *Boston Globe* celebrating the thirty-fifth anniversary of the publication of *The House of God*, Bergman said that he wrote "to resist injustice, and to show the healing power of connection." Harvard provost Dr. Steven Hyman succinctly expressed the local sentiment regarding Bergman in 2008: "He's gone from being a pariah to, despite his best efforts, being acceptable in polite company."

SOURCES

Jones, Val. "Samuel Shem's New Book May Depress You." Review of *The Spirit of the Place*, by Samuel Shem. *Better Health*. February 6, 2013. http://getbetterhealth.com/the-spirit-of-the-place-samuel-shems-new-book-may-depress-you/ (accessed May 9, 2018).

Markel, Howard. "A Book Doctors Can't Close," *New York Times*, August 17, 2009. http://www.nytimes.com/2009/08/18/health/18house.html?_r=0 (accessed April 5, 2018).

"Official Web Site of Samuel Shem." Samuel Shem. 2018. http://www.samuelshem.com (accessed April 5, 2018).

56

DEEPAK CHOPRA

Completeness Trumps Personal Prejudice

The issue of personal prejudice has been addressed by two famous physicians. The French neurologist Jean Martin Charcot wrote, "We eliminate and ignore everything that is not part of prejudice." American surgeon Charles W. Mayo stated, "One of the signs of a truly educated people and a broadly educated nation, is a lack of prejudice." Taking to heart the implication of one of my surgical idols, and in appreciation of the sheer number of widely read books produced by an individual, who, at one time during his career, was recognized as a reputable physician, it would be negligent not to include Dr. Deepak Chopra among contemporary doctors who are popular with a broad readership.

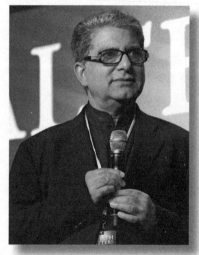

Chopra, the son of a prominent cardiologist, was born in New Delhi, India, on October 22, 1947. He completed his early education at the famous St. Columba's School, and in 1969, he graduated from the prestigious All India Institute of Medical Science. After a brief period as a doctor in rural India, Chopra moved to the United States. He interned at Muhlenberg Hospital in Plainfield, New Jersey, and completed a residency in internal medicine and specialty training in endocrinology at the Lahey Clinic, St. Elizabeth's Medical Center, and the Beth Israel Deaconess Medical Center in Boston.

Following his training, Chopra established a presence in traditional allopathic medicine in the Boston area. He participated as an adjunct member of the faculty at several of the local medical schools, conducted a private practice specializing in endocrinology, and served as chief of staff at the New England Memorial Hospital (currently Boston Regional Medical Center). He is board certified in internal medicine, endocrinology, and metabolism, and a fellow of the American College of Physicians.

In 1981, while on a visit to New Delhi, Chopra became more deeply exposed to Ayurvedic medicine, a system of healthcare with a history of over three millennia in India. The system is based on the concept of universal interconnectedness between the body's constitution and life forces, which are analogous to the bodily humors of classic Greek medicine. Treatment consists of herbs, proprietary medications, diet, exercise, and modification of lifestyle. Chopra took up transcendental meditation, and in 1984, he resigned from his medical commitments to become the founding president of the American Association of Ayurvedic Medicine.

Chopra's alternative medicine attracted several celebrities. In 1989, his first book, *Quantum Healing: Exploring the Frontiers of Mind/Body Medicine*, sold well and enhanced his reputation. His second book, *Perfect Health: The Complete Mind/Body Guide*, was published the following year.

In 1993, he moved to California as the executive director of Sharp Health Care's Institute for Human Potential and Mind/Body Medicine, and head of the exclusive Center for Mind/Body Medicine. That year, Chopra's *Ageless Body, Timeless Mind: The Quantum Alternative to Growing Old* appeared in print. His relationship with Michael Jackson, which was initiated in 1988, led to an interview on *Oprah* that enhanced book sales and made Deepak Chopra a household name. In 1995, he established the Chopra Center for Well Being in Carlsbad, California. Chopra has a medical license in Massachusetts and California.

His literary career has contributed to his recognition and financial success. He has published more than eighty-five books, which have been translated into forty-three languages. Twenty-five of his books have appeared on the *New York Times* best-seller list; *The Seven Spiritual Laws of Success* (1994) remained on the list for seventy-two weeks. In 1999, *Time* magazine referred to Chopra as "the poet-prophet of alternative medicine" and as one of the top one hundred heroes of the century.

Chopra created the concept of "quantum healing," a term that expresses a process by which quantum phenomena are integral to health and well-being.

He argues that an individual's mind and brain are responsible for everything that happens throughout the body. He writes, "Quantum healing is healing from a quantum level. That means from a level which is not manifest at a sensory level. Our bodies are ultimately fields of information, intelligence and energy. Quantum healing involves a shift in the fields of energy information, so as to bring about a correction in an idea that has gone wrong. So quantum healing involves healing one mode of consciousness, mind, to bring about changes in another mode of consciousness, body."

Chopra's consideration that quantum physics, a branch of science concerned with processes involving atoms and photons and other quite small particles of matter, can be allied with well-being and healing forms the basis for his "alternative medicine." That basic concept is vigorously criticized by traditional doctors and scientists. The physicist Heinz Pagel writes, "The claim that the fields of modern physics have anything to do with the 'field of consciousness' is false." Particle physicist Victor Stenger authored a 1994 essay titled "Quantum Quackery" in the *Skeptical Inquirer* in which he states that "quantum mysticism" has no basis in physics or biology and represents a leap of metaphysical imagination. In *The Skeptic's Dictionary*, it is concluded, "What Chopra is peddling is quantum gibberish." In 1998, Chopra was sarcastically awarded the "Ig Nobel Prize."

Chopra has maintained a diversified life as a healer, an educator, and a successful entrepreneur. He is a Clinical Professor in Medicine at the University of California, San Diego, teaches at the Columbia Business School and at the Kellogg School of Executive Management at Northwestern University. He participates at the annual "Update in Internal Medicine" sponsored by the Harvard Medical School and the Beth Israel Deaconess Medical Center. It is intriguing to compare Deepak Chopra's career with that of his younger brother, Sanjiv. Dr. Sanjiv Chopra, who is less than two years younger than Deepak, has been on the faculty of Harvard Medical School since 1979. He is currently professor of medicine and previously the Faculty Dean of Continuing Education at Harvard Medical School. He is a highly regarded hepatologist and the James Tullis Firm Chief in the Department of Medicine at the Beth Israel Deaconess Medical Center, which is divided into four medical firms.

Sanjiv has gained esteem as a medical educator. He has received awards for education from the house staff of the Brigham and Women's Hospital, the house staff and students at the Beth Israel Deaconess Hospital, and the 1991 graduating class of Harvard Medical School. In 2003, he received the

American Gastroenterological Association's Distinguished Educator Award. In 2009, he was elected a master of the American College of Physicians. He has published five books, including *Live Better, Live Longer, The New Studies That Reveal What's Really Good and Bad for Your Health*, and *Leadership by Example: The Ten Key Principles of All Great Leaders*.

In considering the argument regarding the relative importance of an individual's innate qualities as compared to personal experiences, i.e., nature vs. nurture, which side does a comparison of the brothers' lives support?

SOURCES

"Deepak Chopra," Deepak Chopra, https://www.deepakchopra.com/ (accessed April 5, 2018).

"Help Yourself." *Time*. June 6, 1999. http://content.time.com/time/magazine/article/0,9171,26419,00.html (accessed May 8, 2018).

57

PAUL CARSON

Productivity and Popularity Surmount Profound Personal Adversity

In a review of the lives of physicians who established a presence in the literary world, one is unmatched for the personal adversity experienced by the author during a period of productivity. The personal saga of an author, whose works have taken his readers on thrilling roller-coaster rides, highlights his own frighteningly precipitous descents and threatening troughs. And even through periods of dire disability and exhaustion, publications continued to be produced.

Paul Carson, the author of five health books, two children's books, and five best-selling thrillers, was born in Belfast, Northern Ireland, in 1949. He grew up in

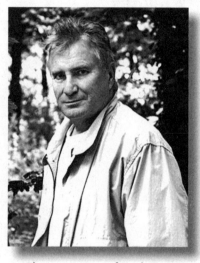

Photo courtesy of Paul Carson.

the seaside town of Newcastle on the east coast of Northern Ireland. After receiving an early education at a local primary school, he spent six unpleasant years at an all-boys Catholic boarding school before he entered Trinity College Dublin to study medicine. Carson remained at Trinity from 1969 to 1975, graduating with an honors degree in pediatrics.

After completing an internship, he moved to Australia, where he joined his brother. In the state of South Australia, he undertook postgraduate studies, worked in a hospital, conducted a family practice, and assisted a journeyman surgeon. In 1984, Carson returned to Dublin and established a clinic that specialized in pediatric allergy. During the ensuing twelve years, while engaged in a busy allergy practice, he published articles in medical journals, magazines, and newspapers in addition to five medical books and two books for children.

Carson's books on health include *How to Cope with Your Child's Allergies* (1987), *Coping Successfully with Your Child's Asthma* (1987), *Coping Successfully with Your Hyperactive Child* (1987), *Coping Successfully with Your Child's Skin Problems* (1988), and *Beat Your Allergies* (1995). His two children's books, *Norbett Bear MD* (1994) and *Norbett's Bistro* (1995), are delightful tales of the bear Norbett and his faithful assistant, Bamber Bear, who open the doors of the first Forest Medical Centre. Beginning in 1996, Carson edited fourteen issues of *Irish Doctor*, a monthly journal for doctors. In a lead article, he explored the health services in Ireland's most dangerous prison, Mountjoy jail. Other subjects of his essays were rehabilitation of sex offenders, care of patients in the detention center for the criminally insane, and care of preterm babies at Dublin's famous Rotunda Hospital. The journal rapidly surpassed its competitors in numbers of readers.

Carson's entrance into the medical thriller genre was in direct response to the request from a literary agent, who sought a medical equivalent to John Grisham. In 1997, Carson's first thriller, *Scalpel*, was published. The tale of an HIV-positive, woman-hating serial killer gynecologist became an immediate *Irish Times* best seller, spending seventeen weeks at number one and thirty-three weeks among the top five. Shortly after the publication, investigation of the author's persisting fatigue led to the diagnosis of a rare autoimmune blood disorder, which later proved to be the immunological harbinger of a lympho-cytic transformation. Despite chronic hemolytic anemia and recurrent infections, Carson published his second novel, *Cold Steel*, in 1998.

In *Cold Steel*, the investigation of the death of a prominent American surgeon's daughter in Dublin leads through a circuitous path that exposes criminal politics, the drug world, and wrongdoings of medical personnel. It was another best seller. In 2000, Carson's neoplastic blood disorder emerged as chronic lymphatic leukemia, accompanying the hemolytic anemia with consequent infections. Before that year ended, his third novel, *Final Duty*, appeared. In that thriller, an Irish doctor moves his practice to Chicago, where he and his family become exposed to a series of suspenseful, life-threatening experiences.

At this point in his life, Carson's energy was drained, and he limited his medical activities, which he totally abandoned in 2003 when chemotherapy and immunotherapy were initiated. He continued to produce thrillers in order to financially sustain his family. *Ambush* (2003) is the action-packed tale of a mild-mannered American doctor who moved to Dublin. His wife is killed in an ambush aimed at an anti-drug justice minister. The physician joins with his Irish cop brother-in-law, who has always hated him, to track the villain and gain revenge.

In 2004, Carson's disease was declared in remission, which has persisted for over a dozen years. His fifth medical thriller, *Betrayal*, was published in 2006. Once again, the protagonist is a doctor, this time the chief medical officer at an Irish penitentiary, Europe's most dangerous jail. The book topped the best-seller lists for six weeks.

Carson gradually rebuilt his medical practice that is now conducted at the Slievemore Clinic, a multidisciplinary medical center in South Dublin. In April 2013, an article in *Writing.ie*, a news periodical for writers, bore the heading "No. 1 Best Seller Paul Carson Is Back!" This announced the release of *Inquest*, which immediately was included on the *Irish Times* best-seller list. It was also short-listed for the Irish Book of the Year. The novel follows an inquisitive pathologist who questions the conclusions of a previously investigated "suicide." In the course of his investigation, he uncovers complex financial intrigue, while he puts his life and the lives of his family members in jeopardy. A reviewer wrote, "Another great thrill-a-page read from Paul Carson."

Carson sees himself, primarily, as a physician. He indicates that he writes "because I enjoy the buzz of the final product and the distraction of story-telling from my daytime job as a medical doctor." He has no plans to retire from medicine. Nor will he stop writing.

SOURCES

"Meet Paul," Paul Carson, http://paulcarson.ie/meet-paul/ (accessed April 5, 2018).

Review of *Inquest*, by Paul Carson. Independent.ie. September 29, 2013. https://www.independent.ie/entertainment/books/review-paul-carson-inquest-29616928.html (accessed May 9, 2018).

58

CHARLES KRAUTHAMMER
Widely Read and Highly Regarded

Charles Krauthammer, who is considered by some to be "the most important conservative columnist" in the United States, is a Pulitzer Prize–winning columnist and best-selling author. His literary reputation evolved after a brief period during which he was identified as a psychiatrist. The career change was, in part, related to a life-altering accident that occurred when he was a medical student.

Krauthammer was born on March 13, 1950, in New York City and grew up in Montreal, Canada. In addition to elementary and high school education, he received Jewish schooling at a Hebrew day school. In 1970, he graduated from McGill University with first-class honors

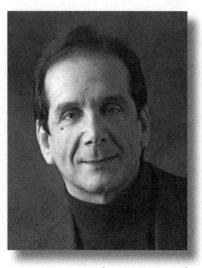

Photo courtesy of
Charles Krauthammer.

in political science and economics. He spent his postgraduate year as a Commonwealth Scholar at Balliol College, Oxford, where he studied politics.

Krauthammer entered Harvard Medical School in 1975. During his first year at Harvard, he struck his head on the bottom of a pool after diving from a board and sustained a cervical fracture that left him paralyzed and dependent upon a wheelchair. Although Krauthammer was hospitalized for fourteen months, he was able to complete his second year while in a hospital rehabilitation unit. He could not handwrite until three years after the accident but graduated with his original class in 1975.

In 1978, he completed a residency in psychiatry at the Massachusetts

General Hospital. While he was a resident, he coauthored a significant article, "Secondary Mania: Manic Syndromes Associated with Antecedent Physical Illness or Drugs," which was published in the *Archives of General Psychiatry*. This was followed by an article on the epidemiology of mania. In 1978, he moved to Washington, DC, to help direct the planning in psychiatric research during the Carter administration.

While working at the National Institute of Mental Health, Krauthammer began contributing articles to the *New Republic*. This led to employment as a speechwriter for Vice President Walter Mondale and subsequently as a writer and editor for the magazine. In 1984, his essays in the *New Republic* won the National Magazine Award for Essays and Criticism. In 1983, he began publishing in *Time* magazine, and, in 1985, he initiated a weekly column in the *Washington Post*.

Krauthammer's column, which is syndicated to four hundred newspapers worldwide, was awarded the Pulitzer Prize in Journalism for Commentary in 1997. The citation reads, "For his witty and insightful columns on national issues." In regard to Krauthammer's journalistic contributions, noted conservative George F. Will, a fellow columnist at the *Washington Post*, wrote, "Krauthammer's columns take journalism to the level of literature."

Krauthammer is also well recognized as a television commentator. In 1990, he began a twenty-three-year tenure as a panelist for the weekly PBS political roundtable *Inside Washington*. For the last decade, he has appeared as an analyst and commentator for Fox News, providing him a platform for his political conservatism. He has been referred to as "the most powerful force in American conservatism." In 2006, the *Financial Times* considered Krauthammer to be "the most influential columnist in America."

Krauthammer's one book, *Things That Matter: Three Decades of Passions, Pastimes and Politics*, was published in 2013. Over a million copies were sold, and the book remained on the *New York Times* best-seller list for fifty-one weeks and at the top of the list for ten weeks. The work consists of an autobiographical introduction followed by ninety-three previously published essays, which are divided into three categories: personal, political, and historical. In the 2015 paperback edition, an epilogue titled "The Age of Obama" was added.

The publication was greeted with great praise. The *Weekly Standard* regarded the work to be "the best of the best." Former secretary of state Henry A. Kissinger wrote, "From personal meditations to learned examinations of history and policy, *Things That Matter* stands as a record of a transformative period in the American experience and a remarkable intellect at work."

In 2002, Krauthammer was appointed to President George W. Bush's President's Council on Bioethics. He is also a member of the Council on Foreign Relations and the Chess Journalists of America. He is a cofounder of Pro Musica Hebraica, an organization dedicated to promoting Jewish classical music.

Krauthammer, who maintains his certification by the American Board of Psychiatry, is the recipient of several awards, including the People for the American Way's First Amendment Award, the Champion/Tuck Award for Economic Understanding, the Bradley Prize for conservative thinking, and the Eric Bendel Award for Excellence in Opinion Journalism. In 2013, he received the William F. Buckley Award for Media Excellence. His sense and sensibility expressed in a superior and engaging literary style have justly assigned to him iconic status.

SOURCES

"Charles Krauthammer." Harry Walker Agency. http://www.harrywalker.com/speakers/charles-krauthammer?ret=search&all=0&pg=1&y=600&term=Charles%20Krauthammer (accessed April 5, 2018).

"Charles Krauthammer Bio." *Washington Post.* https://www.washingtonpost.com/people/charles-krauthammer/?utm_term=.6288893d4297 (accessed April 5, 2018).

Krauthammer, Charles. *Things That Matter: Three Decades of Passions, Pastimes and Politics.* New York: Crown Forum, 2015.

59

JEROME E. GROOPMAN

An Exceptional Exemplar

The living "exemplar" for the current male and female physicians who satisfy the literary appetites of a public that has become informed and interested in medicine is assigned the adjective "exceptional" as a consequence of his research, scholarship, patient care, and role as an educator and mentor. Jerome E. Groopman has superimposed a literary presence on an exceptional career in academic medicine.

Perusal of his curriculum vitae would lead the reader to conclude that his accomplishments in medicine and his success as a writer were to have been anticipated. Born in New York City on January 11, 1952, Groopman demonstrated an

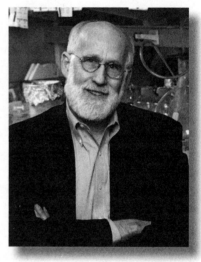

Photo courtesy of
Jerome E. Groopman.

early inclination for scholarship, both as an undergraduate and as a medical student. In 1972, he graduated from Columbia College summa cum laude as a member of Phi Beta Kappa and the recipient of the award for excellence in premedical studies, with a major in political philosophy. Four years later, he graduated from the Columbia College of Physicians and Surgeons as the class valedictorian, a member of Alpha Omega Alpha, and with the Robert Loeb Prize in Internal Medicine.

After completing a residency in internal medicine at the Massachusetts General Hospital in Boston, he spent two years as a fellow in hematology-oncology research laboratories at UCLA and Harvard. His initial faculty position was at UCLA. In 1980, he returned to Boston as an attending physician at the New England Deaconess Hospital, where he has remained. He was the recipient of the Dina and Raphael Racanati Chair in 1992, and designated the chief of the Division of Experimental Medicine at Beth Israel Deaconess Medical Center in 1996.

Groopman's major research interests are immune function relative to cancer and AIDS, the formation of blood, polypeptide growth factors, cytokines, and signal transduction. His name appears on more than 180 scientific articles in peer-reviewed journals, the most recent of which was published in 2015. He served as editor or as a member of the editorial board of several important scientific journals. He is a member of the prestigious National Academy of Medicine, the American Association for the Advancement of Science, the American Academy of Arts and Sciences, and many societies pertinent to his medical interests.

In 1997, Groopman embarked on his literary activity when he began writing stories about his patients. A year later, he became a staff writer for the *New Yorker* magazine. Over the ensuing eighteen years, his essays and book reviews appeared in that periodical and also in the *New Republic*, the *New York Review of Books*, the *New York Times*, and the *Washington Post*.

Groopman's first book, *The Measure of Our Days*, was published in 1997. It was subsequently serialized in the *New Yorker* and the *Boston Globe Sunday Magazine*. The book was the inspiration for the television series *Gideon's Crossing* (2000). Drawing from eight of his own professional encounters with patients afflicted with AIDS or malignancies, disorders that were the focus of his scientific and clinical attention, *The Measure of Our Days* emphasizes the importance of a bilateral, interpersonal relationship between the emotionally devastated patient and an empathetic, caring physician.

Thought processes that form the basis for holistic management are considered, and the importance of dialogue issued by both patient and physician is emphasized. Reviewers assessed the work as "a unique, important and wonderful book" that "offered practical advice to both patients and physicians."

Groopman's next book, *Second Opinions: Stories of Intuition and Choice in the Changing World of Medicine* (2000), follows the pattern of his first book. It considers eight stories about the care of patients with life-threatening illnesses, including his son and his grandfather. The messages that emerge from the author's captivating narrative emphasize that the care of patients is a combination of art and science, that human error is a critical factor, and that the current healthcare system is subject to criticism.

The Anatomy of Hope: How People Prevail in the Fact of Illness (2004) deals with the biologic basis of hope and the effect of that hope in critically ill patients and for the family members of patients. The six cases used as the platform for discussion include the author's personal experience with back pain.

Shortly after its publication in 2007, *How Doctors Think* rose to the top of the nonfiction best-seller list of the *New York Times*, as testimony to the author's engaging style and a growing readership of those interested in and intrigued with medicine care and issues about its delivery. The book, which received both the consumer-driven Quill Book Award in the category of health/self-improvement and the Books for a Better Life Award, appears as a well-worn volume on a shelf of most medical schools.

The essence of the work is a consideration of mental processing that takes place when a doctor is evaluating a patient. Once again, the author employs individual patients' situations as springboards to assess clinical thinking and decision-making. The issue of heurism, self-educating, and exploratory problem-solving techniques is introduced. An epilogue advises patients how to communicate with the physician and establish a vital partnership that facilitates and enhances decision-making.

Groopman's most recent book, *Your Medical Mind: How to Decide What Is Right for You* (2011), was coauthored with his wife, who is also a physician. As stated by the authors, "Medicine involves nuanced and personalized decision making by both the patient and the doctor." Rather than considering *Your Medical Mind* as a sequel to *How Doctors Think*, the authors present it as an enhancement, or a contrapuntal element.

The significance of Groopman's literary contributions is evidenced by the awards that he has received: the John McGovern Medal from the American Medical Writers Association, the City of Newton Appreciation for contribution to the literary arts and in the pursuit of literary excellence, the Council for the Advancement of Science Writing's Victor Cohn Prize for Excellence in Medical Science Reporting, and the Humanism in Medicine Award from the Arnold P. Gold Foundation.

SOURCES

"About." Dr. Jerome Groopman: Author, Physician, & Scientist. 2018. http://
jeromegroopman.com/aboutjerome.html (accessed April 5, 2018).
Levitin, Daniel J. "How Patients Think, and How They Should." *New York Times*,
October 7, 2011. http://www.nytimes.com/2011/10/09/books/review/
your-medical-mind-by-jerome-groopman-and-pamela-hartzband-book
-review.html (accessed April 5, 2018).

60

TESS GERRITSEN

Practicality Trumps Passion,
but Passion Perseveres

T he young daughter of a second-generation Chinese American chef and an immigrant Chinese mother loved to write and produce books. She wrote short stories about her pets and sewed the pages together to create the semblance of a real book. To her parents, who typified the Asian immigrant culture, becoming a writer was viewed as impractical, and instead she was directed to apply her intellectual capabilities toward becoming a doctor. She dutifully complied but subsequently returned to satisfy her literary passion, which proved to exceed the profitability of her profession.

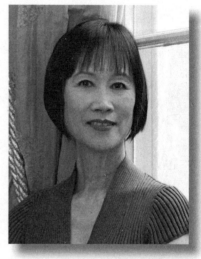

Photo by Leonardo Cendamo, courtesy of Tess Gerritsen.

Tess (née Terry Tom) Gerritsen was born on June 12, 1953, in San Diego, California. She graduated from Kearny High School, which lists her as a distinguished alumnus. She graduated from Stanford University in 1975 with a major in anthropology, having been elected to Phi Beta Kappa. She received a medical degree from the University of California, San Francisco, four years later. In 1977, she married classmate Jacob Gerritsen, who had grown up in Hawaii. The couple completed residencies in internal medicine at the University of Hawaii Medical Center. She joined the Kaiser Permanente Medical Group in Honolulu and also worked at the Rehabilitation Hospital of the Pacific.

Tess Gerritsen continued writing throughout medical school and her residency, generally recording medical experiences. While on maternity leave, she submitted a short story to the magazine *Honolulu* and won the five-hundred-dollar first prize. Subsequently, one of her patients presented her with a bag of Harlequin romance novels, suggesting that the stories might counter the stress of her medical practice. This gift provided an added stimulus to rejuvenate a latent interest in writing. After a few false starts, Gerritsen sold *Call after Midnight* to the Harlequin publishing company in 1986. Over the ensuing years, she produced eight romantic thrillers that were published annually by Harper Intrigue and Harper Paperbacks.

Gradually, Gerritsen decreased her practice, and eventually her literary passion assumed a priority that led her to discontinue her medical pursuits. The family moved to Camden, Maine, where her reputation was established. At the specific suggestion of her agent, Gerritsen published her first medical thriller, *Harvest*, in 1996. James B. Patterson referred to the novel, which reached number thirteen on the *New York Times* best-seller list, as "the best medical thriller I've read since *Coma*." It was followed by three more best-selling medical thrillers: *Life Support* (1997), *Bloodstream* (1998), and *Gravity* (1999). The review of *Life Support* stated, "Gerritsen's pacing is excellent, her writing is very good, and her use of medical/scientific detail is superb . . . what distinguishes this book from Michael Palmer's work [see chapter 50] is a touch of horror."

In 2001, Gerritsen published her first crime thriller, *The Surgeon*, in which she introduced detective Jane Rizzoli, who would be paired with medical examiner Dr. Maura Isles. The two would become the protagonists of Gerritsen's ten subsequent novels. These books inspired a television series, *Rizzoli & Isles*, which premiered in 2010 and presented 105 episodes over seven years. *The Surgeon* won the RITA® Award for the Best Romantic Suspense Novel in 2002. A *Publishers Weekly* critique indicated that "Gerritsen . . . originally a romance writer, had morphed into a dependable suspense novelist whose growing popularity is keeping pace with her ever-finer writing skills."

Among the eleven books in the Rizzoli/Isles series, *Vanish* (2005) received the Nero Award for best mystery novel and was nominated for an Edgar Award® by the Mystery Writers of America and a Macavity Award from Mystery Readers International. In 2007, she published a historical thriller, *The Bone Garden*. The narrative, which interweaves nineteenth- and twenty-first-century protagonists, brings into focus Oliver Wendell Holmes, a notable physician and literary figure (see chapter 17).

One of Gerritsen's most recent publications, *Playing with Fire* (2015), represents a unique departure for the author. Paula L. Woods, in a December 4, 2015, review that appeared in the *Los Angeles Times*, wrote, "As beloved as Rizzoli & Isles may be, they can go on sabbatical more often, if that gives Gerritsen time to craft terrific thrillers like this." The novel includes a unique accompaniment, which is unmatched in the history of literature created by doctors. Tess Gerritsen, an amateur violinist with no formal training in music composition, created a ninety-eight-bar waltz titled *Incendio* for violin and piano. It has been recorded by a world-renowned violinist.

In 2010, Gerritsen had joined with Michael Palmer (see chapter 50) to teach a course in writing thrillers at Cape Cod. More than thirty million copies of her books have been published in forty countries. She currently ranks third in total sales among the contributors to the medical thriller genre. She has been referred to as the "medical suspense queen."

SOURCES

Gerritsen, Tess. "About Tess Gerritsen." 2017. http://www.tessgerritsen.com/about-tess/ (accessed April 5, 2018).

Rogers, Amy. "Latest book review: Life Support by Tess Gerritsen." 2010. http://www.sciencethrillers.com/2010/latest-book-review-life-support-by-tess-gerritsen/ (accessed May 11, 2018).

Harnett, Lynn. "Author Tess Gerritsen's Life Takes an Unexpected Turn." Sea Coast Online, September 18, 2005. http://www.seacoastonline.com/article/20050918/ENTERTAIN/309189973 (accessed April 5, 2018).

Review of *The Surgeon*, by Tess Gerritsen. *Publishers Weekly*. July 2, 2001. https://www.publishersweekly.com/978-0-345-44783-8 (accessed May 10, 2018).

61

ABRAHAM VERGHESE
Medical Humanism and Honed Literature

L ife's pathway for Abraham Verghese can be characterized as circuitous and bimodal. The main roads that
he has traveled transcend three continents:
Africa, Asia, and North America. The two
disparate goals for which he gained recognition and admiration share an overarching
emphasis on humanism and empathy. His
voice as a physician educator champions
the importance of a direct hands-on relationship between the doctor and the patient
in an age of depersonalization, consequent
to the infusion of informatics. His voice as
a nonfiction author expresses concern for
AIDS patients and their families and the
tragedy of drug addiction in medical personnel. And in his crowning production,

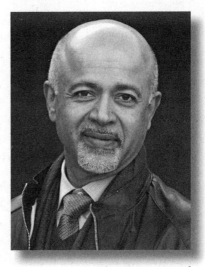

Photo courtesy of
Abraham Verghese.

the most widely read medical fiction of the twenty-first century, the concept of
the importance of "words of comfort" is thematic.

Abraham Verghese was born on May 30, 1955, in Ethiopia, the son of
two teachers, who had been recruited as educators from Kerala in India, where
Orthodox Christianity was the dominant religion. The medical training, which
he had embarked upon in Ethiopia, was interrupted when Emperor Haile
Selassie was deposed in 1974. Verghese spent one year in the United States as
a medical orderly before returning to India, where he completed his medical
education at Madras Medical College in 1979.

After a one-year internship in Madras, he spent the subsequent three years in a newly established internal medicine residency program in Johnson City, Tennessee, affiliated with East Tennessee University. He next completed a two-year fellowship in infectious diseases at the Boston University School of Medicine before returning to Johnson City as an assistant professor of medicine. From 1986 through 1990, he was chief of infectious diseases at the VA Medical Center in Johnson City. In 1988, he received tenure and was promoted to associate professor. Throughout his time on the faculty at East Tennessee University, he oversaw the care of AIDS patients in a rural area, a unique experience that influenced his later writing.

Exhausted by his clinical and academic commitments and with the desire to develop an identity as an author, Verghese made an abrupt change. He suspended his medical activities and enrolled in the Iowa Writers Workshop for two years, graduating with a master of fine arts degree in 1991.

For the next eleven years, he served as professor of medicine and chief of infectious diseases at the Texas Tech Health Sciences Center in El Paso, Texas. The title was deceptive in that, during most of the period, he was the sole provider of care for patients with infectious diseases. While at that institution, his teaching prowess was rewarded when he was designated the Grover E. Murray Distinguished Professor of Medicine.

In 2002, Verghese became the founding director of the Center for Medical Humanities and Ethics at the University of Texas Health Science Center at San Antonio. In that capacity, he held the Joaquin Cigarroa Chair and Marvin Forland Distinguished Professorship. In 2007, he was recruited to the Stanford University School of Medicine as the senior associate chair for the theory and practice of medicine. He later assumed the directorship of the Internal Medicine Residency Program. In 2013, he initiated and became the director of the innovative Program in Bedside Medicine, and his Stanford experience was capped in 2014 when he was designated the Linda R. Meier and Joan F. Lane Provostial Professor and Vice Chair for the Theory and Practice of Medicine.

Verghese is identified as the twenty-first-century's embodiment of Sir William Osler's precepts (see chapter 20), in that he champions the position that the "clinician" should be true to the Latin origin of the word, namely, "at the bedside." Verghese emphasizes the value of the physical examination of patients in establishing a diagnosis and, concurrently, in developing a bilateral doctor-patient, patient-doctor relationship. In addition, he espouses the prominent inclusion of the humanities and ethics in the curriculum, to which medical students and trainees are exposed. These tenets assume added importance in the current environment, which is dominated by an explosive growth of scientific knowledge and a dependence on informatics for dialogues and dissemination of information.

As an academic physician, Verghese published about one hundred articles, which span the spectrum of infectious disease and medical education in peer-reviewed scientific journals. The esteem with which he is held by medical colleagues is manifest by numerous teaching awards, honorary degrees from the Royal College of Physicians of Canada, Swarthmore College, the University of Northern Illinois, the State University of New York, the Royal College of Surgeons of Ireland, and the Royal College of Physicians of Edinburgh, in addition to being elected as master of the American College of Physicians and a member of the National Academy of Medicine.

Verghese's first book, *My Own Country: A Doctor's Story*, was published in 1994. The narrative eloquently interweaves the author's personal journey, which brought him to rural Tennessee, where he provided care for the patients afflicted with AIDS along with their families. The work was chosen as one of the five "Best Books of the Year" by *Time* magazine. It was also listed as a *New York Times* notable book in the year of its publication, and it has been incorporated in the prescribed reading list by medical schools to convey the need for empathy and compassion in an era of technology.

Verghese's second work, *The Tennis Partner: A Story of Friendship and Loss*, an account of the author's friendship with a talented medical mentee who is addicted to drugs, was published in 1998 and reissued in 2009. The sport of tennis represents a metaphor for the two men, both in a stage of significant vulnerability, on opposite sides of the net. The prevalence of addiction in medical personnel is addressed.

Verghese's reputation as a writer soared with the publication of his first novel, *Cutting for Stone*, which appeared in 2009. The book, which sold over one million copies, was on the *New York Times* best-seller list for more than two years. It was among Amazon's and *Publishers Weekly*'s list of "Best Books from 2009." In 2010, it received the Indies Choice Book Award by the American Booksellers Association.

Verghese merits recognition and praise for his contributions to both literature and medicine. In literature, he is to be credited for the great medical novel of the twenty-first century. In medicine, he provides one of the most luminescent beacons to light the road that leads to the goal of providing humanistic care for patients in an age dominated by technology.

SOURCES

"Abraham Verghese." http://abrahamverghese.com/ (accessed April 5, 2018).

"Abraham Verghese, MD, MACP." Stanford Medicine. 2018. https://med
.stanford.edu/profiles/abraham-verghese (accessed April 5, 2018).

Wagner, Erica. "Doctors and Sons." *New York Times*, February 6, 2009. https://
mobile.nytimes.com/2009/02/08/books/review/Wagner-t.html (accessed
April 5, 2018).

62

KHALED HOSSEINI

Indelible Impressions Contribute to Divorce from Medicine

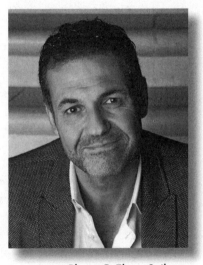

Photo © Elena Seibert.

The impressions of his youth in a faraway land persisted and form the backdrop for the fiction created by a California physician. The personal satisfaction that he associated with writing, coupled with the financial success of his first publication, led to his decision to pursue his literary passion unimpeded by medical obligations. He has formally divorced himself from medicine and identifies himself as a writer.

Khaled Hosseini was born in Kabul, Afghanistan, on March 4, 1965. At the time, Afghanistan was a sovereign state, ruled by a monarch, and Khaled's father served as a diplomat in the Ministry of Foreign Affairs. In 1970, the family moved to Tehran for three years. The Hosseinis were living in Kabul when the monarchy was overthrown in 1973. Khaled's father was assigned by the new republic to the embassy in Paris, where the family was residing when the Communist faction overthrew the government in 1978.

The Hosseinis gained asylum in the United States and moved to San Jose, California, in 1980. The family was destitute, on welfare, and fifteen-year-old Khaled, who initially spoke no English, worked alongside his father in a flea market. Hosseini graduated from Independence High School in 1984 and entered Santa Clara University in preparation for becoming a physician. He was awarded a bachelor's degree in biology in 1988 and an MD from the University of California San Diego, School of Medicine in 1993. He completed a residency in internal medicine at Cedars-Sinai Medical Center in Los Angeles in 1996.

Hosseini began his medical practice in Pasadena and later moved to Northern California, where he joined the Kaiser Permanente health maintenance organization as an internist. He established his family's home in Mountain View. He experimented with writing short stories while he was, ostensibly, focused on scientific studies. After his medical practice was well established, he awoke early each morning to write for several hours. He started his first novel in 2001 with a constant image of his native land in his mind. The al-Qaeda attacks on the United States occurred around that time, and then the consequent launching of Operation Enduring Freedom to remove the Taliban from power in Afghanistan.

Two years later, *The Kite Runner* was published. The story is set in Afghanistan in a time span from the fall of the monarchy, through the Soviet intervention, the exodus of refugees to the United States, and the rise of the Taliban. It is a father-son story and one of friendship of youths from disparate classes. It is also a tale of multigenerational guilt and redemption.

The Kite Runner spent 101 weeks on the *New York Times* best-seller list, four weeks as number one. It returned to that list five years after its initial appearance. It was published in more than forty languages, and the sales have exceeded twelve million copies. The novel received the South African Boeke Prize in 2004 and the Reading Group Book of the Year for 2006 and 2007. Two years after the publication of *The Kite Runner*, Hosseini ended his association with medicine, which he referred to as an "arranged marriage."

Hosseini's second novel, *A Thousand Splendid Suns*, was published in 2007 and became number one on the *New York Times* best-seller list for fifteen weeks and remained on the list for another 103 weeks. Again, the story is set in Afghanistan and relates the entwined lives of two women from different ethnic backgrounds. Both novels portray relationships between parent and child, and extend the narrative over several generations.

The most recent of Hosseini's novels, *And the Mountains Echoed*, was published in 2013 and remained on the *New York Times* best-seller list for thirty-three weeks. The work continues the familial theme of his previous novels, and the plot plays out in Afghanistan, America, and Paris. In this novel, sibling relationships rather than the dynamics between a parent and child are brought into focus.

In 2006, Hosseini began service as a special envoy for the United Nations High Commissioner for Refugees. He has also established a foundation to provide humanitarian aid to Afghanistan, which remains a continuous concern for him.

SOURCES

"Khaled Hosseini." 2018. http://www.khaledhosseini.com (accessed April 5, 2018).

"Khaled Hosseini, MD." Last revised March 22, 2018. http://www.achievement .org/achiever/khaled-hosseini/ (accessed April 5, 2018).

63

DANIELLE OFRI

Humanities and a Human Voice

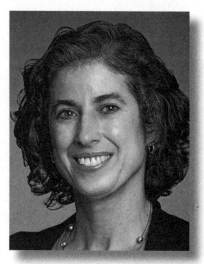

Photo courtesy of Danielle Ofri.

The homepage of the Stanford Humanities Center's website states, "The humanities can be described as the study of how people process and document the human experience." The humanities encompass philosophy, religion, literature, art, history, and music. The cello has been described as the musical instrument that produces a sound closest to the human voice. The conjunction between medicine, literature, and music brings into focus a physician who has achieved acclaim as a literary figure dedicated to humanizing medical experiences and, incidentally, is an accomplished cellist.

Danielle Ofri was born in New York City on August 22, 1965. She grew up in and around the city where she was educated at public schools. She enjoyed writing stories as a child. While in high school, her early desire to become a veterinarian changed to the goal of becoming a doctor. In 1986, she graduated with a degree in physiology from McGill University in Montreal, Canada, where her undergraduate studies consisted, almost exclusively, of the sciences.

Unable to decide between becoming a practicing physician or a scientist, she completed a seven-year MD-PhD program at New York University Medical School. Her PhD in pharmacology was fulfilled with studies of signal transduction by opioid receptors. Reports of her research appeared in peer-reviewed journals, including *Brain Research*, the *Journal of Neurochemistry*, and

Receptor. After graduating in 1993, she spent three years in an internal medicine residency at New York University's Bellevue Hospital. During the next eighteen months, she traveled around the United States, serving as a locum tenens, filling in for other physicians in order to pay off loans, which she had taken to pursue her education.

In 1998, she returned to New York City, where she became a member of the Department of Medicine at New York University and an attending physician at Bellevue Hospital. Shortly thereafter, she published medical journal articles on acne, deep venous thrombosis, and hormonal replacement after menopause. She is currently an associate professor engaged in outpatient medicine and in teaching medical students and precepting residents.

Ofri began writing for a general readership during the interval between the completion of her residency and her return to join the faculty at New York University. The earliest of her over 160 published essays appeared in 1998. In 2001, her essay "Merced" was awarded the Editor's Prize for Nonfiction by the *Missouri Review* and was included in *Best American Essays 2002*, coedited by Stephen Jay Gould. Later that year, the first of her eleven articles to be published in the *New England Journal of Medicine* appeared.

The essay "Merced" was included in her first book, *Singular Intimacies: Becoming a Doctor at Bellevue*, which was published in 2003. The work consists of a series of essays that relate the experiences and feelings of medical students and residents as they care for people in New York City. The reviewer for the *New England Journal of Medicine* indicated that the humility of Ofri's prose transformed "it from mere storytelling into memorable parables."

The first of approximately fifty of her contributions to the *New York Times* appeared in 2005. She has also contributed to the *Atlantic*, the *Los Angeles Times*, and *Slate Magazine*. Her second book, *Incidental Findings: Lessons from My Patients in the Art of Medicine*, was published that year. The work consists of several essays deriving from Ofri's experiences as a locum tenens in small towns and, also, her experiences at Bellevue Hospital. One of the essays, "Living Will," was selected by Susan Orlean for *Best American Essays 2005*, and "Common Ground" was selected by Oliver Sacks (see chapter 48) for *Best American Science Writing 2003*.

Medicine in Translation: Journeys with My Patients was published in 2010 and focuses on issues related to providing medical care for patients in the face of language, cultural, socioeconomic, and religious barriers. Her fourth book, *What Doctors Feel: How Emotions Affect the Practice of Medicine*, was published in

2013. In that work, Ofri emphasizes the significance and importance of *caring for* while participating in taking care of patients. She decries the current perceptible decrease of empathy among students and caregivers. She also considers the emotional consequences on the physicians caring for patients.

Ofri can lay claim to a unique contribution to the literary world related to her role as cofounder and editor in chief of the *Bellevue Literary Review*. As the first literary magazine to be established in a hospital, the journal publishes fiction, poetry, and nonfiction about health, healing, the human body, and illness. Ofri's frequently appearing columns in prestigious newspapers maintain her literary visibility. Her contributions to literature were recognized with an Honorary Doctor of Humane Letters from Curry College in Milton, Massachusetts, which, coincidentally, had been founded as the School of Elocution and Expression, and with the McGovern Award from the American Medical Writers Association.

Ofri indicates that, currently, several novels lay fallow in development, but a new book on doctor-patient communication should be published shortly. Incidentally, she is working on two of the great works in a cellist's repertoire, the Elgar Concerto and the Bach Suites for Unaccompanied Cello.

SOURCES

"About." Danielle Ofri. 2018. http://danielleofri.com/bio/ (accessed April 5, 2018).

Ofri, Danielle, MD. *Well* (blog). https://well.blogs.nytimes.com/author/danielle-ofri-md/?_r=1 (accessed April 5, 2018).

Schwartz, Robert S. Review of *Singular Intimacies: Becoming a Doctor at Bellevue*, by Danielle Ofri. *New England Journal of Medicine*. July 10, 2003. https://www.nejm.org/doi/full/10.1056/NEJM200307103490222 (accessed May 10, 2018).

"What Are the Humanities?" Stanford Humanities Center. http://shc.stanford.edu/what-are-the-humanities (accessed May 10, 2018).

64

ATUL GAWANDE

A Mercury for Modern Medicine

I n mythology, the Roman god Mercury, known to the Greeks as Hermes, was the bridge between the upper and lower worlds, and the patron of messages and communication. It is presciently symbolic that Apollo, the god of medicine, represented by the staff of Aesculapius with a single entwined snake, gave Mercury a caduceus with two entwined snakes, the symbol of commerce. The day of the doctor as a heroic societal figure has been replaced by teams of individuals replete with scientific knowledge and by consortia of medical management—a healthcare industrial revolution.

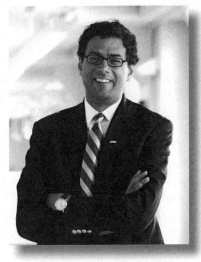

Photo by Kelly Davidson.

A current messenger of medical issues is an active general surgeon with a specific interest in operations on endocrine organs, who has, concomitantly, provided medical professionals and the lay public a canon of literary contributions that constitutes lucid explications of many concerns related to healthcare. For readers, a consideration of Atul Gawande's atypical and uniquely personal path to celebrity and distinction is intriguing and represents a lagniappe or added treat.

Atul Atmaram Gawande, born to a urologist father and pediatrician mother on November 5, 1965, in Brooklyn, New York, is the son of Indian immigrants. His youth was spent in Athens, Ohio, where he graduated from public high school in 1983. He received an undergraduate bachelor's degree in biology and political science from Stanford University in 1987. While a student, he coauthored several scientific articles that appeared in peer-reviewed oph-thalmology journals, and he was also a volunteer for Gary Hart's Democratic primary presidential campaign (1988). After graduation, he acted in a similar capacity in Al Gore's presidential campaign. Shortly thereafter, as a Rhodes scholar, he attended Balliol College, Oxford University, where he studied poli-tics, philosophy, and economics and received an MA in 1989.

Upon completion of those studies, Gawande worked as a researcher for US Representative Jim Cooper on a healthcare reform proposal. In 1990, Gawande entered Harvard Medical School but left after two years to advise Bill Clinton's presidential campaign on health issues. After Clinton's election, Gawande worked on the healthcare proposal, headed by Hillary Clinton, that eventually failed. He returned to medical school and received his MD in 1995.

"Later in medical school, however," he said, "I chose surgery because I thought that perhaps this would make me more like the kind of person I wanted to be. Certainly I loved technique and using my hands and the sheer blood and guts of it all. But what most attracted me was the predicament of surgery—the combination of high stakes and uncertainty—and the character of those who deal with it well." His surgical residency at the Brigham and Woman's Hospital, a training period usually completed within five to seven years, extended from 1995 to 2003, during which time he also satisfied the requirements for a master of public health degree at Harvard.

Over the ensuing years, Gawande has remained an active surgeon at the Brigham and Woman's Hospital and the Faulkner Hospital in Boston, with a concentration on endocrine surgery. He rose through the academic ranks, being designated as the Kessler Endowed Assistant Professor in 2004–2006 and the Samuel O. Thier Professor of Surgery in 2014. In a 2009 interview, he indicated that he performed over 250 operations per year, whereas, with the more recent increase in his extra-surgical commitments, this number has been reduced to about one hundred operations per year on the thyroid, parathyroid, and the adrenals.

Gawande is a fellow of the American College of Surgeons, and an active member of the Association of Academic Surgery, the American Association of Endocrine Surgeons, the Society of Surgical Oncology, the New England Sur-gical Society, the American Surgical Association, and the National Academy of Medicine. His roles as director of the Health Systems Innovation Research Group at Harvard School of Public Health and, more recently, as director of the Ariadne Labs: A Joint Center for Health System Innovation have found expression in his writings. The publications, in turn, have resulted in his high-impact contributions to improve medical care and its delivery.

These innovations include the World Health Organization (WHO) Safe Surgery Checklist, the WHO Childbirth Checklist, a Clostridium difficile prevention checklist, safety standards for resident-attending communications regarding postsurgical patients, and others. As added testimony to his academic surgical presence, Gawande has coauthored a chapter on adrenalectomy in a surgical textbook and approximately 150 articles in peer-reviewed medical journals.

Gawande began his literary career in 1996 when he was invited by a friend to submit material to the online magazine *Slate*. His early pieces on the encounters and challenges of a surgical residency gained the attention of the editor of the *New Yorker*, and he was invited to become a staff writer in 1998. Henry Finder, the editorial director of that magazine, referred to Gawande's style in *Harvard Magazine* as "carefully carpentered, an almost surgical precision," and compared Gawande's style to that of Rachel Carson in *Silent Spring*.

Gawande's first book, *Complications: A Surgeon's Note on an Imperfect Science*, was published in 2002. Many of the chapters had been originally written as contributions for the *New Yorker*. The volume brings into focus the lack of knowledge on which some decisions are made in medical practice, and the psychological issues that confront surgeons. The book was a National Book Award finalist, the recipient of the PEN/Allbrand Award for First Nonfiction Book, and Amazon's Best Nonfiction Book of 2002.

In 2007 came the publication of *Better: A Surgeon's Notes on Performance*, which also incorporated material published in the *New Yorker*. In that book, Gawande stresses the critical elements of "Diligence," "Doing Right," and "Ingenuity" that are embodied in the optimal discharging of medical responsibilities. His next book, *The Checklist Manifesto: How to Get Things Right* (2010), with its evangelical pronouncement, has played a role in policy changes that have been enacted in hospitals and outpatient facilities to minimize adverse experiences in patient care.

Gawande's most recent book, *Being Mortal: Medicine and What Matters in the End*, was published in 2014. The author's messages are in concert with those that emanated from Sherwin Nuland (see chapter 46) and Jerome Groopman (see chapter 59), who wrote for the public. Gawande emphasizes that the goal of medical care, particularly as it relates to the seriously ill, critically compromised, and those waning with age, is to provide for a meaningful life and not just mere biologic survival.

Gawande's literary output, which has been addressed to the general public over the past two decades, is prodigious. It includes almost two dozen contributions to *Slate Magazine* in addition to almost three dozen essays in the *New Yorker* and a dozen columns in the *New York Times*. Many of these writings were selected for inclusion in Best Scientific Writing annual publications. In 2015, he received the Lewis Thomas Prize Award for writing about science.

In 2006, Gawande was selected as a MacArthur Fellow. He has received honorary doctorates from four American universities and honorary membership in the Association of Anaesthetists of Great Britain and Ireland and the Association of Surgeons of Great Britain and Ireland. He was elected a Hasting Center Fellow and a member of the American Philosophical Society.

Identified best by his "carefully carpentered" writing about both current panoramic and focused issues regarding healthcare, Gawande stated in a 2005 Harvard Medical School commencement address that "by putting your writing out to an audience, even a small one, you connect yourself to something larger than yourself. . . . An audience is a community, the published word is a declaration of membership in that community, and also of concern to contribute something meaningful to it."

SOURCES

"Atul Gawande." *New Yorker*. http://www.newyorker.com/contributors/atul
    -gawande (accessed April 5, 2018).
Fink, Sheri. "Atul Gawande's 'Being Mortal.'" *New York Times*, November 6,
    2014. https://www.nytimes.com/2014/11/09/books/review/atul-gawande
    -being-mortal-review.html (accessed April 5, 2018).
Gawande, Atul. "The Character of a Doctor." Commencement address to Yale
    Medical School. May 24, 2004. https://docwhisperer.wordpress.com/tag/
    dr-atul-gawande/ (accessed May 11, 2018).
Gudrais, Elizabeth. "The Unlikely Writer." *Harvard Magazine*, September–
    October 2009. https://harvardmagazine.com/2009/09/atul-gawande
    -surgeon-health-policy-scholar-writer (accessed April 5, 2018).

65

SIDDHARTHA MUKHERJEE

Biographer of Biology

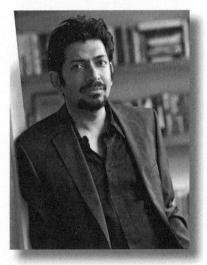

In the mid-nineteenth century, Russian doctor Alexander Borodin gained equivalent prestige in two totally disparate fields: chemistry and classical music. As the chair of chemistry at the Imperial Medical-Surgical Academy in Saint Petersburg, he worked on organic halogens and is co-credited with the Aldol reaction. His musical legacy includes chamber music, two symphonies, the popular symphonic poem *In the Steppes of Central Asia*, and the opera *Prince Igor*. Adaptations of his music remain popular in the songs "Strangers in Paradise" and "And This Is My Beloved." Substituting literature for music, Dr. Siddhartha Mukherjee can be considered as

Photo courtesy of
Siddhartha Mukherjee.

a current analog of Borodin in regard to a presence in two disparate arenas.

Mukherjee, the son of a business executive and a former school teacher, was born in New Delhi, India, on July 21, 1970. He received his early education at New Delhi's famous St. Columba's School, which also lists Deepak Chopra (see chapter 56) among its distinguished alumni. At the time of his graduation in 1989, Mukherjee received the school's highest award, the Sword of Honor, for the best all-around performance. He chose to continue his studies at Stanford University, in part, because several of his cousins were living in California. Mukherjee majored in biology at Stanford, during which time he worked in the laboratory of Nobel laureate Paul Berg on a project to define the cellular genes that change the behavior of malignant cells. As an undergraduate, he was awarded the President David Starr Jordan Merit Scholarship, the Chappel-Lougee Scholarship for Undergraduate Research, and the President's Award for Academic Excellence. He was also elected to Phi Beta Kappa.

Following his graduation from Stanford University in 1993, Mukherjee proceeded, as a Rhodes scholar, to Magdalen College, Oxford, where he spent three years and earned a doctorate (DPhil) in immunology. He graduated from Harvard Medical School in 2000 and remained in Boston to complete a three-year residency in internal medicine, followed by a fellowship in oncology at Massachusetts General Hospital. In 2009, he was recruited as assistant professor and codirector of the Myelodysplastic Syndromes (MDS) Center at Columbia University Medical Center.

Mukherjee is married to the highly acclaimed artist Sarah Sze, a sculptor who incorporates a variety of material and plants in her installations. She has been featured in museums of modern art around the world. She was awarded a MacArthur Fellowship (2003–2008) and was the US representative for the Venice Biennale in 2013.

Mukherjee's scientific interests relate to malignant and premalignant diseases of the blood that arise in the bone marrow. His investigations of the cellular microenvironment of the marrow have led to the discovery of a "novel distinct stem cell" that provides for skeletal formation and repair. Other foci of his laboratory concern the physiology of normal blood-forming stem cells and the pathogenesis and treatment of malignant blood diseases.

The results of his research have been reported in the most prestigious scientific and medical journals, including *Nature, Cell,* the *Journal of Clinical Investigation,* and the *New England Journal of Medicine.* Added evidence of the importance of his research is provided by the support he has received from several private foundations and the National Institutes of Health, including the highly regarded "Challenge Grant."

Among the individuals considered in the current compendium, Mukherjee is unique in that he has published only three works classified as nonfiction literature. But, paucity in numbers has been more than offset by scope and impact. His maiden literary contribution, *The Emperor of All Maladies: A Biography of Cancer,* was published in 2010. It was listed by the *New York Times* among "the 10 Best Books" of that year, and by *Time* magazine in its "Top 10 Nonfiction Books of 2010." In 2011, the book was nominated as a National Book Critics Circle Award finalist and won the annual Pulitzer Prize for General Nonfiction. The Pulitzer Prize webpage referred to the work as "an elegant inquiry, at once clinical and personal, into the long history of an insidious disease." That year, the author received the PEN—E. O. Wilson Literary Science Writing Award and the *Guardian* First Book Award. In 2015, Mukherjee's second literary contribution was published, titled *The Laws of Medicine: Field Notes from an Uncertain Science*. This work, despite its relatively small size, enforces the author's literary stature. Drawing from his scientific and clinical experiences, Mukherjee attempts to determine if medicine has governing laws.

He proposes three laws, which he dubs the "laws of uncertainty, imprecision and incompleteness," but cumulatively they are "laws of imperfection." The three laws conclude that "a strong intuition is more powerful than a weak test; 'normals' teach us rules, 'outliers' teach us laws; for every perfect medical experiment, there is a perfect human bias." *The Laws of Medicine* has been deemed required reading for doctors, patients, and those in a quest of a better understanding of how to achieve personal and societal health.

Mukherjee's third book, *The Gene* (2016), is essentially a biography of genetics, the science with which the author is involved on a daily basis in his laboratory, and one that is also a personal issue related to a familial pattern of mental illness.

The Gene is the logical sequel for an author who has produced a popular work of nonfiction that focus on cancer. Cancer is unrivaled by any other pathologic disorder for priority among medical writers. What is most assuredly a patient (male) with a visible cancer of the breast is described in the Edwin Smith papyrus, the oldest extant scientific document. The writing has been assigned a date of circa 1600 BCE, but is a copy of text written between 3000 and 2500 BCE.

Modern scientists have determined that malignancy is the consequence of alteration or corruption of the anatomic elements or biochemical interactions within the genes that constitute the cells. The science of genetics, the mapping of the human genome, and the application of genetic manipulation as therapy for malignancies are among the most significant achievements of modern biological science.

Mukherjee, a highly regarded oncologic scientist, has also popularized biology for a broad readership. He is the counterpart to the late Carl Sagan, the distinguished professor of astronomy, who popularized astronomy and the cosmos. Ironically, Sagan died in 1996 of myelodysplasia, Mukherjee's specific field of research and clinical expertise.

Both Mukherjee's scientific and literary contributions have generated awards. In 2010, he received the Gabrielle Angel's Leukemia Foundation Award. In 2011, Mukherjee shared the Cancer Leadership Award and was included by *Time* magazine on its "100 most influential list." In 2014, he received the Padma Shri, the fourth-highest award given by the government of India. In 2015, he was awarded the American Association for Cancer Research Prize for Contributions to Science.

The combination of Mukherjee's youth, productivity, and impact evokes the phrase from the apocryphal Acts of Peter, when Peter meets the risen Jesus and asks, "Quo vadis?" What will be Mukherjee's next significant scientific contribution? To what aspect of biology will he apply his engaging prose and wit and inform a broad readership?

SOURCES

"2011 Pulitzer Prize Winner in General Nonfiction," Pulitzer Prizes, http://
   www.pulitzer.org/winners/siddhartha-mukherjee (accessed May 10, 2018).
Gleick, James. "'The Gene,' by Siddhartha Mukherjee," *New York Times*, May 12,
   2016, https://www.nytimes.com/2016/05/15/books/review/the-gene-by
   -siddhartha-mukherjee.html (accessed April 5, 2018).
McGrath, Charles. "How Cancer Acquired Its Own Biographer." *New York
   Times*, November 8, 2010, http://www.nytimes.com/2010/11/09/
   books/09mukherjee.html?pagewanted=all&_r=0 (accessed April 5, 2018).
"Siddhartha Mukherjee, MD, DPhil." Columbia University Medical Center.
   http://cancer.columbia.edu/siddhartha-mukherjee-md-dphil (accessed
   April 5, 2018).
"The 10 Best Books of 2010." *New York Times*. December 1, 2010. www.nytimes
   .com/2010/12/12/books/review/10-best-books-of-2010.html (accessed
   May 10, 2018).
"Top 10 Nonfiction Books." *Time*. December 9, 2010. http://content.time
   .com/time/specials/packages/article/0,28804,2035319_2034029,00.html
   (accessed May 10, 2018).

PATTERNS

Each of the specific paths taken by the sixty-five individuals featured in this volume demonstrates a medical presence or at least exposure to a medical education, and each individual contributed notably to "literature." Considered cumulatively, are there discernible patterns that come to light? Are we any closer to answering the question that stimulated this investigation, as to why this defined group of doctors, who write, had a compulsion to write and be read?

Seven of the fifty-one individuals from the past, whose literary contributions were meritorious, had relatively insignificant relationships with medicine. Although Oliver Goldsmith had a brief exposure to anatomy and wrote that the study of medicine "sharpened sagacity," his possession of a validated medical degree is uncertain. George Crabbe sold a few medical instruments, which he had acquired during his apprenticeships, in order to sustain himself while he pursued his poetry. Also, he is generally associated with the ministry rather than medicine. Friedrich Schiller, who reluctantly completed a medical education and accepted a position as a regimental doctor, almost immediately deserted medicine and never identified himself as a doctor of medicine again.

Although John Keats was licensed to practice as a physician and surgeon when he was a teenager, the remaining five years of his brief life were fully immersed in his poetry. W. Somerset Maugham obtained a medical degree and maintained a lifelong listing in the British medical registry, but the sole evidence of his presence as a physician is a prescription he wrote when he was eighty-seven years old. Vasily Aksyonov went to medical school, specifically, to improve his chances of survival in the Russian labor camps. Michael Crichton became a medical student by default and spent a significant portion of his time as a medical student writing *The Andromeda Strain*. He never entered a residency or engaged in clinical activities. These men are excluded from a determination of patterns.

For those remaining forty-four deceased and fourteen living individuals who are subjects of this work, the timing of their having established a literary identity is of interest. In some cases, their writings occurred sequential to their established medical careers. In that group, occasionally, distinct causative factors were responsible for the transformation to a literary life. In the other individuals, their literary and medical activities occurred in tandem, and were, at times, distinctly intertwined.

The pattern, in which noteworthy writing appeared subsequent to the subjects' concentration on medicine, can be evaluated for the individuals in chronological order. In the first half of the eighteenth century, Cadwallader Colden, who had little success as a practicing physician in London and Philadelphia, became caught up in political affairs in colonial New York. Although he maintained a peripheral interest in medicine, he developed a greater concern for botany, the history of the Iroquois nation, and Newtonian theory, about which he produced a literature, including the first allegedly scientific dissertation to be published in North America. During the same century, Tobias Smollett twice failed to establish a medical practice in England. When his first picaresque novel was acclaimed a success, he never returned to medical practice, although he drew liberally from his medical experience to enhance his fiction.

In the first half of the nineteenth century, Eugène Sue's abrupt transition, at the age of twenty-five, from a military and naval surgeon to an author of popular French fiction, was facilitated by the inheritance of his father's fortune. After a brief period of affluence, Sue squandered his wealth and became reliant on the financial rewards of his publications. Charles Lever, the earliest of the six Irish physicians considered in this work, published his first two novels, including his masterpiece, while he was engaged in a medical practice. But, when he was thirty-six years old and the income he derived from his practice could no longer sustain him, he ended his medical career and, for the next thirty years of his life, supported himself with the income from his prolific publications.

Robert Bridges, the lone physician poet laureate, initially combined the production of poetry with the practice of medicine. But illness forced him, at age thirty-seven, to leave medicine and allowed him to devote his energy to poetry. A year later, he produced his first major work of poetry, and he maintained a long period of literary productivity, which brought him recognition.

During the first decade of the twentieth century, Frederick Treves, at the height of his surgical career, abruptly put down his scalpel and picked up his pen with no apparent explanation. At the age of fifty, shortly after he had successfully drained the appendiceal abscess of the future king, Edward VII of the United Kingdom and the British Dominions, Treves permanently left the medical arena and became famous for his travel books and, ultimately, *The Elephant Man and Other Remembrances.*

Arabella Kenealy, whose first and most famous novel was published in 1894, had to end her medical activity at the age of thirty-four because of illness. She continued to produce fiction and works on feminism and the occult for the next forty years. Her contemporary feminist, Margaret Todd, spent a brief five years as a physician, followed by two decades as a writer.

Spanning the nineteenth and twentieth centuries, after a dismal failure as a general practitioner for eight years and, in spite of the favorable reception of his early writing, including two tales of Sherlock Holmes, Arthur Conan Doyle made one last attempt at medicine as an ophthalmologist, and failed there as well. Consequently, from his midthirties, Doyle devoted his energies to a literary career.

During the same period, Arthur Schnitzler practiced psychiatry contemporaneously with his fellow Viennese Sigmund Freud. When Schnitzler's father, a successful physician, died, the thirty-one-year-old Arthur resigned his hospital post and confined his practice to only a few private patients so that he could pursue his desire to write dramas.

In the twentieth century, Francis Brett Young, who had expressed an early desire to become a writer, divided his efforts between medical practice and literary production prior to World War I. During his service as a physician in the British army, Young suffered from dysentery, malaria, and a badly fractured arm. His compromised health resulted in the end of his medical career and allowed him to focus on literary productivity. Similarly, a serious bout of typhus brought an end to Mikhail Bulgakov's brief and unsatisfying medical career, and permitted him to concentrate on writing. When A. J. Cronin was thirty-four years old, the enforced rest that was prescribed to treat his gastric ulcer provided the stimulus for him to terminate his activities in a profession he never enjoyed, and to become a successful author.

A pattern of authors, whose major literary activity took place subsequent to a medical career, continued among those born in the twentieth century. Frank G. Slaughter, a board certified surgeon, served in that capacity during World War II, but, at the end of the war, he ceased operating and for the remaining fifty years of his life he became one of the most prolific writers of popular fiction. Lewis Thomas's career as an essayist was launched after he had conducted his meaningful research and held administrative positions as professor of pathology, professor of medicine, and dean of the New York University School of Medicine.

Illness played a critical role in the case of three of the more recently deceased writers. Walker Percy's tuberculosis prompted his focus on a literary career. Sherwin Nuland reduced his surgical activities and became an acclaimed author of nonfiction after suffering from severe depression and benefitting from electric shock therapy. Michael Palmer turned to writing after his medical license had been suspended because of his addiction.

Both Ferrol Sams and Richard Selzer deliberately turned away from their active and totally time-consuming general and surgical practices, while in their fifties, to satisfy a long-term desire. In Sams's case, he was spurred on by a remembrance of the encouragement offered by a professor of rhetoric and composition. Selzer, a respected and very active general surgeon, admitted to an epiphany, at age fifty-eight, that stimulated his purposeful transition to becoming an author.

Richard Gordon (Gordon Ostlere) purposefully ended his brief career as an anesthesiologist in order to produce popular humorous literature. A combination of physical incapacity and intellectual inclination contributed to Charles Krauthammer substituting policy, politics, and prose for psychiatry. Robin Cook and Tess Gerritsen, both of whom are identified with medical thrillers, have preferentially substituted their medical careers with literary productivity. Patrick Taylor published most of his Irish tales in the decade after he retired from an active career in obstetrics and gynecology.

The opposite pattern, in which a medical presence was maintained at the same time that significant literary material was being generated, is also evident. This pattern was set and was more prevalent in the distant past, but it has persisted. A notable combination of medicine and literary productivity began with Maimonides, who, in the Middle Ages, published scholarly works on the interpretation of Jewish law, the reconciliation of religion and science, anatomy, and medical practice, while he remained engaged in attending to a multitude of patients, including the sultan.

During the Renaissance in England, Thomas Linacre was recognized for his writings as a great humanist, and simultaneously "restored to life many who during their lifetime were languishing" (see chapter 2). In mid-sixteenth-century France, François Rabelais and Michel Nostredame continued to practice medicine while producing their distinctive literature. Rabelais, as an active physician, generated humorous writings because he contended that laughter and mirth had the potential to heal and regenerate by affecting the humoral balance in the body.

In the middle of the seventeenth century, Thomas Browne was esteemed as the best physician in East Anglia, all the while being considered one of the most highly regarded intellectuals throughout Western civilization based on his meaningful prose. Also in that century, John Locke, who distinguished himself as a physician, was, concurrently, the most profound contributor to the English Enlightenment. His writings encompassed metaphysics, philosophy, epistemology, theology, education, economics, and political theory.

The eighteenth century witnessed the contributions of Albrecht von Haller, "the father of modern physiology," whose impact on medicine, coupled with the appreciation he generated as a poet, earned him the appellation of "the epitome of dual distinction." Erasmus Darwin was, arguably, the most famous physician in Great Britain during the second half of the eighteenth century, and maintained an extensive practice throughout his adult life. He combined his medical activities with an impressive number of scientific publications and poetry, which he also used to popularize science. He was referred to as "the most literary character in Europe."

In the first half of the nineteenth century, Oliver Wendell Holmes emerged as the first citizen of the United States to be held in high esteem for a combination of medical contributions and his reputation as a man of letters with a proficiency in prose and poetry. S. Weir Mitchell, who was slightly junior to Holmes, combined his "fathering" of neurology and scientific medicine in America with the authorship of nineteen novels and some poetry. William Osler, the English-speaking world's premier physician, who spanned the late-nineteenth century and early-twentieth century, produced insightful and oft-referred to literature, which addressed medical history, biography, and education while he maintained preeminence as a clinician.

During the twentieth century, Anton Chekhov penned his plays at the same time that he led the life of a selfless physician with a persistent dedication to the care of his patients. James Johnston Abraham, Fellow of the Royal College of Surgeons in England, had his first book published in 1911, the same year that he received his first appointment to a London hospital staff. He would continue to produce popular literature while he conducted an active civilian practice and also during his time of service in World War I. The popular Dubliner Oliver St. John Gogarty was regarded as a first-class writer of poetry and prose and, continuously, sustained his reputation as one of Ireland's most innovative otorhinolaryngologists.

Geoffrey Keynes stands out as a highly regarded surgeon who was one of the first to champion blood transfusion, and transformed the surgical treatment of breast cancer and myasthenia gravis, while, concomitantly, publishing an unmatched corpus of scholarly and definitive bibliographies of many English literary giants. William Carlos Williams is positioned alongside Keynes as one of the most notable individuals among an assemblage of physicians who divided their energies between continuous care of patients and maintenance of a presence in the literary world. Williams never wavered from his attendance to the medical needs of women and children. As one of America's most highly regarded poets, he stated that "medicine was . . . the very thing that made it possible for him to write" (see chapter 33).

Throughout the twentieth century, the concurrence of medical practice and literary productivity was an evident pattern. During Rudolph Fisher's short life, he established himself both as a practicing physician and radiologist and as an integral participant in the Harlem literary renaissance. No practicing psychiatrist was more prolific than Austin Merrill Moore in producing poetry. Neurologist Oliver Sacks drew from the patients he encountered over a half century of medical experience extending into the twenty-first century as a source for his immensely popular prose.

Several current writers continue to divide their energies between medicine and authorship. Eric Kandel remains active in his research and enlightens the public about the process of memory and appreciation of art. Paul Carson treats allergies in children and satisfies his adult readership with medical thrillers. James Groopman actively continues to advance science in oncology and AIDS, while offering readers a better understanding of the importance of holistic care. Abraham Verghese's academic efforts, the mentoring of students of medicine in the need for establishing relationships between doctors and their patients in order to optimize care, and his popular works that enlighten readers about the practice of medicine have influenced many lives. Danielle Ofri combines an internal medicine practice with championing the importance of the humanities in medicine. Atul Gawande continues to operate on patients with endocrine disorders while informing the public of pertinent issues of current healthcare. Siddhartha Mukherjee conducts basic oncologic research at the same time that he intrigues his readers with the history of cancer and genetics.

In summary, attempts to assess the timing of the literary productivity of the men and women of medicine in the hope of determining whether their writings occurred predominantly as a sequence of their medical career or concomitant with medical activities leads, in the end, to no discernable or distinct pattern. About forty percent of both the deceased and living authors produced the bulk of their publications subsequent to their major medical activities. Although extenuating circumstances, such as illness or the failure to make an adequate living as a physician, were occasional factors, they could not be considered the primary reason for engaging in writing as a career.

Continuing our pursuit for patterns, it is necessary to investigate each genre independently because of its unique factors. If a chart is created to depict a chronological frequency with which doctors who lived during that period published meaningful nonfiction for the public, a fascinating pattern becomes apparent. One peak occurs in the more distant past, and a second peak emerges during current times. The thoughtful literary production of physicians during the more distant past is, mainly, a consequence of the intellectual profiles of the medical authors. By contrast, the recent increase in modern times is audience-driven. An educated, knowledgeable, and concerned readership is appreciative of the multiple ethical and sociological problems that have evolved as scientific and technological advances have been made in medical care. They have called for input, explanations, and solutions, as offered by the experts to whom they have entrusted their healthcare.

From the twelfth to the middle of the eighteenth century, only one doctor under consideration produced fiction: Rabelais, who wrote his ribald tales, which he regarded to be, in part, therapeutic. All the other physicians who published literature for a broad readership during that time frame, namely Maimonides, Thomas Linacre, Michel Nostredame, Thomas Browne, John Locke, Cadwallader Colden, and Albrecht von Haller, contributed nonfiction. They published material that addressed significant intellectual issues, including humanism, grammar, prognostication, finance, education, botany, Jewish law, religious tolerance, political philosophy, the reconciliation of religion and science, and the resurrection of the classics.

It was a time when medicine was considered an integral part of natural philosophy. Physicians were exponents of Renaissance humanism. It was a period of individualism and intellectual inquiry. Marvels of nature were being revealed, and some physicians felt compelled to participate in the concerns and dialogues related to the political, religious, and other attitudinal changes that were taking place.

The second peak for publication of nonfiction by physicians occurred in recent times. The explosive expansion of scientific knowledge coupled with an educated, inquisitive, and receptive audience were factors that stimulated writers to direct their efforts toward providing the public with information and reflections about medical science and medical care. As readers' thirst for becoming informed about well-being and medical matters grew, doctors provided satisfying literature.

Lewis Thomas's essays, which had initially been published for a medical audience in the *New England Journal of Medicine*, constituted the same material awarded National Book Awards for arts and letters. Sherwin Nuland's work, which won the 1994 National Book Award for nonfiction, provided for the general readership a consideration of issues related to death. Oliver Sacks titillated his audience with true tales of unusual neurologic manifestations. Erik Kandel intrigued the public with the new science of the mind and memory.

Abraham Verghese's first two publications, each of which elicited acclaim, were nonfiction and addressed the issues of AIDS and the compromising effects of drug addiction. They were harbingers of the recognition he would gain as a current champion of humanistic care. Jerome Groopman, an eminent scientist, also drew from his clinical experience to bring into focus the importance of a bilateral relationship between doctor and patient. He exposed the public to the thinking of the professionals to whom they entrusted their care.

Danielle Ofri has been an effective champion of including the humanities in the education of future physicians. Atul Gawande has provided the public with an unbiased accounting of the current healthcare system, both the improvements it has effected and the problems that it has created. Siddhartha Mukherjee has enhanced the public's appreciation of cancer and genetics.

Perhaps the most apparent evidence of the public's desire to be kept informed is the growing number of actively practicing physicians and surgeons who are contributing syndicated columns to iconic newspapers and popular magazines on diverse medical issues. The spectrum of issues that are addressed includes AIDS, ethics, end-of-life issues, the problems of an aging population, costs of healthcare, imperfections of physicians and surgeons, and methods to reduce errors that inevitably arise during medical care.

A consideration of patterns associated with the fiction created by physicians requires a more genre-specific analysis. In the category of poetry, there is no living doctor who has gained distinction as a poet. The last doctor to merit consideration in that category was William Carlos Williams, who held a position of prominence among physicians while he produced poetry during the twentieth century.

Over the centuries, relatively few doctors focused their literary skills on the production of poetry. Prior to the eighteenth century, only Nostradamus's quatrains of prognostications, in the mid-sixteenth century, are identifiable as physician-produced poetry. Nothing of consequence within the category of poetry appeared in the seventeenth century. By contrast, the eighteenth century witnessed the publication of several significant poems by doctors. Albrecht von Haller's epic poem *Ode sur les Alpes* (1732) established his reputation as a poet. Two major and four minor poems were published in 1765 by Tobias Smollett, "the father of the English novel." Oliver Goldsmith's long poems—*The Traveller* (1764) and *The Deserted Village* (1770)—and George Crabbe's *The Village* (1783) were well received by critics. The year 1797 was referred to by Friedrich Schiller as "the year of the ballad," during which he produced six ballads as part of a friendly competition with Goethe.

In the nineteenth century, John Keats loomed large during the first two decades as a Romantic poet. In 1872, Oliver Wendell Holmes referenced himself as *The Poet at the Breakfast-Table*. This related to the many years that he produced a multitude of poems, beginning in 1830, when he published "Old Ironsides" and "The Last Leaf," one of Abraham Lincoln's favorites.

A chronological consideration of physician/poets of the twentieth century begins with S. Weir Mitchell, the neurologist and author of nineteen novels, who concentrated on poetry in his later years. In general, his poems were not held in high regard by Mitchell's patient Walt Whitman. Robert Bridges, the poet laureate of Great Britain from 1913 to 1930, published his first volume of poetry in 1889 and his masterpiece, *The Testament of Beauty*, a poem in four books, in 1929.

The 1938 *Oxford Book of Modern Verse* included works by the Irish otorhinolaryngologist Oliver St. John Gogarty, whom the editor William Butler Yeats considered to be "one of the greatest living poets of our age." Toward the end of World War II, Francis Brett Young, who had published a book of poetry at the end of World War I, later published an epic poem, *The Island*, recounting in verse the history of Britain from the Bronze Age to the Battle of Britain. A consideration of physician-produced poetry in the twentieth century includes Austin Merrill Moore, who is unequaled for sheer volume, but his many sonnets, constructed with loose conversational and syncopated rhymes, were more often the objects of derision rather than praise.

John Stone III evidenced his literary capability as a poet before he had completed his training in cardiology. His diverse contributions to the academic excellence of the one medical school he served as a faculty member and administrator occurred at the same time, during the latter three decades of the twentieth century and first decade of the twenty-first century.

The quest to expose patterns that might be ascribed to prose fiction pro-

duced by doctors is complicated. Determinations of the frequency of a dominant medical theme, of the presence and importance of medical characters,
and of the inclusion of background material, which provides evidence of the
author's medical association, constitute subjects to be analyzed for pattern recognition. An additional complexity relates to the fact that there are distinct
subsets of fiction, each of which is associated with intrinsic issues that affect
patterns. The subsets or genres to be investigated are drama, detective stories,
medical thrillers, and general fiction.

The field of drama brings into focus Friedrich Schiller, Anton Chekhov,
Arthur Schnitzler, and Mikhail Bulgakov. Schiller's ten successful plays lacked
reference to medicine, in keeping with his brief exposure to that field. In the
case of Bulgakov, whose medical career was also abbreviated, although his
early stories and ultimate masterpiece novel are replete with medical characters and medical issues, his dramas are generally unrelated to medicine.
A sharp contrast is evident in the dramatic works of Chekhov. No physician
authored plays that bear greater evidence of medicine. His first drama, *Platonov*, tells of a physician's failure to abort a suicide. The drama *Ivanoff* singles
out the doctor, who cares for the title character's dying tubercular wife, as an
"honest man." The title character of *The Wood Demon* holds a doctor's degree.
In *The Seagull*, only the physician, in the play-within-the-play, escapes ridicule.
Dr. Astrov has a central role in *Uncle Vanya*. *The Three Sisters* includes a burnt-
out alcoholic physician. Although there is no medical character in Chekhov's
most popular play, *The Cherry Orchard*, his most frequently invoked medical
quotation, "If there is any illness for which people offer many remedies, you
may be sure that particular illness is incurable," is articulated in that drama.

Arthur Schnitzler's psychiatric and psychoanalytic background is recognizable in many, if not most, of his plays. His first drama, *Anatol*, written in 1893,
focuses on the psychological fear of intimacy. Many of the sixteen plays, which
he wrote in the first decade of the twentieth century, revolve around sexual mores
and encounters. *Professor Bernhardi* (1912), which was modeled on his physician
father, relates a tale of a doctor's care of a patient dying from a septic abortion.

The only theatrical production ascribed to a living physician was authored
by psychiatrist Stephen Bergman (Samuel Shem) and his wife, Janet Surrey,
a clinical psychologist. *Bill W. and Dr. Bob* is a play about alcoholism and the
founders of Alcoholics Anonymous.

It has been suggested that a medical education and medical experience
have facilitated authorship of various detective novels. Medical schooling

exposes the student to both inductive and deductive reasoning, while assembling "clues" from patients' narratives and their personal histories, coupled with physical findings, constitute the initial elements for formulating a diagnosis. A tentative diagnosis is confirmed by the assessment of appropriate tests and selective investigative procedures. The same processes pertain to solving a mystery. It is, therefore, not surprising that doctors would have played critical roles in the evolution of the detective story.

The origin of the detective novel in the English-speaking world is considered to have begun in 1841 with Edgar Allan Poe's publication of *The Murders in the Rue Morgue*, featuring the first fictional detective, C. Auguste Dupin. Forty-six years later, Arthur Conan Doyle created Sherlock Holmes, whose name has become synonymous with "detective." Doyle indicated that the character of Holmes was inspired by surgeon Dr. Joseph Bell, whom Doyle encountered at the Edinburgh Medical Infirmary. Bell was known for his diagnostic acumen and his ability to draw conclusions from observations of minutia and findings that were not generally appreciated.

Dr. John H. Watson, Sherlock Holmes's friend and assistant, is the narrator of all but four of the novels and fifty-six Holmes short stories. In the stories, Doyle's medical knowledge comes through in several of his tales and as he details Watson's biography, namely that Watson received his bachelor of medicine degree from Edinburgh University, Doyle's alma mater, and that Watson had been awarded his medical degree from St. Bartholomew's Hospital and the London School of Medicine and Dentistry.

In 1907, Dr. John Evelyn Thorndyke was introduced to readers by R. Austin Freeman, another physician, who dominated English detective fiction for twenty-five years. Dr. Thorndyke was considered to be "the most scientific detective," and the author was also the innovator of "the inverted detective story," in which the commission of the crime and, at times, the identity of the perpetrator are described at the beginning of the narrative.

Yet another innovation in the detective story category can be credited to a doctor. Rudolph Fisher's *The Conjure-Man Dies* (1932) has been credited as the first black detective story, with a black detective and an all-black cast of characters. Although this is arguable, Fisher was certainly the first African American to have published a black detective novel as a bound book.

The medical thriller subgenre followed the detective story as a more recent development. Robin Cook is credited with starting this type of work, based on the 1977 publication of his book *Coma*. Cook has also been the most prolific author in this category. The deceased Michael Palmer indicated that he followed the lead of Cook, his fellow Wesleyan alumnus, when he embarked on writing medical thrillers. Irish allergist Paul Carson heads the popularity list in Ireland. Tess Gerritsen, who had a brief career in medicine, published her first medical thriller in 1996, and has followed with three more best-selling medical thrillers, which have propelled her to a position among the top five most read in that category.

Perhaps the most intriguing pattern to be analyzed relates to the presence of aspects of authors' medical backgrounds and associations in the general fiction they created. An assessment can be made of the frequency and dominance of medical characters, medical themes, medical issues, and of the use of medical knowledge by doctors who write stories. It is convenient to consider these patterns chronologically.

In the sixteenth century, François Rabelais was the first individual with a bona fide medical education to create notable fiction. The comic nature of his works was considered to be therapeutic, in that laughter was ascribed the potential to heal by affecting the body's humoral balance, which, at the time, was thought to be the basis of disease. Rabelais's *Gargantua* provides evidence of the author's knowledge and experiences both as an ex-monk and a physician. In *Pantagruel* (1532), Rabelais wrote, "[Pantagruel] thought of studying medicine here but decided that the profession was too troublesome and morbid. Besides, physicians smelled hellishly of enemas." The many scatological and genital references in Rabelais's works are in concert with the dicta of Hippocrates and Galen regarding the importance of bodily excretions to define and treat diseases. Pantagruel says, "We entrust our lives to physicians, who, to a man, loathe medicine and refuse to take physics."

Albrecht von Haller's three romances, which were written in the eighteenth century, had no mention of medicine and were focused on comparative political philosophy. By contrast, Tobias Smollett drew from his medical experience to satirize the seamy side of medicine. Medical issues come to light in several of his works, and his quotations related to medicine continue to appear. In *The Expedition of Humphry Clinker* (1771), it is stated, "I have had an hospital these fourteen years within myself, and studied my own case with painful attention," and "The inconveniences which I overlooked in the highday of health, will naturally strike with exaggerated impression on the irritable nerves of an invalid, surprised by premature old age and shattered with long suffering." In *The Adventures of Sir Launcelot Greaves* (1760), Smollett writes, "We have quacks in religion, quacks in physic[s], quacks in law, quacks in government . . . that have blistered, seated, bled, and purged the nation into atrophy."

In keeping with Oliver Goldsmith's questionable exposure as a medical student, there is no evidence of medicine in his fiction. In the first half of the nineteenth century, Eugène Sue drew from his naval battle experiences for his early publications. Neither those stories nor his two major novels, *The Mysteries of Paris* or *The Wandering Jew*, suggest that the author had a relationship with medicine. Similarly, Charles Lever's writings offer no evidence of his medical background, with the exception of the descriptions of cholera epidemics, which he had experienced, in *St. Patrick's Eve* and *The Martins of Cro'Martin*.

S. Weir Mitchell's expertise in neurology is evident in several of his works of fiction. His first short story includes an early description of the phantom limb syndrome. In his first novel, the protagonist is a doctor who becomes temporarily quadriparetic after a bullet wound. In his most famous novel, *High Wynne-Free Quaker*, there is a detailed description of senile dementia. Both of the most notable novels by the female physicians Arabella Kenealy and Margaret Todd in the late-nineteenth century had women as their central characters, one a practicing physician and the other a medical student.

Medical patterns permeate several of W. Somerset Maugham's publications. Given that his association with medicine ended when he graduated from medical school, it is intriguing that he invoked the discipline as an integral element of his fiction. His first major work, *Lisa of Lambeth*, was influenced by his exposure to home deliveries as a medical student. *The Hero* contained a vivid description of enteric fever. A central character in *The Magician* is a renowned surgeon. *The Merry-Go-Round* considers inhumane doctors who allow patients to suffer.

Of Human Bondage (1915) tells of the development of a physician. It contains the memorable quotation "You will have learned many tedious things . . . which you will forget the moment you have passed your final examination, but in anatomy it is better to have learned and lost than never to have learned." Also in that novel, Maugham presents several detailed descriptions of anemia, including, "Her anemia made her rather short of breath, and she held her mouth slightly open." In *The Constant Wife*, the central character is married to an amoral and unethical surgeon. Cholera plays a role in *The Painted Veil*, and the short story "The Narrow Corner" focuses on an unethical doctor.

When Oliver St. John Gogarty was in his fifties, he shifted from poetry to prose. In his first book, *As I Was Going down Sackville Street* (1937), Gogarty distinguishes between the mores of medical practice in London and Dublin: "Here [in London] the doctors are so kind and professional conduct is so nice that they never contradict each other. To maintain this harmony it is taboo to make a diagnosis. In Dublin, where the conspiracy is unfriendly, it is necessary to keep the wits keen if one has to live on his professional brethren's repairs." In *I Follow Saint Patrick* (1938), he wrote, "The telescope, the microscope, and the test-tube have made skeptics of us all. We have changed wisdom for an exact knowledge of stains, precipitants, reactions and refractions, and put it, for this generation, at least, beyond recall." Gogarty incorporated the cavorting of Irish medical students in his work and included the character of a schizophrenic watchmaker.

Francis Brett Young was a prolific writer, who incorporated medicine in many of his books. In 1919, he published *The Young Physician* about the life of a medical student. *My Brother Jonathan* has a general practitioner as its hero. *Dr. Bradley Remembers* is based on his physician father's time.

A. J. Cronin's name has been equated with changes in the British health-care system. From the very beginning of his literary productivity, physicians and medical issues were integral to the narratives he created. In his initial success, *Hatter's Castle*, two distinctly different types of medical personalities are pitted against one another. In *Canary Island*, resentment against the medical world is pervasive. In Cronin's most popular book, *The Citadel*, medical incompetency, inadequacy, and indifference are highlighted.

References to medicine also appear throughout many of Frank G. Slaughter's fifty-eight novels. The first novel published by the accredited surgeon is concerned with the vicissitudes encountered by a young aspiring surgeon. Subsequent works continue to describe the training and development of a surgeon, beginning in the time of Jesus, including contributions from India, and a consideration of changing the process of delivering healthcare from an existent "fee-for-service" system to one based on "capitation."

Ferrol Sams's fiction drew heavily from his personal experiences and the characters he encountered as he consistently relayed homespun tales of the rural South. Richard Selzer's short stories and one novel were all derived from the author's medical experiences, attitudes, and sentiments.

Among the considered living authors who composed general fiction, Samuel Shem's satirical descriptions of the training of doctors are representative of the application of a medical background. Patrick Taylor's Irish tales highlight medicine. Abraham Verghese's *Cutting for Stone*, the twenty-first century's great medical novel, could only have been written by a physician. As John Irving wrote in his review, "I've not read a novel wherein medicine, the practice of it, is made as germane to the storytelling process, to the overall narrative, as the author manages to make it happen here." By contrast, Khaled Hosseini's three popular novels—*The Kite Runner, A Thousand Splendid Suns*, and *And the Mountains Echoed*—offer little evidence that they were written by a doctor.

The next pattern to be considered relates to the question of "Was the literature that was contributed by doctors generally reflective of the times during which it was produced?" The answer is an anticipated affirmative. The nonfiction credited to men of medicine of the distant past flowed from the pens of individuals who regarded their medical knowledge to be part of their intellectual fabric as natural philosophers. The reconciliation of faith and reason, humanism, toleration, government, and education were all central issues of concern between the twelfth and the eighteenth centuries. It was natural that those issues would draw the attention of the thoughtful individuals who had established reputations as physicians.

In the eighteenth century, with the advent of Linnaean taxonomy of plants, inquiring physicians would direct their attention to botany, a science that was integral to their practice. Botany was central to the writings of Cadwallader Colden, Albrecht von Haller, and Erasmus Darwin. And a by-product was the concept of classification, itself, as an intellectual exercise, which merited attention.

In the late-nineteenth century and the first half of the twentieth century, as medicine became increasingly scientific, a few highly regarded physicians delved deeply into nonscientific scholarship related to history, biography, literature, and the humanities. Their implied message was that the romantic past is integral to our present thoughts and activities. In a time of depersonalization, they championed the recognition of heroes.

In the current environment, with a relatively knowledgeable readership thirsty for information about medical diseases, medical care, and the management of health, the production of a large canon of nonfiction has become a major focus of attention.

In the category of fiction, there is also a distinct correlation with the contemporary environment and the circumstances that surrounded the literature. Fiction generally mirrors the time in which it was produced. In the sixteenth century, Rabelais's ribald writings invoked the ethos of carnival and the medical concern with humoral balance and regeneration. By contrast, only the late-twentieth-century fiction could satirize the training of a physician or integrate in a plot the topic of liver transplantation, which was not performed successfully until 1968.

Returning full circle to the question that stimulated and energized this entire scholarly attempt to determine why doctors write and publish for a general readership, we find the number of answers indicates that no one response is adequate. As early as 1481, William Caxton, the first English bookseller and printer to use Gutenberg's movable type wrote, "The spoken word passes away; the written word abides." This suggests that the printed word provides for immortality of a thought and perhaps at the same time the continued remembrance of the writer. Still invoking the ego, writer Joan Didion, known for her novels, memoirs, and literary journalism, stated, "I write entirely to find out what I'm thinking, what I'm looking at, what I see and what it means."

In the seventeenth century, Francis Bacon indicated that he wrote "to think more coherently." In the eighteenth century, James Boswell recorded that Samuel Johnson had opined, "No man but a blockhead ever wrote except for money." Boswell refuted this. In the nineteenth century, Gustave Flaubert, the author of *Madame Bovary*, died penniless but left these words: "Writing is a dog's life, but the only life worth living." In the twentieth century, George Orwell proposed four explicit motives for writing: "sheer egoism, aesthetic enthusiasm, historical impulse and political purpose."

The results of a recent survey of one hundred published authors that was conducted to determine why writers write concluded the following: 30 percent wrote to educate, influence, or help others; 13 percent wrote because they felt compelled; 10 percent found writing pleasurable or therapeutic; 3 percent wrote because it was their profession; 2 percent wrote because they were victims of circumstance; 2 percent wrote to entertain; 2 percent wrote for exposure and fame; and 2 percent wrote to immortalize themselves.

Equally meaningful were the expressions of Somerset Maugham, who stated that he wrote "for sheer solace," or James Thurber, who wrote "to have fun." To be certain, you have your work published because you want it to be more widely read.

SOURCES

Deguara, C. J. "Why Writers Write." *CJ Deguara* (blog). http://cjdeguara.com/why-writers-write/ (accessed May 14, 2018).

Popova, Maria. "Why I Write: George Orwell on an Author's 4 Main Motives." *Atlantic.* June 26, 2012. https://www.theatlantic.com/entertainment/archive/2012/06/why-i-write-george-orwell-on-an-authors-4-main-motives/258955/ (accessed May 10, 2018).

ACKNOWLEDGMENTS

Three individuals have provided invaluable service and support over the past decade, during which I have researched, written, and published three volumes of nonfiction. Steven L. Mitchell, in his role as editor in chief of Prometheus Books, has shepherded *Cadwallader Colden: A Biography* (2013), *The Anatomist, the Barber-Surgeon, and the King: How the Accidental Death of Henry II of France Changed the World* (2015), and this current consideration of sixty-five physicians, who have left a literary legacy, through the process of publication. Gianna Nixon-Saldinger has overseen the selection and visually optimized the illustrative material in all three books. In addition, her organizational skills have been much appreciated. Dr. Marshall Lichtman, an eminent hematologist, medical school dean, and scholar, provided a critical review of every inclusion. Marshall's shared commitment to the importance of the humanities in the education of physicians was a continuing encouragement.